John Crellin assesses popular home remedies from amulets to Zam-Buk ointment, revealing traditional – often ingenious – ways of coping with commonplace health problems. *Home Medicine* is both a comprehensive reference to folk cures and self-treatment and a social history of Canadian pharmaceutical practices and products in Newfoundland.

Based on material from the Folklore Archives at Memorial University as well as other sources, Crellin's catalogue includes such topics as abortion, baldness and hair preparations, blood-letting, cancer, drunkenness, female complaints, Gin Pills, herbs, midwifery and childbirth, Newfoundland stomach, poultices, prepared cures, rheumatism and arthritis, and tonics. Looking at the interplay between mainstream physicians and alternative treatments, and the effect of folk beliefs on today's self-care practices, Crellin examines how the advent of modern medicine has affected self-treatment.

His extensive use of oral and written commentary gives the book a personal dimension that adds to its charm. *Home Medicine* will appeal to those interested in alternative medicine, folklore, and Atlantic Canada, and to medical and social historians.

JOHN K. CRELLIN is John Clinch Professor of the History of Medicine, Memorial University of Newfoundland.

McGILL-QUEEN'S/HANNAH INSTITUTE STUDIES
IN THE HISTORY OF MEDICINE, HEALTH, AND SOCIETY
*Series Editors: S.O. Freedman and J.T.H. Connor*

Volumes in this series have been supported by
the Hannah Institute for the History of Medicine

# Home Medicine
# The Newfoundland Experience

## John K. Crellin

McGill-Queen's University Press
Montreal & Kingston • London • Buffalo

*To JDC for healthy scepticism and much more*

© McGill-Queen's University Press 1994
ISBN 0-7735-1196-2 (cloth)
ISBN 0-7735-1197-0 (paper)

Legal deposit third quarter 1994
Bibliothèque nationale du Québec

Printed in Canada on acid-free paper

This book has been published with the help of grants from the
Social Science Federation of Canada, using funds provided by the
Social Sciences and Humanities Research Council of Canada.

McGill-Queen's University Press is grateful to the Canada Council
for support of its publishing program.

**Canadian Cataloguing in Publication Data**

Crellin, J.K.
Home medicine: the Newfoundland experience
(McGill-Queen's/Hannah Institute Studies in the history of medicine, health, and society; 1)
Includes bibliographical references and index.
ISBN 0-7735-1196-2 (bound) –
ISBN 0-7735-1197-0 (pbk.)
1. Traditional medicine – Newfoundland.
1. Title. 11. Series
R463.N44C74 1994   615.8′8   C94-900618-1

Typeset in Adobe Garamond 10.5/12
by Caractéra production graphique, Quebec City

# Contents

# *Acknowledgments*

Among the many people who have been drawn into the project, Philip Hiscock, archivist of the Memorial University of Newfoundland Folklore and Language Archive (MUNFLA) painstakingly commented on an early draft of the manuscript and facilitated my use of the archive. Some preparatory work in the archive was aided by the V.M. Halpert Cure File, covering 1963 to 1970. Others who have contributed by reading and commenting on the manuscript are Raoul Andersen, Mohammadtakei Kara, Martin Lovelace, Bernard O'Dwyer, Nigel Rusted, and Peter Scott. From the specialties of anthropology, botany, folklore, medicine, pharmacy, and sociolinguistics, their readings ensured that relevant aspects of the disciplines were considered. Material gathered for other projects by the Medical Communications Group (MCG), Memorial University of Newfoundland (of which the author is a member), has been incorporated with permission.

Many people who answered queries from time to time are acknowledged with an appropriate reference. Special thanks go to Captain Peter Troake, who provided this CFA ("come-from-away") with countless insights into Newfoundland culture. Thanks are also due to medical students Lynette Adams and Bill Harvey, whose interviews provided data and context; to Myrtle Champion and Janet McNaughton for permission to print recollections on removing birthmarks; to Chief Michael Joe; and to the many others who answered questions from time to time. Thanks go also to the late Jim O'Mara of the Newfoundland Pharmaceutical Association, who responded to initial queries, and to the association itself, for allowing ready access to its first-class collection of pharmaceutical artifacts. Particular thanks are due to the keen eye of copyeditor W. Dayton and to the courtesies of McGill-Queen's University Press.

*Home Medicine*

Medicine is not only a science;
it is also an art.

# Introduction

*Home Medicine: The Newfoundland Experience* considers many changes and
issues in self-treatment that have occurred during the twentieth century.
Although of special appeal to Newfoundlanders, *Home Medicine* is far from
a parochial account; it is directed toward those interested in medical care
in general, folklore, history, and related areas. Newfoundland, with its
particular social evolution and conspicuous heritage, is a fertile resource for
case studies. This volume reveals a rich tapestry of the many facets of
everyday life and of the countless ways, often ingenious, of dealing or
coping with commonplace health problems.

Confederation with Canada in 1949 foreshadowed many changes for
Newfoundlanders. They faced numerous social changes through, for
instance, mechanization of trawlers and of processing in the fishing indus-
try; new medical and health services; and new roads and the resettlement
of many isolated communities. These and other changes were not without
direct and indirect impact on many of the treatments – homemade and
over-the-counter as well as magical and religious – described in this account.
Most detail is given for the period up to the 1950s and 1960s.

The discussions on ailments and treatments rest on around 3,500 records
of Newfoundland's popular medicines recorded between 1963 and 1989
and deposited, as part of the vivid documentation of an island culture, in
the Folklore and Language Archive at Memorial University of Newfoundland. Structured interviews undertaken recently under the auspices of the
Medical Communications Group, Memorial University of Newfoundland,
elicited further data. Added to this is information from published sources
(much from newspapers), manuscripts, and medical artifacts that illumi-
nates the wide range of treatments, popular beliefs, and social changes.

The richness of the information along with the diversity of Newfoundland's
cultural background raise many issues about past and present health care.

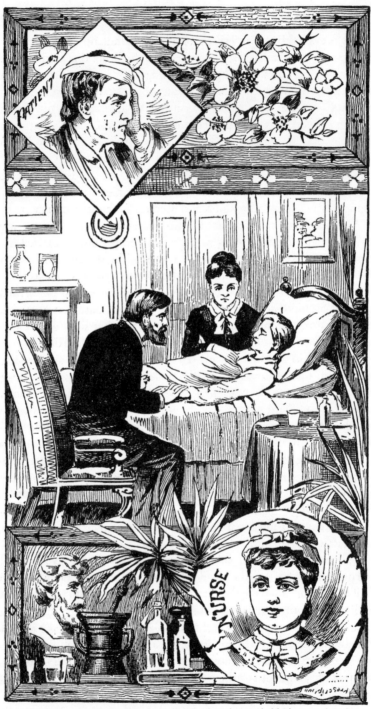

This illustration from Chase's *Receipt Book and Household Physician* (1887) sets the tone for much self-care. It suggests that family care is important, but not at the expense of professional medicine.

Central to the volume is the strikingly wide range of practices and beliefs that have prevailed in twentieth-century Newfoundland. Some, such as the use of sheep manure for treating measles and the belief that fairies can cause harm, may or may not have been widely held. It is clear that Newfoundlanders chose from a pluralistic arena of self-care according to their experiences, existing health beliefs, available advice, and the particular ailment or concern. If one approach did not work, there was always another to try. There is no reason to believe that a person consistently used a particular regimen throughout life, even for a similar condition.

Self-care, in all its variety, has never been static, despite the many elements that persisted over a long period of time. For instance, how do changing attitudes toward religion and medical authority impinge on health care? And do former beliefs about the causes of disease (from "impure blood" to such climatic effects as changing temperatures) as well as past treatment concepts (for example, the use of kidney medicines for "backache") still shape certain individual self-care practices, even for such relatively recently recognized disease states as arteriosclerosis? Unfortunately, the answers are not entirely clear, just as it is unfortunate that many health-care students and professionals may be unaware that such questions concerning their patients' beliefs and their own culture even exist.

As illustrated in this volume, professional or "doctors'" medicine has not been ignored, but, generally speaking, at least in the twentieth century, it has either been sharply differentiated from, or had uneasy relationships with, much lay medical care. At the same time, professional ideas have infiltrated almost all facets of self-care. The tendency to describe a mix of professional medical practices with long-standing lay ideas as "popular medicine" (here called "home medicine") – so as to distinguish it from so-called purer practices of "traditional" or "folk" medicine – recognizes the long-standing sharing of ideas between physicians and lay people. One purpose of *Home Medicine* is to raise questions about present and future relations between professional and lay care, questions which are of current interest as society grapples with the problems of providing equitable health care in all its aspects.

The question is often asked whether traditional or long-standing practices are still employed. Certainly in 1993, many of those popular around 1950 have disappeared from use, if not from memory. On the other hand, innumerable, once-popular herbal remedies and other self-care treatments have recently re-emerged. Increasingly, they are becoming available through health stores, mail-order outfits, pyramid-selling organizations, and alternative practitioners; often they serve to reinforce long-standing, albeit fading, beliefs.

It is hoped that health-care providers will find practical value in this account, for reasons that go beyond insights into social and environmental effects on health which are now receiving more attention within medical education. There is, for instance, a growing appreciation that self-care practices can interact with Western medical care, and that physicians, when taking case histories, should elicit detailed information from patients about self-treatment. The knowledge may not only help to avoid both misdiagnoses through inadequate communication and interference with prescription medication, but also to foster better understanding between physicians and patients. Conversations that are non-threatening or judgmental for patients may thus be encouraged.

Self-care, the most frequent form of primary health care, today prompts much health-policy controversy. In Canada, for instance, discussions abound as to whether certain herbs should be sold on the basis of traditional medical reputations rather than modern clinical trials. Further, Canada has a national policy to preserve multiculturalism and the Canadian mosaic, thereby recognizing that much behaviour connected with health and disease is culturally determined. The demand is that health-care personnel be sensitive to all segments of the population, not just to visible minorities.

At the very least, knowledge of self-care and of cultural attitudes may help a practitioner to assess, for instance, a patient's health-care habits in general; to understand lay views about health and disease; and to shape potentially harmful practices into more acceptable ones. Shaping health practices or encouraging a person's belief in their ability to have control over their health, rather than merely *telling* a patient to follow conventional medical ideas, can be productive.

If readers dismiss many issues raised in *Home Medicine* as of concern only to "the elderly," they must recognize that the growing number of senior citizens challenges society and health-care services. It should also be appreciated that much of the self-care described is, in fact, familiar to countless Newfoundlanders over the age of forty-five, if not to many who are younger, while current interest in alternative or complementary medicine is found in all sections of society.

*Home Medicine: The Newfoundland Experience* is not a definitive study of self-care, for it deals relatively briefly with such matters as psychology and comparisons of self-care practices in various countries, though the relevance of these is made clear. But by drawing attention to a wide range of concepts and behaviours, as well as how individuals cope and limit their medical problems, the account touches on the broader topics of effective health promotion as well as on disease prevention and wellness programs. This account also takes the view that no single theoretical model from the social sciences is applicable overall to the complex arena of self-care. It promotes the approach that health promotion and counselling, in general, must constantly take into account matters of individual behaviour: *this* situation, *this* family, *this* individual. In so doing, sociocultural considerations and how people (whether patients or not) interpret the world around them are constantly kept in mind.

## PART ONE

# Self-Treatment:
# A Kaleidoscope

*The desire to take medicine is perhaps the greatest feature*
*which distinguishes man from animals.*
*Sir William Osler*

Therapy, be it prescribed by physicians or alternative medical practitioners, or employed as self-treatment, has long raised such issues of concern to society as therapeutic fashions and side-effects. The following discussion – intended to provide background to the entries in Part II – covers various issues in self-care, from commercialism to religious influences, all of which will help us to understand the complexity and nuances of what is sometimes called the "silent health-care system."

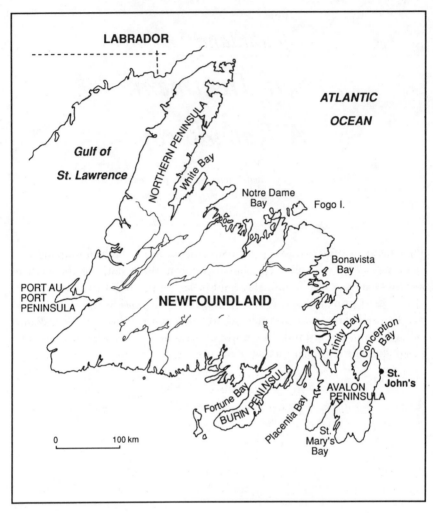

Newfoundland

# Newfoundland Snapshots

The diversity of self-treatment in twentieth-century Newfoundland – a large, rugged island of 43,359 square miles at the mouth of the Gulf of St. Lawrence – is striking. It also reflects such aspects of the island's recent history as changes in the role of the non-market economy and the resulting trends away from self-sufficiency. Above all, it is a reminder of the accounts of stark living conditions and horrendous journeys on medical calls that abound in Newfoundland. Most, however, are but a pale shadow of Wilfred Grenfell's celebrated saga of a house call in 1908 when, with great resourcefulness, which included killing three of his dogs, he survived a life-threatening time on a drifting ice pan. A colleague, physician J. M. Little, wrote in the same year about his own trip:

My next trip was one of sixteen days, on which I saw 135 patients. This was a trip along the west coast of Newfoundland in the Straits of Belle Isle. The inhabitants were in the clutches of severe influenza. There were also scarlet fever, measles and mumps. Owing to the severity of these epidemics, I decided to go along the shore as far as possible; so with my guide I went as light as possible with 11 dogs on one komatik. When we got to a certain settlement, we seemed to 'catch up' with the grippe, for the evening I arrived, 5 people were taken down with it.

The next habitations were fifty miles further along shore. The way we had to go was around a bay which had not frozen solid, consequently, nobody had traveled this route except the mail man this winter. As *we were now farther than any doctor had been along this coast*, my man did not know the way. The mail man arrived that night and the next morning at 5 o'clock I started, using his back track as a guide. We traveled all day over rough ice that lay between the 'landwash' on one side and the woods on the other. Neither one of us could get on the sledge during any of this time, but one in front and one behind were pulling it over, under and through the rough ice. At 7 o'clock, after the hardest day's work I have ever known, we arrived at a habitation and a community of some 300 people. Now the thing that interested me was, that beyond this stretch of almost impossible traveling ... there was not one case of grippe, measles, scarlet fever or mumps, while before it, almost every member of every village had been attacked by one or the other. Moreover, in this community there had just been 2 deaths of cerebrospinal meningitis, two sisters who occupied the same bed.[1]

Difficulties have always existed with regard to providing equitable medical services for rural Newfoundland, with its special geographic and economic problems. This has fostered a belief that, until recently, self-care in the island was largely a consequence of having to do without, or to wait for, professional medical care in one of more than 1,300 scattered and isolated coastal communities or outports. Stories such as told by physician John Olds (died 1985) reinforce this view. After a harrowing journey in response to a call – and a greeting: "Good morning, Doctor. Didn't expect you today, bad on ice, ain't it?" – Olds found the patient had recovered, in part from self-treatment: "She had been constipated a bit more than usual and yesterday she had a pain in the 'back passage' and there was a lump. During the night the fruit salts worked, there was blood on the stool, the lump was practically gone and it didn't hurt anymore! She got some salve and a small bit of sympathy for her ex-pile, and I went down to the kitchen to join Max who had already started to eat."[2]

In many ways, however, the rural situation in Newfoundland merely accentuates aspects of the story of self-care – which is complex anywhere, in urban as well as rural communities. Much of the complexity is because self-care covers numerous diverse regimens that straddle both treatment and prevention; some are accepted by regular medicine, whereas others are vehemently criticized, or prompt ambivalence. Additionally, self-care, with its various beliefs and concepts, has never been static, even in Newfoundland where outports, albeit without access by road, were less immune from outside influences than is sometimes supposed. In large part, however, the striking variety of treatments in the island resulted from the persistence of so many long-standing practices, and for a longer period of time than elsewhere, certainly until the speed of social change gathered momentum from the 1950s onward, thereby providing new frames of reference for health care.

## THE GENERAL STATE OF HEALTH

Lifestyles shaped by, for instance, the fishery, seasonal employment (including the forest industries), business activities, and women's work in managing households and children while their men were away, as well as attitudes toward health and the nature of disease, obviously affected self-care. Newfoundlanders suffered from the same spectrum of serious, self-limiting, and chronic conditions as elsewhere, as well as from an intriguing number of occupational problems from fish hook infections to seal fingers. Notable, too, was a high incidence of tuberculosis (until the 1960s) and a substantial number of cases, relative to elsewhere in North America, of beriberi. Genetic factors have also been (as they still are) a consideration, although of less significance than infections and nutrition disorders. A glimpse of social conditions in Stephenville in the late 1930s is telling: "There was no one in Stephenville for a girl to marry. Before the war came, things were so bad that a girl couldn't get married unless she ended up marrying her first or second cousin. We were all really blood relatives. But what were we to do?"[3]

Just how much self-care was undertaken was undoubtedly affected by the general state of health. In 1945, this was noted to be "far from satisfactory," and malnutrition was said to be "extensive and a major problem."[4] At a medical meeting in 1949, physician Leonard Miller stated: "Just before I left St. John's, a doctor's wife warned me not to be another of those who said that Newfoundlanders were starving."[5] Albeit stated in jest, this was a widespread perception, bolstered by a long series of negative reports and events – beginning around the early years of the century – that focused on nutritional, social, and economic problems in the island. One writer on Newfoundland has described the island as poverty-stricken by the 1930s; a woebegone place, poor and disadvantaged.[6] Such perceptions were fuelled by tangible evidence, including recruitment figures for World War I that showed 47 per cent of Newfoundland volunteers and 57 per cent of conscripts as medically unfit to serve.[7]

Despite many negative views about Newfoundland life, rosy reminiscences speak of the effectiveness of a non-market economy – central to which was gardening, hunting, and bartering – to the life of many Newfoundlanders.[8] Furthermore, the vagaries of the fishery generally meant that not all Newfoundlanders faced economic problems at the same time. It is clear, however, that the non-market economy was not an effective cushion for everyone. There were unquestionably diverse experiences in the way it was handled. Local conditions, including poor soil, inclement weather, illness, and a host of other factors – even whether a mother might sacrifice her own balanced nutrition for the sake of feeding her family – made it difficult for some families to exploit local resources effectively. And "sometimes they'd get so poor they kind of lost interest."[9] This made it even more difficult to escape the formal economy that enmeshed and controlled countless Newfoundlanders via an extensive credit system in which fishermen relied on credit from merchants.

Amid all these considerations – and bearing in mind that some medical statements up to around 1950 about unsatisfactory health on the island reflected misunderstandings of Newfoundland culture – a generally poor state of health often did exist. This predisposed people to skin infections (for example, boils), tiredness, and many other vague symptoms, if not more serious problems.

At times, the unhealthiness of both the non-market and market economies prompted difficult health-care choices. As the following story of the inexorable trend of commercialism in self-care makes clear, there arose many demands for new medicines that usually had to be paid for with credit and undermined self-sufficiency. Perhaps this contributed to some ambivalence toward new products and to the persistence of many long-standing practices that had disappeared elsewhere more quickly. In the end, however, at least following World War II, usage of commercial products had become widespread and commonplace, along with an increased reliance on professional medical advice.

# Commercialism and Change, c. 1900-1950

*Doctor, oh Doctor, oh dear Doctor John*
*Your cod liver oil is so pure and strong.*
*I'm afraid of my life I'll go down in the soil,*
*If my wife don't stop drinking your cod liver oil.*

Why quote from a folksong, "Dear Doctor John," well-known in New-foundland, and with probable origins in the successful marketing of De Jongh's brand of cod liver oil during the second half of the nineteenth century? The song is a reminder that the story of cod liver oil – illustrating as it does a trend away from using home-made oil to reliance on commercial preparations – reflects a striking change that helped to reshape self-care in the nineteenth and twentieth centuries.[10] If it is surprising that commercial cod liver oil preparations became popular when local oil – albeit "unpuri-fied" and less palatable – was readily available at no cost in hundreds of small isolated outports, the 1930 Royal Commission on Health and Public Charities offers relevant commentary: "Although the commission could not obtain exact figures on the subject it appears that at least $250,000 worth of patent or proprietary medicines are used by the people of Newfoundland every year. The obvious conclusion is that a very large portion is used by people who endeavour in this way to make up for what they lack in skilled medical and nursing services."[11] A perception of widespread use of over-the-counter (patent or proprietary) medicines evidently existed. Recent recollections of the use of medicines popular at the time – among others, Carter's Little Liver Pills, Dr. Chase's Nerve Food, and Baby's Own Tablets – and sold by merchants in Newfoundland outports during the 1930s add meaning to advertisements of the time. For example, S.C. Maley, of Bank Square, advertised the following medicines in The *Twillingate Sun* of 19 July 1930: "Philip's Milk of Magnesia, Kidney Tablets, Aspirins, Methol [sic] & Camphor Cream, Boracic Acid, Pazo Ointment, Absorbine J, Castor Oil, A.B.S. & C. Tablets, Neulife Tonic, Anti-Pain Drops, Woodwards Gripe Water, Baby's Own Tablets, etc."[12]

However, the conclusions of the 1930 Royal Commission concerning a close association between over-the-counter medicines and limited medical and nursing services may be debated, for proprietary medicines at the time had considerable sales even where professional help was readily available. Isolation and rural circumstances were, nevertheless, one consideration; studies of Newfoundlanders during the late 1960s, following improvements in medical services in previous years, found that individual anxiety concerning certain symptoms could increase still further the distance from medical help.[13] Even so, it remains uncertain whether such factors as isolation and lack of access to doctors were as significant in Newfoundland in shaping self-care as were such other considerations as the poor state of health, the fear of tuberculosis and many other diseases, and the growing availability of commercial medicines.

## COMMERCIALISM PERVADES, JUXTAPOSING TRADITIONS

Relations between over-the-counter commercial medicines and home-prepared, magical, and religious treatments are intriguing. The ever-increasing usage, high profile, and criticisms of commercial medicines – often relatively expensive – on both sides of the Atlantic from the eighteenth century onward are generally well known.[14] But of special interest to the Newfoundland scene is that the memory, if not always the usage, of home-made and magical treatments has been strikingly persistent – about which more will be said later – even while commercial preparations pushed many of them aside. In many ways, the Newfoundland story is one of consumerism edging out traditional medicines, and with such consequences as diminished self-reliance on self-care among Newfoundland women. Yet at the same time, some over-the-counter remedies reinforced certain long-standing practices, because they used the same ingredients or were promoted on precepts widely known.

The quickening change to over-the-counter products during the first half of the twentieth century – found generally in North America – may have been slower in the outports than in St. John's. Nevertheless, many factors were at play throughout the island, cutting across the different educational levels among Newfoundlanders. For one thing, lay receptivity was fed by the convenience of over-the-counter medicines suitable for men who were away from home for long periods of time (fishing, logging, and hunting) and for women who were constantly active in and around the home and outside helping with the fishery. There was, too, an expanding number of outlets for commercial medicines – some through merchants who supplied them on credit – that capitalized on those intensive and skilful advertisements which exploited concepts and themes linked to popular culture and health reform.

Aside from medicinal entrepreneurs and pharmacists, outlets for people living within Newfoundland's cash economy included mail-orders from

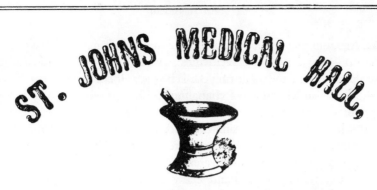

# ST. JOHNS MEDICAL HALL,

# J. J. DEARIN,

PROPRIETOR AND IMPORTER,

Keeps constantly for sale at his Establishment a complete assortment of

## English and American Drugs and Chemicals, Patent Medicines, Perfumery, Dye Stuffs, Spices, Sponges, Hair, Cloth, Tooth and Nail Brushes.
## Preparations for the Toilet, Fancy articles, and articles of every description usually found in a Drug Store.

A few of which may be enumerated as follows, viz:

Logwood, Extract Logwood, Redwood, Cudbear, Pink Saucers, Indigo, Cinnamon, Allspice, Nutmegs, Ginger, Broma, Cloves, Corn Starch, Dubarry's Revalentia, Currants, Raisins, Citron, Genuine Essences, Gelatine, Cleave Soaps and Perfumes. Lubin's first class Perfumes.

Importer of Confectionery; Paraffine, Olive, Sweet, Lard, and Neatsfoot Oils, Garden Seeds, Burning Fluid, Vinegar, Glass Ware, etc.

Physicians' Prescriptions carefully compounded, and orders answered with care and despatch. Farmers and Physicians from the country will find my stock of Medicines complete, Warranted Genuine, and of the Best Quality.

## Paynes' and Ayer's Family Medicines, Johnson's Anodyne Liniment, Sugar Coated Pills, Parson's Rat Exterminator, Brown's Bronchial Troches, Davis' Pain Killer,

and all popular PATENT MEDICINES. Agent for the principal Patent Medicines, both of England and America. Manufacturer of Pure Cod Liver Oil for Medicinal uses, by Wholesale and Retail.

# No. 162 WATER STREET,

# ST. JOHNS, N. F.

Advertisement, 1865. Dearin, who was a conspicuous druggist in St. John's politics, promoted many over-the-counter medicines; he was agent for the successful Ayer company of Massachusetts. Ayer's Sarsaparilla Compound, Ayer's Cherry Pectoral, and Ayer's Cathartic Pills were said to be in great demand.[15]

Eaton's. Newfoundlanders often remember their catalogues – offering many well-known, over-the-counter medicines as well as a range of basic drugs – ending up as toilet paper, but only after being well thumbed.

Some of the outlets reflected changing health-care services. The growth of drugstores – emporia for a wide range of self-care products – even if slow outside St. John's, was significant. One raconteur from the 1930s, noting that "drugs were quite uncontrolled," added "You could write the drugstore and get whatever you wanted."[16] Drugstores, with their variety of health-care and other merchandise and their ease of access, encouraged familiarity with commercial self-care and, as seen in various entries in Part II, mingled commercialism with traditional practices. Further, long-standing home-care activities were increasingly incorporated within the professional pharmacy: by the compounding of family medicines or receipts, the provision of refills for commercially prepared medicine chests, and, as amplified below, the sale (retail and often wholesale) of over-the-counter-medicines

Although over-the-counter medicines had an obvious presence in New-foundland at the time (1860s) of the above Dearin's advertisement, newspaper and other modes of advertising were relatively restrained. By 1900 this had changed dramatically. Additionally, medical entrepreneurs, albeit already noticeable during the nineteenth century, were having an impact. In 1906, E.J. Pratt, Methodist preacher and later a celebrated poet, peddled his "Universal Lung Healer" (containing "spruce tops, wild cherry bark, the rind of fir trees, and sarsaparilla") in the outports. Unfortunately, the precise impact of Pratt's activity is not clear. Nor is the later activity of James Mercer of Shearstown, Newfoundland, and his evocatively named "Arctic Indigestion Cure."[17]

The more conspicuous marketing activities in the early twentieth century centred around the drugstores in St. John's. Both McMurdo and Stafford, typical of countless pharmacies at the time, had popular lines of their own preparations, some manufactured locally.[18] Dr. Bovel's medicines (for example, Herb Tablets for the bowels, liver, and skin) – intensively advertised before World War I, and said to be manufactured in St. John's by the Bovel Manufacturing Company – were also on the market.

### Gerald S. Doyle

Overriding all medicine entrepreneurs was Gerald S. Doyle (1892–1956), one of the most successful in directing the commercialization of self-care

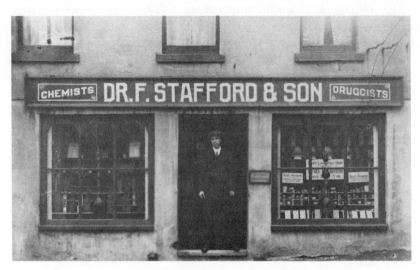

Dr. Stafford developed a line of products popular over many years.
This scene of Stafford and Son was taken in 1910.[19]

in twentieth-century Newfoundland. In 1919, after working as a travelling salesman for a St. John's drug company, Doyle established his own wholesale business for over-the-counter medicines. In ultimately capturing innumerable retail outlets throughout Newfoundland, he developed various ways of spreading his name and distributing manufactured medicines.

Doyle owed his success somewhat to public perceptions that he combined the old and new. Much of *Home Medicine: The Newfoundland Experience* highlights the persistence of beliefs and practices even as many people acknowledged them to be out of date, or even fiction. Although Doyle weaned many Newfoundlanders to his products, he seems also to have encouraged a sense of tradition and community that hardly undermined the traditional remedies that were already part of Newfoundland self-sufficiency.

Doyle's melding of the old and new, which fostered a feeling of familiarity with his medicines, emerged subtly through a range of activities. One of the best known was Doyle's radio "News Bulletin." As the most popular program in Newfoundland – running daily from 18 November 1932 to 1966, ten years after his death – "it nightly plunged the whole island into mute attention."[20] Doyle was probably the most successful entrepreneur in North America to use radio for promoting medicines, partly because listeners tuned in for innumerable personal messages for friends and relatives, such as: "To Mrs Walter Power, Colinet Island, from Dad. Your father had blood transfusion last night, condition about the same. No report from X-ray." (1953)

Also influential, aside from his newspaper *The Family Fireside* (1926–29), was Doyle's *Old Time Songs and Poetry of Newfoundland* (issued for free distribution in 1927, 1940, 1955, and on two occasions following his death). In this songbook, Doyle, as he also did in *Devine's Folk Lore of Newfoundland* (1937), juxtaposed folklore with a plethora of advertisements for his products. The songbook, it should be noted, was not unique as a promotion vehicle for medicines. It is likely, for instance, that Bromo-Seltzer's early commercial success owed something to turn-of-the-century popular songs that mentioned the product; on the other hand, Doyle's activity served more to promote local tradition and feeling.

A legacy of stories about Doyle reveals added elements of showmanship. "One time in Fogo he threw a handful of Tru-Lax packets to a crowd on the wharf and the next day most of them had to stay home 'with the runs' – strong advertising indeed."[21]

Although only advertisements for medicines, rather than advice on treatment, are found in Doyle's songbook and in *Devine's Folk Lore*, these small paperbacks are a reminder of the countless nineteenth- and twentieth-century almanacs, as well as the many substantial home-medicine publications with their obvious purpose of promoting selected brand products. Such publications, popular on the island, straddled the oral tradition and professional medical writings and were a pervasive influence in many ways. In 1951, a medical visitor to Newfoundland noted that the person who then ran the general store at Tilt Cove had some "remarkably good – though old (1912 and 1914) – home medical books. With these he practices very good general medicine – sets fractures, pulls teeth (no anaesthetic), and decides who is sick enough to go to the hospital."[22]

## ALMANACS, HOME-MEDICINE BOOKS, RECIPE BOOKS

One elderly Newfoundlander recently noted that Dr. Chase's Almanacs were sent to every householder free of charge.

On every second page was the date, the weather, and signs. The second page showed the abdomen cut open and the different parts that could be affected by illness ... There were pictures of people who were cured by taking Dr. Chase's medicines. Everyone found their complaints and compared them to the person. There were also jokes and helpful hints, and thirty blank lines to record happenings such as "John Smith died of a stroke" or "a baby boy born to Mary Parsons" or "the Parrots had a boat load of fish."[23]

Chase's almanacs were successful promotional media for company products already established in the nineteenth century. In 1926, just to note one year, the Chase Company told Canadian pharmacists it was distributing 1.7 million copies of the almanac.[24] Even though illiteracy was high in places, information on Chase treatments spread easily. In Newfoundland, aside from intensive advertising, Doyle did more than anyone to make Chase products household-names, indeed a tradition, on the island. Witness, for example, Dr. Chase's Syrup of Linseed and Turpentine, Dr. Chase's Ointment, Dr. Chase's Nerve Food, and Dr. Chase's Cold Tablets. At the end of a Doyle "News Bulletin," the following (from a 1953 broadcast, or something similar) might appear:

Dr. Chase's Nerve Food can help you get natural rest night after night. Start today with Dr. Chase's Nerve Food. Dr. Chase's Nerve Food is a tested tonic thousands use to help improve general health. Dr. Chase's Nerve Food contains blood-improving iron, vitamin B, and other necessary minerals. These work together to help build up your whole system. When you take Dr. Chase's Nerve Food, you can feel better, eat better, have steadier nerves, more restful nights. Take the first step toward better general health with Dr. Chase's Nerve Food. It can help you feel better all day long, rest better all night through.

Say are you catching cold? Reach for Dr. Chase's Cold Tablets now. Dr. Chase's Cold Tablets with four proven fighting ingredients stop miserable cold symptoms in just 24 hours. Be ready for the cold season with Dr. Chase's Cold Tablets.[25]

Doyle also distributed copies of Dr. Chase's recipe books (for example, *Receipt Book and Household Physician*). The medical section of this useful home encyclopedia contained much advice, some of it professionally acceptable, about looking after the sick; such as provide clean air, invalid foods, herb teas for the sick room, and so on. An eclectic range of recipes was also included, such as the well-known "kitchen remedies" kerosene and borax, which probably influenced many Newfoundlanders. Also noted were such commercial medicines as Ayer's Cherry Pectoral (which, although it competed with Chase's products, hardly diminished the overall promotion for the Chase company).

Another domestic-medicine book, almost certainly well known in Newfoundland until World War I, was R.V. Pierce's *The People's Common Sense Medical Adviser*, published between 1875 and c.1941. Unlike Chase's volume, it was limited to medical and health advice, extolling and promoting such medicines as Dr. Pierce's Favourite Prescription and Dr. Pierce's Golden Medical Discovery.

Of the Chase and Pierce volumes – their low price helped with promotion – Chase's was the most influential on the island. Both were akin to countless home- and sea-medicine guides – other texts that may have influenced Newfoundlanders – as well as family collections of medical, culinary, and other recipes handed down from one generation to the next, which illuminate home medicine in the more distant past.[26] Unfortunately, since printed sources of information on self-care in early Newfoundland are scarce, few such manuscripts with a Newfoundland association have been located. This makes one manuscript, Redfearn/Smith, compiled in Britain during the early decades of the nineteenth century, especially valuable.[27]

There is no way of knowing if this manuscript was used much in Newfoundland after its arrival – probably not long after it was written – although permanent settlement in the island was increasing at the time. At least it contains much that is in line with later Newfoundland self-treatment. Linseed, for instance, was the basis of a cough medicine; senna was commonly noted for complaints for which a laxative was recommended, as was Epsom salts; camphorated spirits was indicated for strains; tobacco poultice for the stomach to treat "stoppage" of urine; and turpentine as an application to cuts. There are hints, too, of uncertainties about professional care. It was said, for instance, that a recipe for worms had never been known to fail, though physicians had given up on their patients.

### ADVERTISEMENTS: FAMILIAR THEMES

The impact of domestic medicine books by Chase, Pierce, and others in Newfoundland would have been much less without the intensive advertising of their medicines in newspapers and elsewhere. Various concepts and themes employed in the advertisements illustrate that commercial success in the self-care market owed something to exploiting and sustaining existing popular beliefs, as well as to invoking new science and fashions. Also significant was the use of concepts, particularly cleanliness and nutrition, stressed by health reformers in North America and elsewhere. Like the activities of Doyle, a mix of tradition and newness prevailed. Furthermore, such beliefs as purification, discussed later on, provide insight not only into lay attitudes toward health and disease, which have shaped home medicine, but also into factors that can affect physician-patient relationships.

### Concepts of Purification

Perhaps the most conspicuous advertisement theme in the first half of the twentieth century, possibly more so in the United States than elsewhere, played on concerns about cleanliness, both outside and inside the body. Although soaps and toilet products with their many overtones of improving health and revitalizing the body did reach Newfoundland, their precise impact is uncertain. Of greater influence, however, was the notion of inner cleanliness or purification, both by laxatives (for example, Epsom salts "cleans the blood they tells you") and blood purification. These regimens were intended to free the body from "poisons" or "toxins" and thus prevent or treat disease.

Although the latter concepts encouraged the long-standing use of laxatives and blood purifiers, added credibility came in the early decades of the twentieth century through the new theory of "autointoxication" accepted and used by many physicians. In part, associated with the notion of visceroptosis – that is, kinking in the intestine considered to produce stasis – autointoxication alleged that absorption of toxins led to chronic poisoning. In the early 1900s, the theory was promoted and disseminated not only by establishment medical figures, such as London surgeon Sir William Arbuthnot Lane, but also in novels, plays, and popular medical works. One character in Bernard Shaw's *Doctor's Dilemma* said: "Ninety-five percent of the human race suffer from chronic blood-poisoning and die of it. It's as simple as A.B.C. Your intestine is full of decaying matter – undigested food and waste products – rank ptomaines."[28]

While popular medical works such as Charles M. Campbell's *The Lazy Colon* (1924) also helped to cement new ideas of toxins among the English-speaking public, countless appendectomies, tonsillectomies, and teeth extractions – in the belief that alleged sites of focal infection (autointoxication) were being removed – probably had a greater public impact. In St. John's, one medical practitioner even viewed the cervix as an infection site and, for this reason, sometimes removed it surgically. The St. John's *Evening Telegram* told readers during March 1921 about Nujol, a laxative to control autointoxication in "thirty-five feet of danger." By the 1930s, when professional medical criticism of autointoxication emerged – for instance, "it must be [said] that the 'autointoxication' bugaboo ... may be speedily dismissed" – it is doubtful whether the criticism had much immediate public impact.[29]

Among advertisements for medicines in the St. John's *Evening Telegram* during the 1930s that undoubtedly sustained lay notions of "purification," "poisons," and so on was Cystex, recommended for the kidney and said to clean out "acids and poisons," to purify blood, and to bring new vigour within forty-eight hours. Another was Sal Hepatica, a "saline cocktail," promoted to cleanse the whole system, sweep out toxic wastes, and purify the blood stream. The long popular Dodd's Kidney Pills had a similar message: "Healthy kidneys filter poisons from the blood. If they are faulty and fail, poisons stay in the system and sleeplessness, headaches, and backaches often follow. If you don't sleep well, try Dodd's." And there were other concepts such as Listerine for a "new" disorder – halitosis or bad breath.[30]

Such promotion reinforced popular concepts about the causes of disease. Aside from bolstering opinions about toxins, they underpinned the views of those who saw purification as tinged with religious overtones. Almost certainly, too, there was support for various concepts linking blood with disease. Apart from the fairly common idea of "thick" and "thin" blood, it was said (in 1936) that Newfoundlanders thought insanity was caused by a "turning of the blood" as a result of a fight or a quarrel, though it is not known if this was widely believed. In a similar manner, the nightmare of the old hag – often noted in Newfoundland records – has been attributed to "stagnation of the blood."[31]

### Foods as Health Products

The passionate promotion of food products for better health, prominent on both sides of the Atlantic from 1900 onward, exploited many beliefs and fears. Although criticisms in the early decades of the century as to unwarranted nutritional and medical claims for numerous cereals and beverages were justifiable (some called it "nutritional quackery"), the claims underscored the rampant nature of nutritional problems. This probably had a special impact on many Newfoundlanders, who were being increasingly subjected to "messages" about health issues.

In Newfoundland, as elsewhere, many people were influenced by such notions as "strengtheners," tonics, and energy. Even before 1900, numerous medicines (for example, Dr. Pierce's Golden Medical Discovery) were promoted in this manner, and it seemed natural to read that Grape-Nuts was a "rebuilder of brain and brawn." Cod liver oil, which came to be promoted essentially as a food, was said to help "correct nature's failure. For bones, teeth, malnutrition." And there was Guiness: "no beverage in the market is possessed of the recuperative qualities of Guiness." In a sense, many foods were also viewed as a "fuel" for the body as engine. Seeing the body in mechanical terms, a long-pervasive analogy, has been conspicuous in the twentieth century. In fact medical language still embraces the analogy in many ways, using such terms as "run-down," "worn out," "fix my plumbing," and so on.

Other concepts were also at play. Products such as Epps's Cocoa, in being "specially grateful and comforting to the nervous and dyspeptic," may have had a special appeal to Newfoundlanders, since both conditions ("nerves" and stomach problems), as noted later, were prevalent.

By the 1920s, another factor had become significant. Food product manufacturers were pushing relatively new scientific thoughts about the importance of vitamins, with often overly optimistic therapeutic claims. Dr. Chase's Nerve Food gained a new lease on life. Advertisements in Doyle's 1940 songbook catalogued numerous symptoms for which the product was to be employed – "jittery nerves, irritability, pallor of skin, weariness, lack of pep, sleeplessness, indigestion, gloomy feelings, headaches" – all implicating vitamin $B_1$: "This food treatment contains Vitamin $B_1$, which along with mineral substances present in the Nerve Food, make this an outstanding restorative of the blood and the nerves. With new rich, nourishing blood coursing through the arteries, nervous energy is restored and with it

the confidence and well being which is reflected in new poise and personality." Chase's product, in fact, not only promoted a vitamin, but also
offered another way to manage two long-standing considerations: nerves
and impure blood.

## Mother and Baby

A conspicuous feature of food and health promotion was (and is) catering
to the mother and baby market. Perhaps as much as anything, this promotion both fostered and exploited a sense of comfortable tradition, inasmuch
as it stressed new developments. Many products – from Allenbury's "food
for infants" to preparations of malt (for example, Virol, which stressed, in
1900, "vital principles essential for growth and development"), as well as
Chase's and other medicines – often wove motherhood and healthy families
into their advertisements. During the 1930s, even "Grandma's nerves"
became well again with Chase's Nerve Food. Much promotion reflected a
theme that extended back to the eighteenth century, namely linking many
health issues with the woman and her family.

The extent to which commercial products were used as an alternative to
breast feeding in Newfoundland, at least prior to World War II, is not
entirely clear. The growing use of condensed milks, which emerged in the
last decades of the nineteenth century, reflected increased promotion on
both sides of the Atlantic. By the 1920s, thanks to the newspaper advertisements, Newfoundland mothers must have often been told that Carnation
milk – which is still a popular product on the island – was "safe milk for
your baby." Its use for the celebrated Dionne quintuplets in the 1930s
influenced mothers worldwide.

An especially well-known product in Newfoundland, Cocomalt, also
played unabashedly to family centredness and became widely known to
children in Newfoundland, especially those who received it as a school
drink. A 1937 advertisement warned Newfoundland women who were
"sailing happily into motherhood" not to leave this important event to
chance, but to consult a physician. "Wise mother! Lucky babe! And the
physician will always stress the importance of diet." The need for vitamins
and minerals (vitamin D, iron, calcium, and phosphorus) was stressed.
Cocomalt – "The Protective Food Drink" – was, of course, the answer.

Various entries in Part II make clear that an especially difficult aspect of
child care was choosing from countless children's medicines, many of which
underscored mothers' fears about infant diseases. There were fears, too,
about certain medicines. Concern existed, for instance, in the early years
of the twentieth century about the opium (or the isolated morphine)
content in a number of medicines for children. Even in 1940, Baby's Own
Tablets were still being said to "contain no opiates or stupefying drugs."

That much traditional self-care is, as will become clearer from later sections, a melded collection of diverse beliefs contributes both to making certain elements resistant to change, as well as to making it easy for new practices to be incorporated. Newfoundlanders were undoubtedly as receptive to new over-the-counter medicines and their promotion as were people elsewhere. Although there is little overtly distinctive to the Newfoundland commercial medicine story, the role of Doyle and the tradition – here meaning long-standing familiarity – that enveloped certain medicines (for instance, Chase's products, Minard's Liniment, and cod liver oil) is striking. It is no paradox that a small core of over-the-counter products melded into New-foundland self-care, emerging as part of its tradition.

### CHANGE AND CONTROLS

Advertisements for medicines from the first half of the twentieth century, when read nowadays, serve as a sharp reminder of the considerable changes that have taken place in recent times. Any understanding of this change must recognize the backdrop of countless medical, scientific, and social developments in the nineteenth and twentieth centuries.

Developments that included X-rays, insulin for diabetes, other hormones, vitamins, antibiotics, and surgical advances contributed significantly to the growing authority of the medical profession during the first half of the twentieth century. Much of this authority was reinforced by the expanding role of hospitals in Newfoundland, as elsewhere, and, indirectly, by the increasing role of government (and the physicians it called upon) in health matters. Significant, too, was the community involvement, ranging from the Newfoundland Association for the Prevention of Consumption to "Fish Appeals" for the Notre Dame Bay Memorial Hospital. Fish were given to raise proceeds: "Maybe a fish a day will keep the doctor away."[32]

All such developments are frequently viewed as helping to make twentieth-century life increasingly dependent on professional medicine. Certainly, along with the commercialization of over-the-counter medicines, the changing medical scene did undermine many existing home remedies. But this was not always because of the latter's ineffectiveness. Many, which had long-standing European or North American origins and well-estab-lished reputations for providing relief for minor complaints, were increasingly seen as "old fashioned" or "quack medicines" and pushed aside. Indeed, many elderly Newfoundlanders now say that the greater reliance placed on doctors contributed to the decline of home remedies as well. One said recently (1992): "First you'd have to believe that they [have] made no progress in medicine, but they have, so I can't push that in the back, all the new technology. I'd have to be taken to the Waterford [mental hospital] to get my head examined if I started using home remedies today."[33] Yet

change was slow. By 1900, the claims for countless over-the-counter remedies were being challenged by the medical profession on the basis that they
misled a gullible public. Much advertising, certainly striking for its extravagant therapeutic claims (see many entries in Part II), became the butt of
public jokes and satire. One early twentieth-century song poked fun at all
treatments:

> I've swallowed tons of doctors pills
> Of black draughts had my share, too
> I've every potion, lotion, drug in the pharmacopoeia
> That medicine is all humbug is now my firm idea ...
>
> The patent medicine advertised I have got tired of swillin!
> I've tried bay rum, Taraxacum, and likewise Podophylin
> The list of remedies I've used would fill a tidy vollum.[34]

Reform of medicines was conspicuous amid such a climate; efforts grew
to make the disclosure of certain ingredients (opiates, for example) man-
datory and to curb excessive therapeutic claims in the United States, Britain,
and Canada, particularly during the first half of the twentieth century.
Newfoundland, despite its first Pharmacy Act in 1910 – putting in place
controls over the sale of certain drugs and poisons – had no specific impact
on the proprietary medicine market. However, since most medicines were
imported, they reflected controls elsewhere.

Even so, excessive claims remained commonplace throughout the first
half of the twentieth century. Since the 1950s, alongside the growing
number of prescription-only products not advertised to the public, advertising of over-the-counter medicines has become increasingly restrained and
increasingly focused on analgesics, laxatives, cold and cough medicines,
stomach preparations, and vitamins. Nowadays, much of the local advertising focuses as much on low prices (compared with a competitor's) as on
medical claims.

In 1949, through Confederation, Newfoundland came under Canadian
jurisdiction. The result was a more limited range of available preparations.
Under the jurisdiction of the 1934 amended Food and Drug Act, Canada
had established a list of medical conditions for which it became illegal to
advertise treatments directly to the public, thereby reducing available preparations from some 60,000 to 6,000 or so. Even so, countless questions
continued about the advertising and safety of both prescription and over-
the-counter medications.[35]

# Physician and Patient: Attitudes and Interactions

One facet of the changes in medicine and the growing authority of physicians from 1900 onward was the professionals' attitude to self-care. Were Newfoundland physicians as critical about proprietary medicines and other aspects of self-treatment as countless physicians elsewhere? In fact, many historians consider that the professionalization of medicine from the nineteenth century onward contributed to self-medication being increasingly viewed as "unprofessional," as well as to a sharpening of the differences between self- and professional care. Unfortunately, insufficient evidence has been uncovered to provide a clear picture of attitudes in Newfoundland. The following remarks make clear, however, that a variety of factors helped to shape (as they still do) lay and professional attitudes toward self-care practices.

## MEDICAL AUTHORITY AND THE PUBLIC

Various remarks by physicians who wrote on nutrition problems in Newfoundland (c. 1910–50) suggest that there was little professional sympathy with "non-scientific" medical practices.[36] These writers, however, were a select few. Others may have been sensitive to local beliefs, or at least relatively non-judgmental, and employed them in their everyday practice. Wilfred Grenfell was generally positive about the basic lifestyles of fishermen and their families as he tried to create healthier conditions in Labrador and northern Newfoundland. From today's perspective, however, he had a paternalist attitude ("doctors know best"), commonplace among physicians at the time. In 1919, Grenfell tried to "explain" away superstitions among Christians of devout and simple faith: "The superstitions still found among them are attributable to the remoteness of the country from the current of the world's thought, the natural tendency of all seafaring people, and the fact that the days when the forebears of these fishermen left 'Merrie

England' to seek a living by the harvest of the sea, and finally settled on those rocky shores, were those when witches and hobgoblins and charms and amulets were accepted beliefs."[37] Perhaps in this context Grenfell humoured patients who followed superstitious practices: "Charms were worn by many, and time after time Grenfell was asked to 'charm' away a pain. He grinned and waved his hand and said, 'meenie Mini Mo,' and [then he] got to work properly."[38]

Even if condemnation of local self-care practices by some physicians in Newfoundland – who often came from Britain and America where quackery aroused strong emotions – was conspicuous, it did not necessarily influence Newfoundlanders. Certainly, it is unclear at present how rural communities accepted "modern" medicine: readily and quickly, enthusiastically, or with elements of suspicion or questioning. A story by Grenfell suggests the latter, at least on occasions.

A colleague of mine was visiting on his winter rounds in a delightful village some forty miles south of St. Anthony Hospital. The "swiles" (seals) had stuck in, and all hands were out on the ice, eager to capture their share of these valuable animals. But snow-blindness had attacked the men, and had rendered them utterly unable to profit by their good fortune. The doctor's clinic was long and busy that night. The following morning he was, however, amazed to see many of his erstwhile patients wending their way seawards, each with one eye only treated on his prescription. The other (for safety's sake) was being doctored after the long-accepted methods of the talent of the village – tansy poultices and sugar being the favourites. The consensus of opinion obviously was that the risk was too great to venture both eyes at once on the doubtful altar of modern medicine.[39]

That physicians' prescriptions did not always help was a common occurrence, and it is noteworthy that oral reports of self-care often proclaimed triumph over professional medicine. Yet whether or not this justification contributed to the reluctance of many Newfoundlanders to consult professional help is unclear. ("Jim has never been to a doctor in his life and doesn't intend to start now" is a frequent statement.) Certainly other considerations existed, such as fear of losing work, particularly if one was a fisherman (see, for instance, entries on *appendicitis* and *seal finger*).

Many other issues probably at times affected physician-patient relations, some of which are noted elsewhere in this account. They included illness behaviours of Newfoundland women linked to their busy lives and particular health concerns, men's perceptions of manliness and independence, religious beliefs, and the oft-noted fatalism among Newfoundlanders (a ready acceptance of what life brings). There is, too, Newfoundlanders' diverse attitudes to authority; for instance, they were often less respectful of "government" physicians (for example, salaried physicians in the cottage hospitals) than of private practitioners.[40] Today, older physicians remember that such horrendous pathology as tumours among Newfoundlanders was once more common than nowadays, because of failure to consult professionals early.

Against such a background, Newfoundlanders probably rarely worried about professional medicine's concerns and frustrations about self-care, particularly that serious problems curable by scientific medicine might be masked. Even with such striking changes in Newfoundland health care during the 1920s and '30s as the emergence of the Newfoundland outport-nursing program, government-sponsored cottage hospitals, prepaid health-care schemes (reflective of earlier "book" practices in Newfoundland) and new therapies – all developments that helped move self-care closer to professionally accepted practices – numerous Newfoundlanders still accepted the positive testimonials of family and friends about countless old-time remedies.

Yet, at the same time, Newfoundlanders were swayed by the subtle and less subtle promotion of the over-the-counter medicines already considered. Aside from the role of pharmacists and advertising, encouragement to use commercial products came from the apparent imprimatur of certain doctors, some of whom had their own lines of products. From the 1890s onward, the distinction between medicines advertised to doctors (sometimes called "ethical proprietaries") and medicines specifically for self-care became blurred. As doctors and their patients welcomed the convenience of more and more packaged remedies, manufacturers saw a market to exploit on both sides of the Atlantic. Indeed, the first prescription written by a doctor for products like Fellows' Syrup of Hypophosphites was apt to be the last. Many a sufferer, from the printing on the carton and the pamphlets packed within, found enough medical advice – and in vigorous, down-to-earth, and frightening prose – to dispense with a doctor.[41]

PERSONAL HEALTH AND ATTITUDES, LIFESTYLES, AND PUBLIC HEALTH

Lay attitudes to medical authority can affect the success of health programs, especially those which depend on personal and home hygiene. Professional and commercial emphasis on inner and outer cleanliness, good nutrition, and so on has already been noted, though how Newfoundlanders translated these into practice, as with other medical ideas, depended on many interacting factors. These might include personal beliefs about the cause of a disease (for instance, germs, sins, or imprudent living), severity of the condition, perceptions and advice of friends and relatives, social pressures (the authority of a physician), as well as general cultural issues such as the local availability of alternative healers and long-standing concerns about, say, the environment.

Despite cultural "norms" – known in any community – that stressed health as central to the happiness of mankind, and the necessity of fresh air, hard work, careful attention to diet, peace of mind, moderation in sexual habits, and so on, the influence of published discussions on, for instance, "damp cellars" and "dust and disease" in reinforcing existing ideas is unclear, even among the literate. Some health precepts, it seems, received relatively little reinforcement at times. As noted in entries in Part II, references to disinfectants and germs were hardly mentioned in the New-foundland press until around 1900. Elsewhere, even by the 1880s, disinfectants were often promoted as a principal precaution against germs. Did the lack of commercial pressure make Newfoundlanders less receptive, less prepared, for new public-health messages based on germs?

Until at least the 1950s, long-standing ideas, well-established prior to the modern germ theory concerning the impact of the environment, especially changes in temperature ("You'll catch your death of cold") certainly per-sisted. There were also concerns about health at critical life-stages, such as when giving birth, breast-feeding, or in old age. One story is that a Newfoundland mother died as a result of handling cold cabbage after giving birth; another Newfoundlander recalled that in 1975: "I had abscess of breasts, both; they took the child out to be baptised. This is what I blamed for it. When they came home she was warm, and when they laid her along side of me, I thought I felt a chill."[42] This, of course, implied an awareness that there were some behaviours to avoid. Nevertheless, despite public-health education programs on sanitation and other matters, and particular concerns about such infectious diseases as tuberculosis and scarlet fever, it is not clear that a consciousness about prevention was widespread. The notion, for instance, that "an ounce of prevention is worth a pound of cure" can be found in the oral tradition, but there is no certainty that it was a guiding principle for Newfoundlanders in general.[43] The oral record contains few specific suggestions on prevention that reflect the teachings of regular medicine at the time, aside from concerns about such children's diseases as measles, and quarantine measures for diseases ranging from influenza to tuberculosis. Although it is, of course, hard to know how many people took cod liver oil regularly, carried charms to prevent rheumatism, or even carried a piece of bread into the woods to make the fairies friendly, elderly Newfoundlanders nowadays remember little discussion about health in the "old days."[44]

Twentieth-century writings on Newfoundland public health, while point-ing out that health problems on the island have been difficult to deal with because of poor economy and isolated communities, have generally painted a picture of continual improvement. In many ways this is justified, but it skates over the idiosyncrasies of individuals who may not look kindly on authority and who often create personal and domestic situations far different from those advocated by medical texts. This makes it difficult, if not impossible, to answer many questions. Was immunization implemented as recommended throughout the first half of the twentieth century? To what extent were culturally accepted recommendations about sleep, diet, and fresh air heeded? Did the use of charms, and so on influence attitudes toward these health maxims? Were various "health" sayings generally known and taken seriously, such as "carrots improve your sight" and "give you curly hair" or "it is bad luck for two people to dry their hands on the same towel?"[45] And what were the attitudes toward "germs"?

In fact, many Newfoundlanders, at least when looking back, hold the view that an outdoor life with much hard work and rough food was all that was necessary for good health: "Just never had a day's sickness; I was right in the bloom of health. But somewhere down along the road probably I abused myself and picked up that germ, see – that was the weak spot."[46] The concept of a weakness or carelessness that is difficult to avoid is still current.

It is well known that perceptions of health and illness may reflect socio-economic status and contribute to differences between precept and practice in preventive medicine. Unfortunately, such factors are little explored *vis-à-vis* Newfoundland. For instance, what, in fact, did women consider as a sufficiently healthy meal in times of shortage? Did this mean more attention was paid to healthful cod liver oil? And how widespread was resistance to eating brown bread, which had a stigma of poverty?

An amusing, telling example of the difficulties of public-health education was told by Dr. Rutherford in Bonavista when delivering a health-education lecture in 1909. His account to a lay audience about the problems of getting people to use a spittoon is a reminder of the difficulties of public health and of the idiosyncrasies found time and time again in the story of self-care:[47]

My first experience with a highly decorated cuspidor showing birds and tropical plants gracefully wandering round its mouth impressed upon me the necessity of choosing for public use at any rate, only those of the plainest patterns. Some years ago, I placed on the floor of the surgery well in the centre, so that the most erratic workman could hardly miss it, a very pretty little cuspidor. It was a handsome article ... with the willow pattern painted on the bowl and some botanical freaks dipping down into the well. After some days' bombardment, I was much puzzled to know how it was that, though the surrounding floor was a foaming sea of sputum, the cuspidor floated bravely high and dry above the waves, without shipping a drop of water. At length I enquired of a particularly energetic marksman

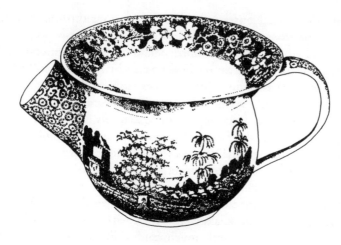

Blue and white spittoon, 19<sup>th</sup> century

if he didn't think that with a little more practice he could hit the cuspidor once out of three times at any rate. To my surprise he promptly fired a shot plumb into the centre without touching the sides. Upon my mildly suggesting that he might have found the mark earlier, he looked at me reproachfully and said, "Sir, I was a feerd I'd hit them flowers what's marked on the thing!"

## MEDICAL INTERFACES AND MATTERS OF COMMUNICATION

The interface between professional medicine and self-treatment has always been complex. The medical profession's disquiet over much home care remained at a high level during the first half of the twentieth century and helped to sustain, and perhaps sharpen, the view that self-treatment was second-class medicine. This was just one factor that encouraged certain practices to be viewed as fringe medicine. Another consideration was (and is) a person's failure to act consistently in a totally rational way; this tendency – sometimes reflecting the co-existence of magic, religion, and science as part of an individual's world view – can complicate physician-patient interactions by shaping attitudes and beliefs often at variance with scientific medicine.

Among specific aspects of popular culture that affect physician-patient relations, effective communication is of particular importance. Elderly Newfoundlanders have often noted that their revered physicians always found time to talk. Language issues are especially significant in the island, for illiteracy has long been relatively high and dialects contributed to a clash of cultures between Newfoundlanders and the many immigrant British, Irish, and American physicians.

Recent studies from many countries have highlighted widespread communication difficulties between physicians and patients, especially in rural areas and places where ethnic differences exist. Noticed are 1) the persistent popular use of medical terms after their disappearance from professional medicine; 2) a misunderstanding of medical terms because of a change in meaning over time or the existence of more than one meaning; 3) euphemisms for pregnancy, genitalia, menstruation, defecation, urination, and so on; 4) words and phrases used to describe a symptom – sometimes purely descriptive even if obsolete, and sometimes metaphorical – that may disguise the severity of symptoms; 5) "folk illnesses" or diagnoses that have no counterpart in current professional medicine; 6) the complexity of medical terminology such that it is often oversimplified by physicians; 7) malapropisms in which a lay person confuses the pronunciation of medical terminology; and 8) different communication patterns in general, reflecting class, educational differences, and much more.[48]

The recently recorded Newfoundland oral tradition contains many examples of medical and related expressions rarely known by younger physicians, even those brought up on the island. In fact, many terms are now obsolete even to older Newfoundlanders, although the editors of the *Dictionary of Newfoundland English* (1990) have noted their surprise at finding "terms, long absent from the printed record, on the lips of contemporary Newfoundlanders."[49]

If only because of the uneven usage of many Newfoundland words and expressions, it is appropriate to give a sampling here; others are illustrated in Part II. Diagnostic terms such as "grippe," "stomach flu," "liverish," "biliousness," and a "fester" (also a "gathering" or "rising") were once commonly found in the professional and lay medical literature of the past. When used today, they may be correctly understood – even if unfamiliar to a health-care worker – from the clinical context, as, for instance, such terms as "dropped palate." On the other hand, pitfalls in interpretation can exist for a variety of reasons, aside from what are described as popular or ethnomedical (rather than biomedical) diagnoses. Recently "grippe" has been used to describe "griping," rather than flu, and "stomach flu" has been used to refer to vomiting. At the same time, expressions reported as malapropisms may embrace persistent popular concepts; for instance, "roaches of the liver" may point to a belief in animalcules as well as cirrhosis (see entry on liverishness).[50]

The accounts as a whole – the narratives – of Newfoundlanders describing their conditions and treatments raise various issues. The language is commonly expressive, with its telling metaphors, analogies, and resonances, all of which often help, along with other factors mentioned later, to retain memories and experiences. In a personal communication, one Newfoundlander related in 1992 about a childhood event: "She said, 'I'm going to cure your lips for you now and you'll never have it anymore.' So she said: 'Are you a good hand to dance?' I said, 'Yes.' 'Well,' she said, 'You're going to dance now,' because she put vinegar on my lips." The informant remembers well "dancing lips" and still carries the vinegar for whenever the trouble occurs.

Feelings and sensitive issues difficult for some to make explicit are noticeable too. One Newfoundlander told a story of a patient describing a "wonderful pain" in her stomach. Aside from "wonderful" meaning bad, the pain was actually in the breast; there was a reluctance to use the word breast and the stomach was a respectable area nearby.[51] This is just one example of "coding," or ways in which people refer to issues and feelings they do not want to make explicit.

Particular issues surround certain diagnostic terms used by Newfoundlanders (for example, "nerves"; see entry), which often have no precise match with a professional medical diagnosis. This is also a reminder of a caution (first raised in 1980) that some people interpret hypertension as hyper-tension; that is, as a condition characterized not by blood pressure, but by excessive nervousness and untoward social stress.[52]

Many other words and phrases in popular speech, such as "bun in the oven" (pregnancy), are commonplace throughout the English-speaking world and are thus unlikely to be misunderstood. This also applies to the Newfoundland expression being "up the stump again" (pregnant again), although "stumping the baby" is the change from long to shorter clothes after the first six weeks of life. Just as signs of pregnancy may help health-care workers extricate themselves from pregnancy euphemisms unknown to them, so clinical and other contexts can aid in interpreting the following selection of terms and phrases recently remembered in Newfoundland, even if rarely used today. (Omitted are those commonly known throughout English-speaking countries).[53]

- bazzom (purplish coloured bruise)
- bladder (pimple, blister from burn)
- boo (louse)
- brew a cold (develop a cold)
- browal (a swelling on the head, often the forehead or brow)
- burned (frostburn, frostbite)
- cow out (to be exhausted physically)
- crit (in cramped position, kink in back)
- dead-eye (sore or callus on the hand)
- dead-man's pinch (small mark or bruise appearing without apparent cause)

- dishy (pale or sickly in complexion, perhaps also known as "shortage of blood")
- going out to squeeze my brews (going to the outhouse, to the toilet)
- jaw-locked (unable to talk from cramped muscles or dislocation)
- scutters or scuts (diarrhoea)
- split your spraddle (injure the pelvic area)
- west or wis (for styes)
- yuck (to vomit).

Additionally, various descriptive terms exist, which although rarely completely misunderstood by health-care workers can give the unwary a false impression of a patient's own perception of his or her symptoms. New-foundland usage of "smart" can mean in good health or to have a pain, while "awful" can mean bad or exceptional (also with regard to pain). Even words like "rampsing" – fooling around like children – may need to be assessed when reviewing injuries. For instance, how much fooling was involved?

As indicated, most of the expressions noted above are rarely, if ever, heard nowadays, at least by health-care workers. It is well known that when patients talk with health professionals (especially physicians), they tend to switch from vernacular speech to what they perceive as medical language. Yet if vernacular terms are used, the health-care worker must not only be sufficiently sensitive to ensure the patient freedom from embarrassment, but also to understand the concepts behind the words.

A significant communication issue is that although certain words and phrases may have largely disappeared, the concepts behind them remain a living force, albeit sometimes modified. "Dirty blood," for instance, may no longer be mentioned in the presence of a health-care worker, but there is renewed interest nowadays in blood purifiers and tonics (see entries). All this is helping to re-establish wide interest, although partly under the concept of "balanced blood." The persistence of concepts, of which other examples are noted in the following section and elsewhere, serves to caution health-care workers about the counselling of patients; they are reminded to elicit all the concerns of their patients, not just ones about the biological lesion. Persistent concepts also serve as a reminder of the problems of health promotion in physicians' offices.[54]

# Self-Care:
## Effectiveness and Community Roles

The ascendency of commercial preparations (already described) and their contribution to edging out many long-standing practices, along with the scepticism if not opposition of physicians, prompts various questions about the effectiveness of both the old-time practices and the newer products. There is a question, too, as to whether Newfoundland self-care had a social role that has been lost to the changes in recent years.

### QUESTIONS ABOUT REMEDIES: BELIEFS AND EFFECTIVENESS

Despite testimonials supporting numerous traditional home-regimens and a belief that since they were used they must work, many were generally ineffective, at least if assessed by current pharmacological knowledge. Why then did they persist or continue to be known, even some that were generally recognized as of little value? A striking range of factors and lay concepts in fact contributed to the belief in, and probably the persistence of, many practices. One elderly Newfoundlander, when asked in 1992 about "old remedies," said: "I suppose it is foolish, but I believe in it." Behind this attitude may be such considerations as 1) experience, testimonials, and familiarity; 2) the attitudes of a physician; 3) religion and magic; 4) symbols; 5) concepts of diseases; 6) environmental beliefs; and 7) faith. Such factors are not to be seen as mutually exclusive, for as they interact they contribute to an individuality of explanation and, during transmission, changes in the ideas occur. These factors also reflect shades of meaning and reality for individuals, thereby helping them to reinforce, undermine, or justify practices and beliefs to suit their particular circumstances. Interaction of ideas also contributes to inconsistencies in explanations and uncertainty about causes of disease and treatments, all of which seems to encourage disquiet with professional medicine as well as tendencies to try non-professional treatments.

Nowadays, Newfoundlanders over 65 years of age often vividly remember positive experiences and testimonials about old-time remedies. They remember a readiness to try out a "new" regimen, especially if recommended by "grandmother."[55] Among those in a family or community who spread testimonials, grandmothers were often perceived as a fountain of empirical evidence and of "common sense" in medical and other matters. For many in Newfoundland this is still the case today, but, as elsewhere, families are increasingly dispersed and children commonly live in distant communities. Grandmother is now more likely to live in a seniors' or nursing home with relatively little contact with grandchildren. Nevertheless, common sense in matters of health and illness continues to justify many treatments. Although common sense means different things to different people, it has long tended to refer to regimens that are viewed as natural rather than artificial.

Despite the overall negative views among physicians about traditional self-care, "orthodox" medical ideas have commonly served as both a "testimonial" to, and a reinforcement (perhaps with some modification in detail) of, the long-standing popular beliefs so readily documented in Newfoundland. Aside from physicians recommending many of the treatments (for example, poultices), there were, in the early decades of the twentieth century, for instance, such theories of disease as autointoxication (already noted) or acidity as a cause of many ailments, both of which reinforced in a general way certain existing lay beliefs about blood and disease. And these beliefs have continued in the popular medical culture long after becoming unacceptable to professional medicine. Further, a professional theory often reinforced a popular belief found under different guises (for example, treating "dirty blood" and the need for "balanced food"), which for some Newfoundlanders helped form coherent patterns of medical ideas. Notions of bad blood, for instance, could justify the use of blood purifiers, liver and kidney medicines, as well as tonics and laxatives. As for the expression "fix my plumbing," although heard less frequently nowadays, it still reflects the concept of the body as an engine and pipes and encourages concepts of cleaning, purifying, and balancing. In fact, such notions are part of the recurring theme of balance and equilibrium in the history of health care, as well as an idea that a lack of balance leads to ill-health.

Long-standing religious beliefs such as "God provided herbs," that God's healing power is transmitted through the clergy or others, and that religious transgressions are a cause of illness have been as significant in Newfoundland health care, if not more so, as elsewhere. Recollections are not so much concerned with what might be called "miraculous healing" as with a need to pay attention to religious matters (for example, by praying, counting the rosary, wearing a religious medal, and adding drops of holy water to a medicine); unsuccessful treatments might be blamed on a lack of faith rather than failure of the medication or regimen. Moreover, there were beliefs that rested on notions of mysterious forces, and on harmful activities of fairies, witches and, in some parts of the island, on the "spells" of Micmac Indians.[56] Although Newfoundlanders have long had doubts about, if not frankly disbelieved, many of these notions, recent studies on Newfoundland folklore raise questions about their persistence.

Another, albeit somewhat intangible, factor behind certain persisting practices was the reinforcement of a medical reputation through a product's overall value and symbolism to Newfoundlanders. For example, the key role of both the spruce tree and salt in the Newfoundland economy may well have encouraged confidence in medical usage (see entries).

Some concepts dealt with providing an explanation for an illness. Indeed, patients generally need to have their illness removed from the unknown; they also need help in coping in a society that sometimes readily accepts sickness but at times also casts a stigma on the sufferer. That does not mean that such concepts did not shape treatment. For instance, in the recent Newfoundland oral tradition notions still exist concerning the once wide-spread concept of small organisms (animalcules), perhaps loosely reinforced by talk of germs. One story is that "yellow jaundice" is caused by a living organism (called a "jaunder") like a jellyfish, which lives in the stomach.[57] There is also a tale about a charmer who, to treat a "cancer" on the hand, drew out "maggots."[58] The latter story echoes others about fairies inflicting "blasts," as discussed under the entry on cancer. A biological rather than, say, a moral or magical cause of an illness comforts many a patient.

Particular environmental beliefs must not be ignored when the persistence of certain practices is considered. Dampness, getting one's wet feet, and similar examples of "imprudence" have often justified the so-called catching of a condition. Such factors could be "weakening" to the system, especially for those with a delicate disposition. In Newfoundland, however, this reasoning has not been linked explicitly to the need to strengthen a life-force, although such a notion, common elsewhere, hovers in the Newfoundland record.[59]

All the above factors, or rationalizations, can be viewed as contributing to an individual's faith in a practice. Students of traditional medicine, as well as many physicians, have long recognized the importance of faith. Indeed, the words of physician Sir William Osler expressed in the early 1900s still resonate for many: "Nothing in life is more wonderful than faith – the one great moving force which we can neither weigh in the balance nor test in the crucible." Nowadays, the viewpoint is that, even if medical science does not accept past treatments as scientifically effective, they often worked because of the person's faith in them.[60]

Evaluating the many issues at play in therapy requires, as a baseline, an accurate assessment of the physiological effects of past practices. Unfortunately, this is now extremely difficult, for the type of proof required by modern medicine (for instance, the gold standard of randomized, controlled clinical trials) is simply too expensive to be undertaken for most traditional treatments. Controlled trials of treatments on single individuals may be acceptable in certain circumstances, but these are rarely done. In the absence of modern trials – and there are some who consider that, anyway, they do not assess the everyday conditions of self-care – much self-treatment of the past must be evaluated indirectly. This is done largely from an assessment of the constituents, dosages given, and overall usage over a long period of time, as well as the social factors, including the use of such treatments in, say, Britain, Ireland, and North America.[61] Certainly one cannot rely on just a few selected testimonials.

Without really going into the complex topic of placebo action – of significance in all therapies – it must be said that many factors encourage such actions. Faith in both practitioner and treatment is especially significant. Generalizations made from unrecognized, inconsistent placebo actions, or from instances of the natural healing power of the body, may also have contributed to the reputation of a particular treatment. These generalizations, as with mistaken analogies between one medicine and another, can be especially relevant to practices which, ultimately, did not stand the test of time.

Some commentators assume that because over-the-counter remedies became so widely used they were (or are) more effective than traditional remedies. This, however, can be far from the case, as already indicated. Aside from the extravagant claims for many of these remedies and the justifiable public disbelief, the consumer was often unaware that the composition of many changed from time to time. In 1936, an account was given of alterations to the formula of Cystex – widely advertised to Newfoundlanders – along with the professional medical opinion that: "the objection to Cystex is simple and fundamental: There is no legitimate place for the self-treatment of pathologic conditions of the kidney and bladder. It is sheer madness for persons who have the symptom-complex described in the Cystex advertisements to attempt to treat themselves and waste what may well be vitally valuable time before seeking competent treatment based on a rational diagnosis."[62]

Many other, certainly not all, over-the-counter medicines deserved the same stricture.

Despite uncertainties and negative assessments, the evidence suggests that much Newfoundland self-treatment in the past – home-made and commercial – helped to provide relief from many symptoms, although rarely a

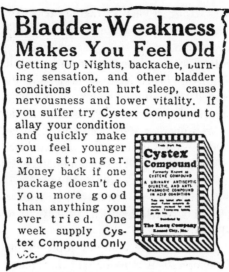

Advertisement for Cystex

"cure" in the way antibiotics cure infections. Some symptom relief almost certainly resulted from psychological (placebo) factors, and it is helpful to remember a distinction often made today between "disease" and "illness." The former is viewed as the biological aspect of an ailment, and illness as a person's individual response. The latter depends more on personality and cultural characteristics, which might include stoicism and fatalism, qualities linked with Newfoundlanders.

One reason why the disease-illness axis attracts attention nowadays is that lay people often question a strictly "biomedical" approach to treating many ailments. The latter range from "rheumatism," long recognized as a difficult problem; to chronic fatigue syndrome, a recently identified condition which is spawning countless self-care and alternative medical practices. Many people look, even if unconsciously, for a characteristic of medicine conspicuous in the past, namely treatment tailored not just to the disease, but also to the constitution, faith, feelings, and experiences of the patient. This was especially evident prior to the establishment of the germ theory toward the end of the nineteenth century, when it was commonly believed that each individual possessed a specific constitution; in consequence, individuals were thought to react to disease and treatment in different ways. Although generalizations about the effectiveness of tailoring treatment should be treated with caution, they at least catered to the illness component of an ailment. In fact, many physicians believe that sensitive caring and relieving of symptoms can quicken the healing process.

SELF-CARE FROM HERBS TO MIDWIVES: SOCIAL
ROLES AND NEWFOUNDLAND DISTINCTIVENESS

Any assessment of the impact of self-care on a community as a whole raises
questions about rural health in Newfoundland in general. First, it would
be helpful to make summary comments about non-commercial self-care in
the island and the fact that, despite the "import" of most if not all self-
care practices, certain features were distinctive to the island. One characteristic is the comparative lack of interest, at least in the twentieth century,
in the various plants that grow in Newfoundland and are widely known
and used medicinally elsewhere. Although sometimes that is because the
plant is uncommon on the island (for example, *Mitchella repens*), that is
hardly the case with blueberry and yarrow (see Part II entries). Having said
this, Newfoundland self-care – in line with traditional herbal medicine
everywhere – does reflect some of the local flora; witness, for instance, the
popularity of juniper and spruce products.

What the record suggests is that medications commonly known as
"kitchen physick" or "kitchen remedies" (many of which were, and are,
readily made from ingredients also used in cooking), as well as treatments
that rest on magical or religious concepts, were more often employed than
plant remedies.

The extent to which Newfoundlanders have used kitchen physick is
striking, and usually reveals a preference for products other than locally
available herbal medicines. Although the common recommendation, for
example, for treating smelly feet in many societies – to bathe in an astringent herbal tea – has not been recorded in Newfoundland, there are
suggestions to rub with sodium bicarbonate; to go down to the sea when
the tide is rising and dip the feet in the water, letting them soak for a while;
or, merely, to dip the feet in brine used for salting meat.[63]

On the whole, however, kitchen physick has contributed less to specific
characteristics of self-care in Newfoundland during the twentieth century
than have the relatively extensive and persistent magical and religious
treatments. It has often been noted that magic tends to prevail where
uncertainty exists in a society and is juxtaposed against a perceived lack of
control over events in the world. This can be said of many aspects of life
in Newfoundland, if only because of the vagaries of the fishery. Although
it seems fairly clear that many Newfoundlanders, until the 1950s, did not
make sharp distinctions between non-natural and kitchen or herbal treatments and accepted all, this area needs more study. After all, disbelief in
many treatment suggestions obviously existed, just as there was a general
recognition that many segments of society – particularly professional medicine and science – saw non-natural practices as primitive, superstitious,
and unacceptable.[64]

In Newfoundland, such dismissal of practices has for some time extended to treatments with strong religious elements, such as the still well-known practice of making a sign of the cross over a stye. Yet many Newfoundlanders undoubtedly felt the practice catered not only to the medical problem, but also to the need to bring religion into everyday living in ways that went beyond the intervention of the clergy. Such interventions might range from giving blessed water to banish fairies to blessing someone who has met them.[65] Such religious and magical considerations, an aspect of belonging to a community, can still be a real need for many people, especially in societies like Newfoundland where religion remains very much a basis of order in life. Religion is pervasive in many ways not easy to document; it is not clear, for instance, that everyone saw the three knots in certain treatment recommendations as a sign of the Trinity rather than as magical medicine. And how many added three drops of holy water to a poultice recipe?[66]

The link of spiritual and bodily needs prompts the question whether self-care in Newfoundland has had a general social role beyond one of serving individuals. Although the question can be asked of any community, it is especially pertinent to Newfoundland with its countless isolated outport communities. The question has particular relevance, too, because of the contradictory ways in which Newfoundlanders and their communities have been viewed. Not only have they been seen as disadvantaged and exploited, stigmatized for high illiteracy rates, but also as a people possessing core values such as belief in the importance of family, hard work, self-sacrifice, and stoic endurance. Newfoundland society has certainly been molded by common experiences and customs, and as such it has prompted much debate over what is traditional and what is modern. And how much is Newfoundland society changing? One recent study of a Newfoundland outport, Calvert, indicated that these questions can be overly simplistic.[67] In Calvert, new possessions, for instance, may change lifestyles, but insofar as long-standing social relations continue, these possessions do not threaten the lifestyle. It is not appropriate to see the community merely as one in transition, caught between the forces of old and new, for accommodation of the new with the old does exist.

It is within such a context of accommodating change and the role of social relations that self-care in Newfoundland's recent past should be viewed. Self-care has contributed to a sense of sharing and self-sufficiency. Although Newfoundland self-care can be viewed as a collection of diverse beliefs in much the same way as is found elsewhere, much of it mirrors such local considerations as available medicaments (often from the kitchen), beliefs in the non-natural; and the use of religious ideas to "connect" the body in illness with the outside world and to encourage self-awareness about such other community-rooted issues as the stigma of disease and social taboos. Further, self-care was not only part of the informal economy that, as already noted, offered some measure of independence from the cashless credit system, it also allowed for independence from the authority of the medical profession, which, as already noted, could arouse lay uncertainty, if not suspicion. Nevertheless, as reflected in the quotation of J.M. Little (p. 11), this independence was sometimes forced upon individuals because of the lack, or relative lack, of physicians and nurses.

Even without such professionals, however, a community was generally supported by a spectrum of lay practitioners. Women, in addition to managing their families and communities, played a role of considerable significance in health care. This becomes clear in numerous entries; see especially *charmers* and *midwifery*). Many women, for instance, extended care and treatment beyond their immediate family by sharing information through their community networks of church groups, women's dart teams, women's lodges, and so on, all of which encouraged (as they still do) families to integrate into a community as a whole. And many applied their knowledge. Rhoda Piercey recalled recently: "An old woman, who was extra gifted with the talent in dressing cuts, was kept busy in the summer with all the fishermen's infected hands or boils. When my father was six years old ... a nail stuck in the middle of his forehead [as he ran under a rail] tore the skin and hair right through to the back of his head. The old lady took blobs of turpentine picked from the green fir wood at the wood pile and stopped the bleeding and kept the cut together."[68] There were also granny midwives who offered more than help with birthing, particularly in terms of postnatal advice and care, and many women who, by serving as charmers and healers, were recognized as the possessors of special gifts. The latter group did include some men, but apparently not the Tilt Cove storekeeper who practised medicine (mentioned above) and members of the clergy (some providing "orthodox" medicine), all of whom added to the pluralistic health-care scene.[69] Not all Newfoundland communities had such a wide range of practitioners, but their availability was part of a general sense of self-sufficiency.

Self-care, then, and its roles in twentieth-century Newfoundland can be viewed not merely as part of the history of the island, but also as a continuing presence that extends the social role by strengthening a sense of place and self-sufficiency. Even though the latter has been undermined by commercialism, some of the products have themselves become part of the island culture. Molasses, Carnation milk, and Minard's Liniment are in no way unique to the island, but their long usage has become part of many a Newfoundlander's lifestyle. Although far less conspicuous than many more obvious features of Newfoundland life, self-care and self-sufficiency meld into an overall sense of belonging for the islanders. The sense is shaped primarily by geography, language, lifestyles associated with the fishery, disasters at sea and memories of them, economic problems, as well as many political considerations including colonial status.

Given these factors, some people consider that the Newfoundlanders' sense of identity embraces a feeling of distinctiveness, of self-consciousness. Although this has not been stereotyped to the same extent as has the distinctiveness of, for instance, the southern United States, William Faulkner's comment, "You can't understand it. You would have to be born there," is as apt for Newfoundland as for the southern United States.[70] Feelings of distinctiveness rest not only on the obvious considerations already noted, but also on the overall impact of relatively minor facets of everyday life, especially when identified by outsiders; included are the saltbox houses and the popularity of Carnation milk, and of fish and brewis. There is also a collective memory of self-care, laced not only by molasses and Minard's as mentioned above, but also by a host of other items that Newfoundlanders see as associated with the island, from cod liver oil to spruce beer.

PRACTICES AND BELIEFS TODAY

Some readers may be uncomfortable with the view that self-care makes a specific contribution to a distinctive culture and heritage in Newfoundland, at least one that persists. They can point out that many well-known island practices, at least until the 1950s, have since faded. Depending on their age and background (be they native Newfoundlanders or "come-from-aways"), readers of this volume may resonate more with vibrations of change, rather than with continuity and a sense of heritage, in the story of self-care.

Yet even readers who see in many of the entries on diseases and treatments in this volume merely gullibility, quaintness, and a legacy of minimal education, and who become more firmly convinced that the present is better than the past, must appreciate that at least some practices persist today.

Clearly, even after the demise of certain practices, beliefs justifying them often persist, implicitly or explicitly. As already noted, some – ranging from personal experience to faith – are still remembered. And there is also a resurgence of interest in many long-standing ideas through the growing interest in alternative medicine. Although no studies are available on the present role of past practices and beliefs in Newfoundland, a recent investigation in a rural region of southern United States is salutary. In an area with certain cultural similarities to rural Newfoundland, "thirty-five percent of the population surveyed is actively using some form of traditional or alternative medicine, most often in conjunction with some form of biomedicine."[71] Similar studies would help us understand the diversity of self-treatment practices in Newfoundland, the extent to which they are currently part of lifestyles and attitudes, their relevance to physician-patient relationships, and the way they can account for fuzzy shifts in a person's beliefs. For instance, if belief in fairies as an explanation for a swelling is later superseded by a concept of infection, this "modernization" may not entirely obliterate older beliefs, particularly when an illness is not progressing favourably.[72] Such circumstances, as also occur with puzzling diseases like the acquired immune deficiency syndrome (AIDS), may foster beliefs in non-natural factors or sins – whether in one's personal behaviour or in that of one's parents.

Nowadays, the general state of health on the island is not considered to be as poor as it once was. Many problems nevertheless remain which may well encourage diverse self-treatments.[73] People who use traditional treatments and newer forms of alternative medicine, as well as their health-care professionals, need to know whether these medications are safe and whether they can be taken with prescription and over-the-counter medicines. Unfortunately, reinforcement or re-establishment of many long-standing practices does not mean that all are harmless or used appropriately, as sometimes implied.[74]

Various studies in places other than Newfoundland have tried to correlate current self-care practices with general socio-economic considerations and more specific issues, such as gender and sceptical attitudes toward doctors. Although all such factors can be relevant, researchers find it difficult to make firm generalizations because different circumstances apply to different people. A recent study of self-care in Winnipeg concluded that "in view of the diverse nature of self-care behaviour, it seems unlikely that a single set of factors will be able to explain all forms of self-provided health care."[75] This hypothesis is certainly in keeping with the varied information that is part of the Newfoundland story.

## AFTERWORD: TRENDS IN SELF-CARE AND THE FUTURE

*Home Medicine: The Newfoundland Experience* appears at a time when changing attitudes toward self-care are becoming increasingly conspicuous. Amid dire concerns about rising health-care costs, a preoccupation with wellness, nutrition, and lifestyles is emerging. In fact, this trend owes relatively little to professional medicine, except as a consequence of public concerns about, for instance, side-effects of drugs and medical technology. Health-food stores and a range of alternative or complementary medicine practitioners are being increasingly used by a broad section of the population, many well-educated.[76] At the same time, the medical profession and underwriters of health care (governments, insurance companies) are increasingly stressing that "orthodox" self-care will help to reduce health-care costs. The call is for healthy lifestyles; the use of self-administered medical tests in the home, supermarket, and pharmacy; and other considerations.

Various questions arise from these trends concerning the place of self-care in the future health-care system. One question is whether self-care will be closely tied to professional medicine or whether, as many supporters of alternative medicine want, patients will acquire a larger role in medical decision-making as part of a pluralistic health-care scene. Already in Newfoundland today, even if less so than elsewhere, a widening array of alternative health care practices is becoming available. Recent legislation in the province has given additional authority to chiropractic, for example, while some medical practitioners include acupuncture (in its various forms) in their armamentarium. Nutrition stores, pyramid-selling enterprises, and mail-order firms offer many herbal and other preparations.

Given the backdrop of self-care considered in this volume and its contribution to self-sufficiency (a reminder of present-day emphasis on "personal control" in health matters), as well as the many beliefs that still have a cultural presence in Newfoundland, new trends are likely to find fertile soil. Newfoundlanders who seek their own ways to adapt to a changing world – amid, among others, consumerism, feelings that civilization is producing more and more health problems, and an increasing incidence of chronic morbidity – may find comfort in both long-standing and newer, alternative practices. The latter – sometimes seen as a justification and revitalization of past ideas – can also, as elsewhere, provide avenues for the expression of self-sufficiency, spiritual needs, and newer social issues such as women's rights.[77]

## Self-Responsibility and Choices

Will current trends mean a re-emergence of greater self-responsibility in health care? As various entries in the present account imply, self-responsibility was particularly evident when individuals were actively involved in preparing their own treatment, especially prior to reliance on over-the-counter medicines. Nowadays, there are calls for more and more patient involvement in medical decisions, even beyond matters of self-care. Yet responsibility today in self-care involves choices that may be more difficult to make than in the past, especially amid a vast amount of published, sometimes contradictory, information. Any perusal of popular self-care journals reveals a startling range of suggestions for the treatment of numerous conditions. For psoriasis, for instance, homeopathic practitioners may offer arsenium album in strengths of 3x to 30x; hydrotherapists may suggest sauna treatment; and nutritionists may recommend an increase in consumption of soybeans, tofu, vegetables, fresh fruits, and so on. Undoubtedly, many sufferers try various treatments at one and the same time.

Difficulty in making treatment choices is compounded by perplexing uncertainties over many areas of regular medical care in general. Choices, especially for chronic and other conditions not particularly well managed by regular medicine, depend on a raft of considerations that include the philosophical outlooks of both the patient and the health-care professional consulted. Most physicians dismiss as quackery all therapy not generally accepted by regular medicine. That, of course, can be sound advice for conditions where there is a *cure*, but is often arguable when only *symptoms* are relieved. Indeed, many lay people have become convinced that alternative medical practices and the self-care associated with them offer safer care and necessary choices, while providing the same symptom relief as regular medicine.

The question then becomes: How much individual choice in health care is appropriate? Should medical pluralism and the flexibility that has become somewhat restricted for patients by twentieth-century developments in medicine, commerce, and social custom be reasserted and accepted by the health professions? This would encourage more personal responsibility, especially for the countless medical problems – many considered in this volume – still taken to doctors without a resulting "cure."

Some people see that developing (or redeveloping) the patients' personal responsibility is one of the challenges of self-care, even as certain trends place aspects firmly within the framework of professional health care. Promoting responsibility is a challenge for medical and other health professionals as they educate society about health care and begin to study current self-care practices.[78] Part of the challenge is to acknowledge the limitations of modern medicine and to decide on the extent to which it should confront the apparent irrationalities of individuals, even communities, which may merely reflect ways people struggle for coherence in their world. The Newfoundland self-care story – to reiterate – suggests that the health system needs to recognize fully how various people call upon various beliefs and practices in self-care, how a sense of place and self-sufficiency may be significant to some individuals, how attitudes toward medical authority can be culturally bound, how significant the roles of community support are, and so on.

As medical technology places more and more strains on such considerations, the government, the health professions, and the public must respond in practical ways. Clearly, there is considerable room for lay involvement in a wide range of health-care issues beyond the aspects of wellness and health education that are currently fashionable. Strategies for this cannot be discussed here, aside from making one suggestion. Could Newfoundland, with its quota of problems of access to, and equity in, health care, establish a Council for Self-Care?

That council would be a public forum, where lay people (including those with such serious problems as AIDS and cancer, which so often prompt interest in a wide range of alternative treatments) could interact with representatives from the many "orthodox" and "unorthodox" approaches to health care, as well as from the legal profession, business, and other segments of society. In reviewing and advising about, for instance, the many facets of health promotion and disease prevention linked to professional medicine, about alternative medicine and its roles in different social contexts, and about lay responsibility and many other matters, the council could critically serve the government, the public, and individuals in matters of self-care across a broad range of issues.[79]

## PART TWO

# Ailments, Treatments, Concepts

# Introduction

The arrangement of the entries that follow is an alphabetical mix of accounts of ailments and treatments used or known during the the first half of the twentieth century. Numerous practices, however, have a much earlier origin, many continuing beyond 1950 and some being of recent introduction. If at first sight this appears to be a reference guide rather than a book to be read as a continuous story of home care, a straight reading of the entries or of selected themes, such as diseases or herbs, will clearly illustrate the kaleidoscope, choices, and complexity of health care, and in ways that conventional accounts often fail to do.

## INTERPRETING THE RECORD

Making firm generalizations about the popularity of many self-treatment practices in Newfoundland is not easy. Indeed, some interpretations suggesting that a particular practice was more commonplace than another might need revision when further information becomes available. As noted, the Folklore and Language Archive at Memorial University of Newfoundland has been a principal source of information. The collection was begun in the early 1960s – hence its designation in the entries as the "recently recorded" oral tradition – although many informants remember that similar practices extended back to at least the early years of the century.

Although students who gathered the archival data followed guidelines, the amount of probing done to elicit complete information was variable. This sometimes accounts for the limited detail on recipes as well as the uncertainty about the veracity of some recommendations. Moreover, it is well known that many Newfoundlanders are suspicious of giving personal information to anthropologists, folklorists, and perhaps some students. There is strong evidence, however, that the countless students involved in this collection were seen as non-threatening and certainly not as strangers;

they were able to elicit information readily. What has not been pursued, then, is the possible differences between one community and the next, between Anglicans and Catholics, between merchants and the rest of the community, between women and men, and between generations.

Nor have particular ethnic groups such as the Micmacs on the reserve at Conne River been considered, apart from occasional comment. By the early 1990s, when this volume was being written, attempts by a core of Micmacs to uncover and revive traditional knowledge of health care had been underway for some time. It is noteworthy that this Micmac traditional knowledge differs relatively little from that found throughout Newfoundland. Whether it will ever be possible to distinguish original Micmac self-care from that of European immigrants is unclear.[1]

Also largely omitted is information from Labrador (part of the province of Newfoundland) and the native inhabitants who live there. There is, however, little evidence that the self-care of the European settlers in Labrador was significantly different from that of Newfoundland; at least some of the lore derives from Newfoundland fishermen going to Labrador for the summer fishery. Generally speaking, available evidence does not suggest that major regional differences existed in the province throughout the time period we are considering. Even the information contrasting St. John's with the outports suggests few major differences, although reliance in the capital on drugstores was probably for greater. As one person noted: "Now you'd go to the drugstore for [your] ailments; all the Southside went to the same druggist. He'd ask you what was wrong, whether you had a cold or husky throat or something else, swelling, discharge, a sore or anything, you'd tell him and everything was mixed in the drugstore then."[2]

Another issue associated with the oral record is that of uncertainty about diagnoses. A biography of a nurse-midwife, Myra Bennett, who worked on the west coast, highlights the issue:

Often she would be told that a child had scarlet fever ... Upon seeing the child she might discover nothing more than a nettle rash. One elderly man to whom she was called, had had some bleeding and had been persuaded by the experts of his community that he had a lung haemorrhage. He was so convinced of this that he set his house in order and prepared to die, for ... a bleeding of the lungs meant consumption in an advanced stage and it was something that almost invariably preceded death. When Myra arrived, however, she discovered that he was suffering from a ruptured gastric ulcer. At first the man refused to believe her but he did take her medicines and treatment nonetheless and complied with the diet she mapped out for him. The man lived for many years and Myra's reputation in that community went up considerably.[3]

Various entries raise questions about lay and professional differences concerning diagnoses and treatment. Lay people generally focus more on symptoms than do physicians, who also search for signs and other data from physical examinations and tests. It is noteworthy that one symptom (for example, a cough) can, in fact, be a "label" for a spectrum of conditions; it may even hide a suspected diagnosis. For example, in Newfoundland, a "cough" has been used euphemistically for tuberculosis.

A further consideration is that the entries do not cover every treatment employed in Newfoundland, especially for, say, burns, coughs, cuts, stomach problems, and warts (for which the variations of basic approaches are legion). Also, references to religious practices (counting the rosary, wearing the medal of St. Ann, using holy water, and so on) are generally omitted to avoid giving any sense that religious considerations were limited to a few conditions. An observation, recorded in 1967, that "most people of St. Mary's have a strong belief in the healing power of a priest" is just one testimony to the pervasiveness – as already noted – of religious notions.[4] Added to this are the religious overtones connected with many charmers and charms, and perhaps the role of the Pentecostal church, which has a special concern with healing. Commonly bound up with religious healing, too, is the belief that an ailment arises from some religious transgression. Although the extent to which this belief – as well as the belief in the role of the supernatural, fairies, black magic, and spells in causing disease – holds true in Newfoundland is unclear, it seems evident that, where relevant, the ailments may well have been attended to spiritually or with charms and spells, as well as with medicaments.[5]

Another limitation is that few of the recommendations in the oral record consider the supportive care commonly given with specific remedies. The old adage "feed a cold, starve a fever" may be a case in point.

Throughout Part II, as already mentioned, the Folklore and Language Archive material has been supplemented by much additional material. Historical background is noted where relevant, though space limitations mean that fuller details must be sought elsewhere. Although some entries are fairly comprehensive, additional data on such topics as abortion, the use of herbs such as bogbean and beaver root, the management of failing eyesight, and the quantities of over-the-counter medicines sold to people in isolated outports are still required to provide a firmer picture of both the changing character of self-care in Newfoundland, and the interaction between professional and lay approaches. To overcome this, in part, we have included plentiful quotations, though this is only a substitute for an extended narrative that gives a fuller sense of the way a person learned and used the information.

Despite such caveats, these entries make clear the eclecticism of self-care, the impact of commercialism, the changes in self-sufficiency and lifestyle, the difficulties of making choices, and the sundry other issues that make up the matrix of self-care in Newfoundland. The myriad of elements – a kaleidoscope of changes – reveal patterns, individual idiosyncrasies, and features in the past that may or may not still be current.

NOTE ON CITATIONS

In addition to references at the foot of each entry, citations are given to the Folklore and Language Archive, Memorial University of Newfoundland (MUNFLA) files. These refer to representative examples of the treatment noted, to quotations, or to specific discussion. Citations to MCG refer to the files of the Medical Communication Group, Memorial University of Newfoundland. Although specific citations have not generally been attributed to the many Newfoundland newspaper advertisements noted, they are taken from the *Evening Telegram* and the *Daily News,* unless otherwise indicated.

# From Abortion to Zam-Buk Ointment

No estimates are available of the incidence of illegitimate births or non-professionally induced abortions in Newfoundland, except for recent times. Anecdotal information suggests that the latter were fewer than illegitimate births, at least in many communities – Catholic and Protestant – until the 1940s. Aside from shot-gun marriages, a commonplace observation was that "if a girl got pregnant before she was married, no one saw her for months before or after the baby was born. If she did not marry the man, she lived with her parents until she could find a job as servant girl to support herself." There was also infanticide: "The Iron Ore Company [on Bell Island] had horses to pull the old carts. Pits were made, into which manure was thrown. Every spring these pits were cleaned out and they revealed just as many infants as manure." The intensity of the stigma of being an unmarried mother – one was "marked for life" – must have often encouraged such extreme measures. At the same time, few hints about inducing abortions are noted in the Newfoundland record, including whether the women were married or not. Indeed, it has been said that, in Canada during the early decades of the twentieth century, most women seeking abortions were probably married.

It is unclear to what extent abortion knowledge was part of a woman's information network; certainly when, in 1992, Newfoundland women aged sixty-five years and over were asked about abortion, few said they knew anything about it in the "old days." Yet practices ranging from physical interventions, such as using scissors or jumping from a loft, to administering substances by mouth or vaginally were tried at times.

All Western cultures have had a reasonably extensive knowledge – much of it extending back to classical times – of reputed plant abortifacients. In Newfoundland, two plants have been readily available: tansy (q.v.) and juniper (q.v.). Aside from drinking tansy tea, Newfoundlanders could at times purchase manufactured Tansy Pills. In 1898, they were advertised in the St. John's *Daily News*: "Never Fail. A safe, easy and positive ladies relief."

Two species of tansy grow in the province, *Tanacetum huronense* (of limited west coast distribution) and *T. vulgare*, but only the latter is widely documented in professional and lay medical literature as an emmenagogue (see *female remedies*) and an abortifacient. Maternal fatalities have been reported in the older literature, but these resulted from taking the isolated tansy oil rather than a home-made "tea" of the leaves or flowering tops. No evidence exists that *T. huronense* has significantly different chemical constituents or pharmacological properties.

Juniper, at least the oil from *Juniperus sabina*, has long been reported as an abortifacient, although other junipers (for example, *J. communis*) have also been known. Suggestions exist that an extract can also serve as a contraceptive when taken orally or applied vaginally. The story of juniper in Newfoundland is bound up with the term "saffron": "Saffron is not very common. The old people use it for young girls who got pregnant before they were married. They used to steep the roots and have the girls drink the tea." Additional information suggests that it had to be drunk over a period of time to be effective. The saffron has been identified as *Juniperus horizontalis* as well as savin (*Juniperus sabina*), which does not grow in Newfoundland (although perhaps the savin oil was purchased); it seems clear that *J. communis* was also used. (For other meanings of saffron, see *measles*.)

Another natural product, the commercially available quinine, which had become widely known as an abortifacient on both sides of the Atlantic by around 1900, was certainly employed in St. John's during the 1930s. It was used alone or, commonly, in combination with castor oil. The two items were often purchased separately from drug stores and mixed at home in quantities not reported in the oral tradition. In 1939, a committee investigating abortion in England viewed quinine, along with pennyroyal and apiol (a constituent of parsley, see below) as favoured abortifacients.

On the subject of commercial preparations, pennyroyal oil (generally from *Mentha pulegium* rather than from "American" pennyroyal *Hedeoma pulegioides*) was certainly very well known. It could be an

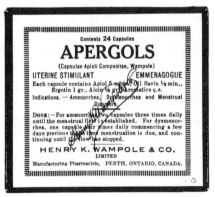

Apergols box label

effective abortifacient as well as dangerously toxic to the mother; no evidence is available about usage in Newfoundland.

Another commercial preparation, apiol (extracted from parsley), was probably readily available – at least in St. John's – in the form of over-the-counter Apergols.

These capsules were prepared from various uterine-active compounds besides apiol and sold in Newfoundland during the 1930s and 1940s. Although promoted for such menstrual problems as amenorrhea and dysmenorrhea, oral evidence indicates some physicians prescribed Apergols for abortion, and pharmacists provided it "under-the-counter."

Apiol preparations were undoubtedly effective abortifacients if used in appropriate dosage. The reasons for their decline during the 1940s are unclear. One suggestion, at least for Canadian women, is that they were "able to get instrumental abortions from doctors and paramedical abortionists with relative ease" compared with earlier times and stopped using drugs. But this was not the case in Newfoundland.

The use of the popular laxative, Epsom salts, was almost certainly tried on occasion to promote abortion; one Newfoundland report stated: "Take a double or triple dose of Epsom salts between six weeks and two months of pregnancy." Although abortions using laxatives have long been attempted, there was probably an appreciation that their effectiveness was only occasional. Such usage of laxatives is obviously not to be confused with recommendations for senna tea (another laxative) to induce labour "if the baby was late."

One plant, "maidenhair" (almost certainly *Gaultheria hispidula*, see *creeping snowberry*), was noted in an eighteenth-century account of Newfoundland as an abortifacient. However, it has not been generally known as such, although emmenagogue properties (to promote menstruation) have been reported from time to time. Aaron Thomas observed in 1794:

The Maidenhair Plant is a humble but insinuating production, creeping through the moss and just showing its head ... The poor people constantly make use of it. I myself have made use of it and by no means am dispos'd but to speak favourable of its pleasing flavour. The importation of this tea into England is prohibited and the reasons given by the common people are curious. They say that the Maidenhair Tea or the Leaves, bruis'd and eaten by the fair Sex when pregnant occasions abortion. How far this is true I know not.

Thomas was apparently incorrect about the ban on importation; it is not known how long the reputation as an abortifacient persisted in Newfoundland.

Other vegetable preparations, the formulae of which are uncertain or unknown, have been suggested as abortifacients in Newfoundland. One is "Polly Pitchum," which according to one report, was a "home brew made from ingredients picked off rocks or trees." Some people think it was prepared from a fern, perhaps *Polypodium vulgare*. Another unidentified preparation was "a black liquid from a Bell Island drugstore."

At least one reference exists to the use of "blackberry bush and herbine bitters;" the composition is uncertain, but the herbine bitters was probably the commercial "Dr. Wilson's Herbine Bitters" (containing dandelion, mandrake, burdock, along with alcohol, according to newspaper advertisements in 1920.) The purgative action of the mandrake (presumably *Podophyllum peltatum*, not found in Newfoundland) is well known, but may not have been sufficiently potent in the quantity present and because of other ingredients. If the blackberry bush was a species of *Rubus* (as the name suggests), its astringency (particularly if the root was used) could limit any laxative effect of other ingredients. The possibility exists, however, that the "blackberry" was the plant *Empetrum nigrum* which, with its black berries, is better known to Newfoundlanders as "blackberry heath" (and sometimes "crowberry".) One hint exists in the Newfoundland record that this has been used to facilitate childbirth (see *midwifery*), though no reports have been found that it possesses pharmacological activity.

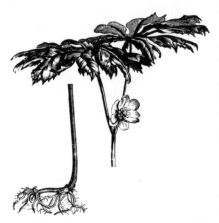

*Podophyllum peltatum* (mayapple, mandrake) a potent purgative and an ingredient in many proprietary medicines (for example, Stafford's Mandrake Bitters, see *bitters*) is a well-known medicinal plant. Its drastic purgative action has been tried for abortion.

The general impact of commercial over-the-counter medicines in twentieth-century Newfoundland is reflected in a suggestion that a "large quantity of Radways" could be taken to induce an abortion. Radway & Co., an American company, produced many proprietary medicines of which the best known in Newfoundland, and elsewhere, was probably Radway's Ready Relief (RRR); this – either applied externally or taken internally – was generally viewed as a stomach medicine and painkiller, so that the Radways Pills for female complaints was the likely candidate for abortion attempts. There were also other "female remedies" (for example, Dr. Pierce's Favourite Prescription), which, in sufficient doses, were commonly viewed as potential abortifacients.

The sketchy abortion knowledge just outlined, probably richer in practice, has faded in recent decades because of changing medical knowledge and new medical services for abortion and contraception. As abortion emerged as an issue of public controversy, past Newfoundland knowledge did not obviously shape current attitudes, although past silence has made it difficult for many to welcome the new openness. It is perhaps unwise to assume that past practices have disappeared, never to be used under certain social, psychological, and other circumstances.

No clear picture emerges about birth control, for which abortion was one method. Unfortunately, both male and female attitudes toward contraception in Newfoundland prior to recent times are entirely unclear, although religious influences were considerable. One commentator, however, has suggested that large family size, high illegitimacy rates, early marriage ages, high unemployment levels, and low-income per capita made prospects of fertility regulation appealing when the legalization of contraceptive advertising started to have an impact and more methods became widely available. Tubal ligation rapidly became the preferred means of modern fertility regulation among young village women. The notion of being "on the pill" also brought social changes to the island.

The lack of a Newfoundland record on contraception is not altogether surprising, not only because of natural reticence and the influence of the Catholic church, but also because of feelings that artificial methods were not "natural." The only approach suggested in the Newfoundland oral record – to get a girl to drink whisky – was probably not taken seriously. Coitus interruptus (the husband "hauls out") was undoubtedly known, as was belief in the contraceptive value of breast-feeding. The latter, however, has been an uneven practice on the island; one wonders if the belief that a baby should be taken from a mother's breast after nine months, because the milk then became poisoned, was widespread.

Despite the relative silence about contraception, veiled suggestions existed in home-medicine books and were almost certainly part of the popular culture. Long-standing knowledge of barrier methods such as sponges soaked in vinegar must have been known to some. Vaginal hygiene products sold through Eaton's catalogues were also relevant, although questions about the effectiveness of all such approaches must be borne in mind.

Until recently (1970s), latex condoms were not readily available in Newfoundland, and no evidence has been found as to the use of those made from intestines. The arrival of American servicemen during World War II is said to have encouraged a "black market" that lasted until the change in Canada's criminal code (public display or advertisement of contraceptives had been forbidden). The background of comparative silence on sexual matters is just one of the many cultural considerations in current issues concerning AIDS in the province.

NOTES

See: Benoit (1990), for information on stigma and punishment concerning pregnancy prior to marriage, stomach salts, and jumping from a loft to procure abortion; Piercey (1992) 62, on pregnancy in the unmarried; Shorter (1982) 213–24, on apiol and other abortifacients; McLaren and McLaren (1986) 40, on abortion among married Canadian women; Ness (1976) and Davis (1983b and 1988), on social and contraception changes in the 1970s, tubes tied and so on, coitus interruptus, continued breast feeding; MCG (1992), for various files indicating lack of knowledge of abortifacients in the "old days;" Davis (1983b) 60–1, for a report on an Anglican outport that suggests acceptance of having to get married (studies on Catholic communities unavailable for comparison); *Dictionary Newfoundland English* (1990) 426, on saffron; Thomas, A. (1968) 141, on maidenhair; Grindstaff (1980) 60, on advertising condoms.

Representative MUNFLA references: 63-120 (Polly Pitchum), 66-11/73 (whisky after intercourse), 76-249 (Radways, tansy), 78-211 (infanticide and "haul out"), 78-249 (Radways), 78-195 (blackberry and bitters), 82-121 (Epsom salts and tansy), 82-122 (poisoned milk).

Personal communication: N. Stowe (1992), on apergols and contraceptives.

## ABSCESSES, BOILS, CARBUNCLES, RISINGS

The terms "boil" (a circumscribed swelling caused by localized infection, commonly on the back of the neck), "carbuncle" (like a large boil, or collection of boils formed closely together but spread more deeply), and "abscess" ( a local collection of pus found in various sites of the body) have all been used loosely in popular medicine. In Newfoundland, however, a carbuncle generally implies a more serious condition than an ordinary boil. A "rising" refers to boils or carbuncles, as well as more generalized infections of, for instance, the finger and hand (see also *cuts and minor wounds*).

Poultices (q.v. for details) – once a common treatment in Newfoundland for all these conditions – have been widely employed on both sides of the Atlantic and in both professional and domestic medicine. Until toward the end of the 1800s, specific poultices were often earmarked for

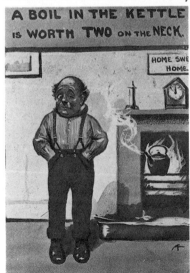

The commonplace nature of boils is reflected in this early twentieth-century comic postcard.

specific conditions; however, with declining interest in this form of care within regular medicine the use of special and medicated poultices faded. Nevertheless, "simple" poultices persisted, especially in home medicine.

One of the best known, the soft-bread poultice, was frequently applied in Newfoundland for boils, and so on. In 1908, Dr. J.M. Little wrote about Newfoundlanders: "Of boils and abscesses, superficial and deep, there are many, and the only care they get is bread and molasses poultice from the beginning to the end, whatever that may turn out to be. In consequence, some horrible cases of suppuration are seen." Hard bread (to be softened) was occasionally recommended, perhaps because of its ready availability, as was turnip poultice. The fact that the "turnip" grown in Newfoundland is the related rutabaga is of no consequence, since the rationale of poultices is merely to apply and retain local heat to facilitate the release of pus and to encourage the healing process. Much testimony exists that poultices gave ease and were effective for boils and local inflammation.

One problem with poultices is that the skin around the boil or carbuncle can quickly become sore through moistness. A sensible Newfoundland recommendation was for an "old-fashioned plaster." For this, a clean, if not sterile, white cloth with a cut-out hole (the same size as the boil), was placed over the boil so that the latter protruded. A paste made from scrapings of Sunlight soap, molasses, and flour was applied over the boil and covered with brown paper. A variation involved protecting the surrounding skin with burnt cloth.

In view of the use of many animal products in Newfoundland, it is perhaps surprising that relatively few references exist to the application of fat pork (q.v.) or meat to boils. This is a fairly common recommendation elsewhere.

Newfoundland suggestions for poulticing boils – different from those generally described in professional and lay medical literature – include adding juniper (q.v.) or tansy (q.v.), both of which are locally available plants. Warm cow-dung applied directly, although long viewed as distasteful, is also noted. A specific suggestion for treating carbuncles was to use dragon's blood (q.v.) poultices.

A variant of the soap poultice or "plaster" (which sometimes incorporated sugar) had the consistency of a salve (or ointment), and was spread over the boil. Perhaps this was viewed as a home-made, easy-to-use version

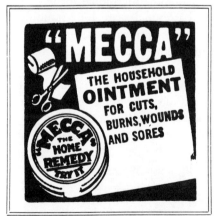

By 1955, advertisements for Mecca Ointment had dropped specific reference to boils. But as a "household ointment," it was used for all manner of ailments, including boils.

of commercial salves, which made some headway in pushing aside the use of poultices, even before the availability of antibiotics in the 1940s, and despite uncertain effectiveness. Mecca Ointment was specifically promoted for boils prior to World War II, although at least one competitor, Antiphlogistine, also became popular.

Occasional references exist to ways of managing boils other than by messy applications. One was to warm a small-necked bottle (perhaps with hot water) and to place the neck over the boil. As the bottle cooled, the core of the boil was drawn out. Another suggestion – to suspend a nutmeg around the neck – was perhaps intended more as prevention than cure. (For a general discussion, see *amulets, necklaces*.) Much self-treatment (for almost any ailment) embraces suitable ready-to-hand items; perhaps that was the reason for tying a piece of tacker – waxed thread used by cobblers – around the neck, rather than suspending a nutmeg. In line with traditional confidence in the number nine, a tacker that had nine knots and was tied nine turns around the neck was viewed as especially helpful.

Any account of boils, minor infections, and skin ailments should note that, until around World War II, blood purifiers (q.v.) were commonly recommended for internal use, along with the employment of external applications. Sulphur and molasses (q.v.) were probably the best known in Newfoundland. Furthermore, during the 1930s, as knowledge of vitamins was established, Newfoundlanders were told that products such as Fleischmann's Yeast, which gained notoriety for excessive claims, was good for "*boils*, indigestion, poor appetite, headaches, [and as a] blood cleaner." Commercial yeast was one item that helped to displace traditional blood purifiers.

Current professional medical recommendations (1992) for treating boils and carbuncles are long-standing, with antibiotic usage replacing many practices (at least for severe cases) after penicillin became generally available during the 1940s. Magnesium sulphate paste continues to be suggested, as do hot fomentations, while yeast (as well as sound nutrition) is still reported "to be of value," albeit not as a blood purifier. Popular self-care manuals today do sometimes recommend treatment of "internal impurities" with long-standing blood purifiers (for example, burdock, q.v.). At times the blood purifiers are promoted as nutrition products, implying that they are not "medicines." This partly reflects legislation that prevents medical claims being made without accepted scientific proof.

NOTES
See: Little (1908b); Brown Collection (Hand 1961, vol. 6) 129–34, for many examples, including poultices, fat pork and fat meat, nutmeg as charm, and blood purifiers; Havard (1990) and Bricklin (1990), for current practices.

Representative MUNFLA references: 66-2/79 (tacker), 66-2/80 (soap salve), 67-4/8 (protective plaster), 68-11M (fat back), 68-19/3 (cow-dung), 68-21/4 (nutmeg), 69-7Ms (blood purifier), 69-26/5 (turnip and other ingredients), 76-249 (warmed bottle, soft bread), 78-195 (soap, flour, and molasses), 78-200 (fat pork), 78-205 (Sunlight soap and sugar), 82-218 (dragon's blood), 82-238 (tansy).

## AFTERSHAVE LOTION, ALCOHOL RUBS

A recommendation to apply aftershave lotion to cold sores reflects the lotion's alcohol content and its astringent (drying) property. In fact, many commercial cold-sore lotions have long been alcohol-based. Although there is no sense of a permanent cure (everyone with a cold sore knows it comes back), the frequent application of alcohol provides relief by promoting "drying" of the blisters.

The use of alcohol as an application to painful muscles and other aches and pains (including "rheumatism" and "fibrositis") appears in many records of self-treatment, including those of Newfoundland, where one suggestion is to rub it on the ear for earache (q.v.). The "alcohol" may have been rum, whisky, and so on, although "rubbing alcohol" has long been commercially available. This preparation of denatured alcohol, *not* to be taken internally, is generally recommended as an application to the skin for painful muscles, and general aches and pains. It is thought to act as a rubefacient; that is, to have a reddening and warming action on the skin.

NOTES
Representative MUNFLA references: 66-18/47 (cold sore), 68-10/7 alcohol rub.

## ALDER

Two native alders (*Alnus crispa* and *A. rugosa* – sometimes called *Alnus incana* ssp. *rugosa*) are common in Newfoundland, although the latter is not on the Avalon or Northern Peninsulas. That relatively few references to medicinal uses of alder exist in the recently recorded Newfoundland oral tradition seems to suggest a lack of usefulness. In fact, theory may be at the core of its reputation. The Newfoundland recommendation to drink one or two mouthfuls of an infusion of alder "cones" or "buds" (fruits) two to three times a day, for about two weeks, to treat boils sometimes invokes a blood-purifying reputation rationalized by the astringent (drying) property. It should be noted that much past treatment of skin conditions commonly included taking so-called blood purifiers (q.v.) by mouth.

Other recommendations were to use a tea of the cones for rheumatism (probably also viewed as blood purification), the buds for itch (q.v.), the flowers ("catkins") for fevers, and an application of a strong "tea" to chancres. Although only one suggestion for treating diarrhoea has been found, it carries an enthusiastic testimonial, typical of those that accompany many Newfoundland self-care recommendations: Alder "would seize you right up."

One external usage may reflect ready access to the plant more than any other justification. Recent Micmac informants remember well: "Alder leaves, yes they used that for headache. Put it on the forehead and tie the rag around." A "cooling" property was utilized, and the leaves might be replaced by others after a short while.

In general, Newfoundland beliefs about alder – except for the headache treatment and a reference to treating warts (q.v.) which has a magical association – conform with information published in professional and domestic medical texts up to the early years of the twentieth century, although the latter generally refer to the similar *A. glutinosa* indigenous to Europe and not found in Newfoundland. It is noteworthy that at least one Newfoundlander is using alder leaves for headaches in 1993 by placing them inside a cap.

NOTES
See: Introductory note to bibliography for general history and information; Bergen (1899) 110, decoction of alder bud for itch and water in which alder buds have been steeped for rheumatism; MCG (1993) 2, for Micmac usage.

Representative MUNFLA references: 69-7/Ms (boils), 69-13/10 (arthritis), 77-87 (fever), 84-295B (diarrhoea).

ALUM

Newfoundlanders' recommendations to suck on alum for a sore mouth or a sore tongue are in line with published information on medicinal usage of the astringent mineral, best known as a mordant in dyeing. Mixed with honey, the alum was more palatable to take. Commercial alum preparations were also promoted for sore mouths, as aftershave lotions, and so on. Surprisingly, no Newfoundland reports have been found for using alum for thrush (q.v., also called "thrash" or "whites") in children, since this is a common recommendation elsewhere.

One must wonder if the comparative silence in the Newfoundland record reflected the public impact of many pre-World War I advertisements in St. John's newspapers for Baking Powders (for example, Emerald's and Royal) that stated "alum is a poison," or "Alum baking powders are the greatest menaces of the present day." Acme Baking Powder even stated (*Daily News* 19 January 1906) that stomach troubles and so on, were caused by inferior baking powder. No doubt, too, some found the alum too "caustic" or astringent to use comfortably.

NOTES
Representative MUNFLA references: 76-249 (sore mouth), 82-146 (sore tongue).

## AMULETS, NECKLACES

Suspending aromatic substances and other items around the neck, which has a long history, was a well-known practice in twentieth-century Newfoundland. Apart from asafetida – one of the best known aromatics in many parts of the United States, but apparently unrecorded on the island – many others (for example, nutmegs, mothballs) were well known. They were employed (sometimes wrapped in a small bag) to ward off infectious disease, to prevent or to control chronic conditions such as rheumatism, and even to treat colds.

A well-known chapter in the use of strongly aromatic substances in Europe is highlighted by elegant gold and silver pomanders of the sixteenth and seventeenth centuries. These seemingly had their origin in *pomum ambrum* or ointmentlike masses hardened by resin and hung around the neck. The use of pomanders meant that at least the scent could be readily changed. There is little doubt that pomanders served as jewellery and perfumery containers, as well as for health considerations, until the eighteenth century, when the popularity of aromatic substances slowly gave way to the use of vinegar as a general preventative. One common way of using vinegar in the first half of the nineteenth century was to soak it into pieces of sponge, which were then placed in small containers called "vinaigrettes" hung around the neck or from items of

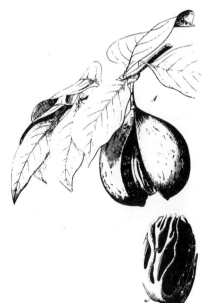

Nutmegs (shown with mace still on the outside) were a well-known exotic spice and medicine in Newfoundland. Not only were nutmegs worn as amulets, they were used internally for indigestion and externally in poultices.

clothing. As these became popular so did smelling salts, used by Newfoundlanders up to World War II (if not later) for headaches and fainting.

Suspending a pomander or vinaigrette had overtones of wearing a protective amulet (or charm), which has often taken the form of a dried medicinal root or other parts of a plant. Like almost everything in self-care, these have been promoted commercially at one time or another. It has been said, for instance, that a "savage war was going on for the domination of the [anodyne] necklace" in early eighteenth-century London, which helped to popularize these and other necklaces. Perhaps such commercial reinforcement of the oral tradition contributed to the persistent popularity, until the nineteenth century, of their use with teething children. It is not overly speculative to suggest that such influences filtered onto the Newfoundland scene as well.

A wide range of items, sometimes carried, sometimes suspended, have been accorded healing properties through magical and religious associations. The recent Newfoundland record includes innumerable examples. One recent reminiscence states: "Charms used for various disorders were legion in number. There were charms against migraines, nosebleed, toothache, warts, moles, freckles or summer moles, bleeding, cramp colic, rheumatism and the ague." Many so-called charms were, in fact, employed to transfer a disease from a sick person; for example, the potato, lodestone, and hazelnut for treating "arthritis" and "rheumatism" (q.v.), and rocks, earthworms, and other items for warts (q.v.).

Carrying charms (even good-luck charms such as a rabbit's foot) is less openly acknowledged nowadays, but variations on this practice are found among certain ethnic and social groups. Nevertheless, usage and beliefs persist which, even if they do not interfere with physicians' medications, can create contentious issues in overall treatment.

NOTES
See: Grenfell (1920) 116, for one view on continuing customs; Schmitz (1989), on pomanders; Doherty (1990), for quote on anodyne necklace, also Doherty (1992).

Representative MUNFLA references: 63-6/21 (nutmeg for cramp), 69-7/MS (fish doctors or fish heads in cloth bag for rheumatism), 78-195 (charm for toothache; mothballs in bag around neck for cold; nutmeg in bag for boils).

Personal communication: J. O'Mara (1990), on smelling salts.

ANALGESICS (PAINKILLERS)

Discussions about relieving general aches and pains are not found in the Newfoundland record and even specific treatments (for example, for headache q.v.) are limited. G.L. Saunders recently wrote: "To my recollection there was no painkiller [in the 1930s] except the headache powder sold over the counter; there was no aspirin as such, but you could 'take a powder' – a small package, wrapped in paper like a stick of chewing gum that contained the equivalent in powder form." Although this suggests a measure of stoicism, no clear evidence exists about a reluctance to use painkillers or to indicate whether or not Newfoundlanders were pleased to read in the *Evening Telegram* (25 February 1957) that the "use of pain-easing drugs is permissible, says

Pope." The newspaper reported that there was nothing immoral or unchristian in the proper medical use of anaesthetics or pain-easing drugs.

There had been no shortage of commercial painkillers in Newfoundland since 1900. Such "powders" or packages mentioned above, of which Hoffman's Headache Powders was one of the first to be advertised in Newfoundland (1898), commonly contained such coal-tar derivatives as antipyrine, phenacetin, and acetanilide. These plus aspirin (q.v.) – all products emerging in the 1880s and 1890s – had an increasing impact in Newfoundland (commonly as such compounded preparations as APC, containing aspirin, phenacetin, and caffeine), just as they did elsewhere in the home treatment of fevers and pains.

Growing awareness of toxicity of phenacetin – as late as the 1970s and 1980s – led to the disappearance of the "old guard," except for aspirin. New concerns about the safety of these products, even after long periods of use, have contributed to current fears about many chemical drugs.

Another painkiller, opium – a key part of Newfoundland medicine ever since settlement of the island – was sold over the counter in many communities until well into the twentieth century. It, or the active ingredient morphine, also spawned many commercial preparations. Collis Browne's Chlorodyne became one of the best known by the second half of the nineteenth century, although other chlorodynes were marketed as well. Another popular narcotic-containing preparation advertised in the St. John's newspapers was Perry Davis' Pain-Killer ("The Home Remedy. Take for Cramps, Colic, Diarrhoea. Apply for Bruises, Sprains, Sore Throat"). All such preparations had had their formulae changed by the 1930s or had disappeared because of legislative controls on opium and morphine, as well as use of the "safer" aspirin and other synthetic analgesics that came to dominate the self-care market. Concern about taking opiates, especially for infants and children, is reflected in many advertisements for Fletcher's Castoria (for example, in 1925: "Absolutely harmless, no opiates").

Any discussion about ways of relieving pain must recognize the use of hot compresses (for example, a rag soaked in hot water), home-made and commercial poultices, and liniments and rubs to relieve painful joints and muscles. As well, some Newfoundlanders may have tried such alternative magical approaches as transference of pain to rocks, at least for a stitch (see *pleurisy and stitch*).

Nowadays, the demand for analgesics for minor pains is perhaps even greater than in the past. Some are noted under the entry on *headache*.

NOTES
See: Saunders (1986) 136, 137.

Representative MUNFLA references: 78-205 (compress).

Personal communication: N. Rusted (1992), on aspirin.

ANIMAL PARTS AND EXCRETIONS, URINE

Animal organs, excreta, and blood have been conspicuous in the oral record of twentieth-century Newfoundland self-care, although knowledge rather than usage may have been more the order of the day. While knowledge has obviously faded since the 1930s, it may be (though detailed studies are needed) that the persistence and extent of the practices in Newfoundland were more commonplace than in other parts of rural North America.

Although the thought of using animal parts generally evokes distaste if not horror nowadays, recent (and some current) usages are legacies of a time when animal preparations were widely employed in medicine. A seventeenth-century author, noting that there was probably no part of the human body that could not offer some advantage to the sick, reflected a substantially different attitude toward the body and mind and their treatment than nowadays.

Although employment of animal products by physicians declined in the eighteenth century, standard textbooks indicate that experience and theory rather than magical or other reasons lay behind the use of some items. Usage coincided with times of relative intimacy with nature and an acquaintance with animal products in a variety of ways. Some preparations, like excrement, were viewed as hot and penetrating. These same concepts were mentioned recently by an elderly Newfoundlander when explaining the effectiveness of cow-dung poultices (fresh or warm dung was preferred.) It would be wrong, however, to assume that recent Newfoundland usage was consciously based on, or justified by, theory.

Medicinal use of dung was probably disappearing in Newfoundland by the 1930s, although it was reported then that cow-dung was employed for bruises, sprains, and frostbite, and sheep-dung for ulcers and for measles (q.v.).

Animal liver – and to a lesser extent, heart – may have played a significant role in managing night-blindness in the island. In 1928, W.R. Aykroyd noted that the inability to see in dim light was "practically confined to men, and its seasonal incidence is the summer." Aykroyd added that the condition was "singularly disconcerting to navigators on the dangerous Newfoundland coasts." He indicated that promptness was necessary in dealing with it, but that a doctor was rarely consulted: "The most popular remedy is birds' liver, cooked or raw. Birds' hearts, rabbits' livers, or cod liver oil are sometimes taken; the last more rarely, having small honour in its own country." Aykroyd rationalized this empirical tradition on the basis that the animal parts were sources of vitamin A.

The beaver deserves special mention if only because it is a memorable part of Micmac traditional lore. As one informant said in 1993: "Beaver gall was good too. We always drink that. That's good for anything too. You get a beaver and kill him and he's warm ... takes it all out, out it in a cup and drink it warm, and anything you got wrong with you it gets better." Beaver testicles ("pride") or castor (a reddish-brown unctuous substance with a strong smell and bitter taste, obtained from the beaver) are also known as applications for sores and used to promote healing, as was the fat.

Knowledge about the use of many animal products persists in twentieth-century Newfoundland; jaybird brains for frostbite, for example, or black cat's blood for a sty. And these are in addition to such remedies as bear's grease (q.v.), goose grease (q.v.), and fat pork (q.v.). Generally, they are viewed as legacies of magical concepts, but studies are still needed to evaluate the physiological value of many animal products as medicine.

Still another facet of animal treatment should be mentioned – passing a child under or over an animal. That constitutes a form of "passing through" (q.v.), commonly reported in many folklore traditions. P.K. Devine wrote in 1937:

When whooping-cough, measles, croup, and other infantile ailments become epidemic, they can be cured or averted by passing the child three times underneath and over the back of an ass and uttering the name of the Blessed Trinity. This was witnessed frequently in the streets of St. John's seventy years ago, and a full description is given in the newspapers of the time. A man named William Dawe of Pouch Cove had an ass with a white cross on its back – an essential feature – and did quite a business whenever he came to town, whether for money or charity the record does not say. One of the doctors of the day took up an argument against it, but he got nowhere. The mothers got the results they sought in their simple faith, and that settled the argument.

Human products generally faded from medicine before many animal parts. Urine, more popular than animal-dung, was a notable exception, although by 1936 it was reported to be little used in Newfoundland, at least on the east coast. Recent recollections from various parts of the island nevertheless suggest a strong collective memory for employment of urine on various skin conditions (sunburn, water pups, sore hands, chapped hands, pimples, chilblains, freckles) and for sore eyes. Two methods – urinating directly on the skin or applying urine via wet diapers – were commonly suggested. Some see urine from babies as a symbol of purity and innocence; perhaps, however, the convenience of using a wet diaper was at times more relevant. There is some scientific evidence that urine can be beneficial in certain skin problems. (For comments on blood, see *blood purifiers*).

NOTES
See: Camporesi (1988) and Bourke (1891), for background; Parsons (1936), on urine little used; Aykroyd (1928), on night-blindness (Aykroyd noted that the preference for fish over bird and mammal liver was scientifically sound); Devine (1937b); Hand

(1980) 12, for symbolism of purity and innocence of a baby; MCG (1993) 2, on Micmacs and beaver.

Representative MUNFLA references: 65-1/80 (urine complexion), 67-4/11 (cow-dung for frostbite), 67-20/31 (jaybird brains), 67-20/29 (urine chilblains), 69-17/3 (urine chapped hands), 68-26/16 (sheep-dung for measles), 72-53 (pig's liver used in 1930s).

## ANTISEPTIC OINTMENTS

Although Newfoundlanders do not seem to have favoured many home-made salves, "antiseptic ointment" does appear in the oral record. This – for cuts (q.v.), sores, and infections such as come from a nail in the foot – could refer to many products, but a strong possibility is Chase's Ointment. Chase products, as noted earlier, became a veritable tradition in Newfound-land. By the early 1900s, the ointment was widely advertised for eczema, haemorrhoids, and children's inflamed and stuck eyelids. It is still available with such promotion as: "For more than sixty years, soothing, antiseptic Chase ointment has brought fast relief to cuts, bruises, minor burns, abrasions, and sunburn. It even relieves the misery of itching piles." Ingre-dients include zinc oxide (long used as an empirical basis for various skin ailments) and phenol (well known as an antiseptic).

Zam-Buk, another popular antiseptic ointment during the first half of the twentieth century, became especially well known through successful advertising and widespread interest in germs (see *germs*). In 1915, an adver-tisement promoted Zam-Buk as an apparent cure-all: "Quickly kills all germs, stops the bleeding, prevents suppuration and blood poison and heals quickly." Later, in 1945, the Zam-Buk promotion was moderated and the ointment was now said "to soothe and heal that foot trouble" and also to relieve "chafing, skin eruptions, cuts, burns and bruises." Captain Troake, who had all the prestige of a Newfoundland sealing captain (as well as being the renowned skipper of the *Christmas Seal*), credited Zam-Buk ("a good salve") with saving his leg following an accident. Testimonials have always been central to successful self-treatments and Troake, a fine storyteller, probably did much to reinforce public confidence in the product.

NOTES
See: Chase's (1993) *Almanac* for current promotion; Troake (1989), 38.
Representative MUNFLA reference: 69-27/7 (antiseptic ointment).

## APPENDICITIS

Surgical treatment for appendicitis was only firmly established in the early 1900s, and hence medical recommendations for home management might be expected to have faded quickly from memory. On the other hand, making a correct diagnosis was worrisome, even for medical practitioners. As one surgeon remembers, typhoid fever and tuberculous peritonitis were always strong diagnostic possibilities in the 1930s, as were other conditions still common today.

Amid diagnostic uncertainties (and tales of recovery without surgery), it is not altogether surprising that Newfoundlanders might see "a touch of appendicitis" as little different from a stomach ailment, especially if there was a possibility that the "touch" would keep them from a fishing trip and their essential income. This possibility led some physicians to readily remove appendices from patients living in rural areas, even if there was only a slight chance that appendicitis was the correct diagnosis. Such "preventive" operations were said to be for "geographic (or geographical) appendices," a term once fairly well known in Newfoundland.

At home, many treated what was possibly an appendix with painkillers or as a bad stomach. The belief that it was "inflammatory" led some physicians to recommend ice packs over the abdomen, especially if difficulties emerged in getting surgery done quickly.

One suggestion found in the recently recorded Newfoundland oral tradition is "cupping" for appendicitis. A small cuplike vessel (which had been warmed over a flame to produce a partial vacuum) was placed over the painful area. As the cup cooled, a mound of flesh was drawn into it. Relief of pain, when it was obtained, was generally explained on the basis of the theory of counterirritation – the theory of a therapeutic action produced at a distance by a "reflex" action. At times, cupping was used to let blood.

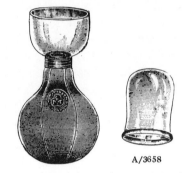

A/3658

Cupping glasses advertised in *Maw's Catalogue of Surgeons' Instruments* (1925).

Cupping, which other Newfoundlanders suggested as a means to relieve any pain, had a major place in professional medical treatment until toward the end of the nineteenth century. It is not surprising that its use faded slowly. Recollections exist of cupping equipment in the General Hospital, St. John's, during the 1930s. In recent times, cupping has attracted renewed interest as a form of alternative medicine.

Another Newfoundland recommendation regarding appendicitis, commonly known elsewhere, was to avoid apple seeds or grape pips altogether – prevention rather than cure. How many felt that constipation predisposed to appendicitis – a thought not unheard of today – is impossible to say. At least one advertisement (1906) for Cascarets told Newfoundlanders to "take a Cascaret whenever you suspect you need one. Thus you will ward off appendicitis, constipation, indigestion ..."

NOTES
See: Fizzard (1988), on concerns of health for fishermen; Brown collection (Hand 1961, vol. 6) 118, for seeds bringing on appendicitis.

Representative MUNFLA references: 69-6/16 (cupping), 66-8/13 (apple seeds, grape pips).

Personal communication: N. Rusted (1991), for background, use of ice and cupping; P. Warwick (1991), on geographic appendices.

## APPETITE RESTORERS

Appetite "restorers" (or appetite "builders") are not usually specifically described in professional or domestic medical texts, but instead are viewed as "tonics" (q.v.), especially bitter tonics. Poor appetite, however, is always of concern to lay people as a sign of ill-health, and it is perhaps surprising that there are relatively few specific references in the Newfoundland record.

Recommendations for stimulating appetite include imbibing teas made from cherry tree bark (wild cherry q.v.), "raw" dogberries (q.v.), and wormwood (q.v.). Another suggestion is to soak "blackberry herbs, boil until the water is black and drink." Of these, only wormwood is bitter, although the astringency of the other herbs may have contributed to their reputation. Although for much of this century usage of non-bitter herbs was contrary to the prevailing theory behind ways to stimulate the appetite, they may well have served as nutritional supplements when given over time. (The many nutritional problems in Newfoundland have been noted.) This suggestion seems more plausible, however, vis-à-vis the use of robin soup for improving the appetite.

No Newfoundland reference has been found for using the crackerberry (q.v.).

NOTES
Representative MUNFLA references: 67-4 (cherry bark and dogberry tree), 73-150 (said to be boiled for an hour; needles and berries of ground juniper might also be added), 69-17/20 (robin soup), 76-249 (dogberries, wormwood), 84-371A/B (dogwood).

## APPLES

Apples – mostly imported into Newfoundland in barrels and known as "barrel apples" – are recorded on the island for the treatment of both diarrhoea and constipation, an apparent contradiction of usage. One recommendation for diarrhoea is to scrape out and eat a raw apple with a spoon. For constipation, on the other hand, two unpeeled raw apples are suggested. The medical literature (professional and popular) generally noted only the use of apples and apple juice as a laxative, although this covered recommendations for "upset stomachs" as well.

A sense of some of the general nineteenth-century (and twentieth) popular interest in the apple is reflected in *Hall's Journal of Health*. It advised American families (1860) to maintain a supply of at least two to ten barrels of apples: they have "an admirable effect on the general system, often removing constipation, correcting acidities, and cooling off febrile conditions, more effectually than the most approved medicines." It was also said that if Americans substituted apples for pies, cakes, candies, and other sweets, "there would be a diminution in the sum total of doctors' bills in a single year." The commonplace adage, "an apple a day keeps the doctor away," has long been recognized in Newfoundland, as elsewhere. The household hints, published in the St. John's *Daily News* (23 January 1906), said that everybody knows the "tonic value of apples." One recent reference to the use of apple cider vinegar and honey "for the kidneys" reflects the widespread "health food" promotion of the vinegar since the 1950s.

Because of the limited number of apple trees in Newfoundland, the absence of any reference to the use of apple tree bark is not surprising, even though it once had a modest reputation (more so during the nineteenth century) as a treatment for fevers.

Contradictory information concerning usage for diarrhoea and constipation has been noted for other plants. This can reflect misinformation, information derived from the use of different parts of a plant; or, in fact, deliberate use of a laxative for diarrhea, in part as a cleansing role. (See *diarrhoea*.)

NOTES
See: Introductory note to bibliography for general history and information; Levenstein (1988) 5, for quote from *Hall's Journal of Health*; MCG (1992) 009, on apple-cider vinegar.

Representative MUNFLA references: 69-23/30 (constipation), 76-249 (diarrhoea).

## ARROWROOT

At least one Newfoundland report exists for the employment of "arrowroot" for treating diarrhoea, although there is uncertainty about the nature of the product, since it is said to have been obtained from the root of the raspberry bush. This is not the genuine arrowroot, a starch, generally derived from the West Indian plant *Maranta arundinacae*. Arrowroot became an invalid food of choice, at least for much of the nineteenth century. Even window displays in British pharmacies sometimes included large display or specie jars labelled arrowroot. *Dr. Chase's Receipt Book and Household Physician (1887)* gave the following recipe: "Mix 2 table-spoonfuls of arrowroot to a smooth paste with a little cold water; then add to it 1 pt. of boiling water, a little lemon peel, and stir while boiling. Let it cook till quite clear. Sweeten with sugar, and flavor with wine or nutmeg, if desired. Milk may be used instead of the water, if preferred."

Arrowroot was, in fact, fading in popularity toward the end of the nineteenth century, at least in British medicine, when one writer described it as "nothing but starch and water." Nevertheless it continued to be available in Newfoundland stores and elsewhere. In recent times, it is again being promoted as a health food.

Any suggestion that arrowroot stopped diarrhoea is not generally supported by the relevant literature, although as a bland food (it was not always made with wine and spices as noted by Chase) it was appropriate supportive care for many gastrointestinal complaints, and was in line with recommendations of gruels for diarrhoea. It is noteworthy that the Newfoundland record notes the use of cornflour mixed with boiled cow's milk for diarrhoea. It should be added that the astringency of raspberry root could be useful for managing diarrhoea.

NOTES
See: Chase (1887), 31–2.
Representative MUNFLA reference: 70-14/56 (root of raspberry bush).

ARTHRITIS (SEE RHEUMATISM)

ASPIRIN

Only one report has been found in the recently recorded Newfoundland oral tradition recommending the ubiquitous aspirin (for earache [q.v.]) perhaps in conjunction with other treatment. This is largely because aspirin is not viewed as a folk remedy and collectors of folklore often fail to ask specifically about commercial preparations. Nevertheless, aspirin, constantly advertised in Newfoundland, was widely used by the 1930s. One physician recollects that demand in the outports during the 1930s was such that in 1935 one entrepreneur was selling aspirin tablets for five cents each. Advertisers made clear which aches and pains (especially headache; for example, "early morning headache") and feverish conditions aspirin should be used for.

Soon after the introduction of acetylsalicylic acid in 1899, the name "aspirin" was trademarked by the Bayer Company, a trademark upheld in Canada, but not, for example, in the United States and Britain. But, even before Confederation, Bayer "genuine" aspirin was the brand most commonly, although not intensively, advertised in Newfoundland. Recent advertising wars involving newer, closely related products such as acetaminophen (Tylenol) and ibuprofen (Advil) have reached Newfoundland, as elsewhere. These wars and the new reasons for taking aspirin (for example, small regular doses to prevent heart attacks) have hardly lessened lay uncertainty over what product to use.

See also *analgesics, headache.*

NOTES
See: McTavish (1987); Mann and Plummer (1991). Representative MUNFLA reference: 68-10/7.

ASTHMA

Recommendations for treating asthma are extensive both in the printed and "oral" traditions of self-care and on both sides of the Atlantic. Perhaps one reason is that, in the twentieth century, lay diagnoses have often been imprecise, more so than those made by physicians; for instance, chest wheeziness alone (perhaps associated with bronchitis) has been self-diagnosed as asthma.

The relatively modest Newfoundland record of asthma partly reflects the fact that general remedies for colds (q.v.) were often used. "There would be colds and I used to get tightness on the chest, then they'd put the linseed meal on me, back and front. My father was asthmatic and he had to wear like a bib, red flannel inside his shirt, tied around him. Then when he'd get a cold, heavy cold, he'd get so tight as a jar and mother would put the linseed meal on him and put him to bed for a day or two." There were, however, specific recommendations for asthma. These included (for internal administration) Friar's balsam and sugar, kerosene and molasses, magnatea berries or leaves made into a tea, and Minard's Liniment and molasses. At least some of the regimens using these products may have relieved symptoms for pharmacological reasons (for instance, the airways were opened, perhaps by loosening phlegm).

*Friar's balsam* (q.v.), an alcoholic preparation of benzoin, aloes, storax, and balsam of tolu, was available by at least the seventeenth century; it has been best known as an application for cuts (q.v.) and sores, for which it is still used. Widely sold in Newfoundland, it is also well regarded as an internal preparation (with sugar to improve the palatability), as an expectorant to bring up phlegm. This probably explains its recommendation for asthma (as well as for bronchitis in another Newfoundland record: a few drops placed in hot water).

*Magnatea berries* or *leaves* are, in Newfoundland, collected from *Gaultheria hispidula,* also known as manna-tea or maidenhair (see *creeping snowberry*). *G. hispidula* (and *G. procumbens*, wintergreen) are characterized by a sharp odour when crushed, due to the presence of the volatile oil of wintergreen. This has long been known for its rubefacient (reddening and warming) action on the skin and other medicinal properties. Although such properties are not generally employed in treating asthma, the oil (commercial oil was purchased) was sometimes rubbed on the chest, thereby helping to "clear the passages," a property of the mild aromatic properties of the berries of *G. hispidula*.

Yet another Newfoundland suggestion – to put "everlasting daisies" (presumably *Anaphalis margaritacea*, not *Armeria maritima* which has a limited distribution on the west coast of the island) under the pillow – hardly seems well founded. Perhaps it is based on an analogy to another plant, life everlasting (*Gnaphalium* spp.), known for asthma elsewhere – which is rationalized on the basis of aromatic, albeit mild, properties.

*Minard's Liniment* (q.v.) has undoubtedly been one of the principal commercial cure-alls employed in Newfoundland where, like Chase products, it has become a tradition. It is not surprising that asthma sufferers tried the camphoraceous odour to ease the chest and clear the passages.

An old record (1899) notes the Newfoundland use of "Andromeda polifolia" as a remedy for asthma. This probably refers to *A. glaucophylla* (bog rosemary), the only species found in Newfoundland. (*A. polifolia* is reported as growing only in Labrador). The medical reputation is slight, but nineteenth-century medical texts at least noted (for *Andromeda speciosa*) the use of the powdered leaves and buds as an errhine; that is, a medicinal used to promote sneezing to clear respiratory passages. If this applies to the Newfoundland species noted above, there may have been some symptomatic benefit.

Many asthma treatments generally rationalized as magical have been touted in Newfoundland. For instance, it is said that boring a hole in the wall at the same height as an asthmatic child will cause the asthma to disappear when the child grows taller than the hole. (Variations of this measurement regimen, also recorded on the island, include filling the hole with the child's hair and plugging it with wood, or placing a lock of the child's hair in the seam of a door). The fact that some children grow out of their asthma only encouraged such beliefs.

Although hanging a small bag of mustard around the neck served as a protective charm for some, the reputation of mustard (q.v., for example in plasters) in treating chest complaints may have reinforced confidence for similarly treating asthma. Whether or not eating green worms or caterpillars from cabbage, another suggestion, rests on empirical or on magical ideas (or both) is unclear. Cabbage caterpillars have not been noted in other folklore records, and since the only two Newfoundland records found are from Twillingate, local considerations may be at play.

Increasingly in the twentieth century, commercial preparations (additional to Minard's noted above) have pushed aside traditional asthma treatments. One long-standing proprietary medicine still promoted in Newfoundland is "Buckley's." Newfoundlanders in the 1920s witnessed claims for W.K. Buckley's asthma and bronchitis remedy as the "world's only two bottle remedy" for "Coughs, Colds, Bronchitis, Asthma, Lung troubles." The 1991 promotion of Buckley's Mixture harks back to "old time" med-icines, or at least one view of them: "It tastes awful and it works." It is also said (1991) to be "reliable and effective for the relief of coughs due to colds, chronic bronchitis, asthma, laryngitis, hoarseness and crouping cough."

Other over-the-counter preparations frequently promoted among New-foundlanders for asthma included Raz-mah (In 1927: "$1 at all St. John's druggists and outport stores" – "No Smoke, No Sprays, No Snuff Just Swallow RAZ-MAH capsules"); it remained well known until at least the 1960s. If Raz-mah contained only aspirin mixed with a little char-coal and caffeine, as once stated, its physiological action was minimal. The ingredients in another popular preparation, Stafford's Phoratone, are unknown, in contrast to many sub-stances used for inhaling (for example, Vapo-Cresoline, Catarrho-zone), often singled out for asthma and based on menthol and camphor. Catarrhozone, drawn in from a cig-arettelike inhaler, used promotional statements (in 1910) such as "No treatment is simpler or more pleas-ant, No remedy so free from pernicious drugs."

One wonders how many of the countless commercial inhalers mar-keted during the nineteenth century and subsequently ("it is difficult to select among them") had a place in Newfoundland homes, or whether a bowl of hot water with added medicament for inhaling and a cloth over the head was generally used.

Advertisement (1910) for Catarrhozone, one of a number of preparations prompting concern if not worry over catarrh (see *colds*).

Special cigarettes or smoking mixtures were also tried; these were either prepared by a local druggist or were commercial preparations such as the well-known Potter's Asthma Cigarettes. The broncho-dilating action of these – to ease breathing – was commonly due to the presence of either stramonium or lobelia herbs, which could be purchased separately from druggists. Recollections of "asthma cigarettes" in Newfoundland may also cover the use of locally available herbs, such as the everlasting daisy noted above.

During the 1960s and 1970s, home asthma treatments were increasingly challenged by a new range of prescription products shown to provide more consistent symptom relief. However, concerns have often been expressed by patients about potential side-effects of the new compounds. Anecdotal evidence exists that some "oldtime" remedies are still used in the hope of reducing the amounts of prescription products needed, situations that can lead to inappropriate mixing of medications.

NOTES
See: MCG (1992) 109, quotation on linseed meal; Bergen (1899) 110, "Andromeda polifolia;" Cramp (1936) 4, for Raz-Mah formula; Creighton (1968) 194–5, for some non-commercial treatments, particularly measurement and smoking (The latter includes mullein, well known for asthma although not recorded in the Newfoundland oral tradition); *Encyclopedia of American Popular Beliefs and Superstitions* (in press 1994), for entry on asthma that provides a general overview of an extensive number of treatments.

Representative MUNFLA references: 68-19/2 (measurement), 68-19/1 (suspended bag of mustard), 76-249 (magnatea berries or leaves, green worms), 82-218 (Minard's and molasses, Friar's Balsam and sugar, kerosene and molasses).

BACKACHE

Suggestions for treating backache (or a "bad back") in the recently recorded Newfoundland oral tradition include: iron over a thin cloth placed on the back; apply dragon's blood (q.v.); or be walked over by "Jim White" who had webbed feet. The limited record – perhaps surprising since heavy lifting has long been part of daily life for most Newfoundland men and women – at least suggests some usage of home-made plasters to provide a rubefacient (reddening and warming action). Bergen (1899) probably refers to one when noting an application of "cabbage kelp" (a seaweed) for a lame back. Commercial back plasters (for example, belladonna plaster) were frequently employed until at least the 1940s; the discomfort of removing such plasters is graphically illustrated in the following early twentieth-century postcard.

There have been many other over-the-counter items available for external or internal use. Among highly regarded liniments (external applications or "rubs" for backache and other pains) were Minard's (q.v.) and Sloan's. (The latter, believed by some to be stronger than Minard's, was reported in 1936 to contain oil of kerosene or turpentine with sassafras and red pepper, but to give inconsistent analytical results.)

A conspicuous feature of backache treatment was the use of "kidney" medicines (q.v.). Low backache had been linked with kidney problems long before manufacturers of commercial preparations exploited the association. By the 1930s, kidney trouble was called backache. Numerous advertisements rein-

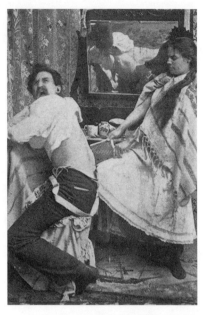

This Parting Gives Me Pain!

forced this by sometimes implying that *all* backaches were linked with the kidney, although this was only the case for some. In 1945, Newfoundlanders were being told that "Gin Pills for Kidneys" (q.v.) helped to "remove the excess acids that are often the cause of the stiff achy back." Cystex (see pp. 40–1) was being promoted in the post-World War II years for "pains in back," and Doyle advertisements in 1966 promoted Dodd's Kidney Pills (q.v.) for "nagging backache" and Dr. Chase's Kidney-Liver Pills for backache.

Although legislation has now stopped such claims for medicines, the association of the kidneys with backache and other problems is still common and may even encourage the sale of backache medicine once associated with the kidney (for example, Dodd's and Gin Pills). Further, amid the vast current health-care literature on self-care for backache – with and without medicines – one finds promotional material that encourages imprudent treatments, such as the use of juniper (q.v.).

NOTES
See: Bergen (1899) 112; Cramp (1936) 185, for analysis of Sloan's; Tizzard (1984) 83, for recollections of kidney trouble being called "backache" in the 1930s.

Representative MUNFLA references: 66-2/58 (bad back), 78-195 (ironing back), 82-146 (dragon's blood).

### BAKEAPPLE

The bakeapple (*Rubus chamaemorus*, known elsewhere as cloudberry, baked apple, knotberry) is commonplace throughout Newfoundland, especially in boggy areas on coastal cliffs. The edible, amber berries have long been an important crop – both for home use and the commercial market – and their employment by Micmac Indians for "consumption, cough and fever" has been reported. It is uncertain, however, whether this latter usage has been long-standing. Certainly, it did not become generally known throughout the island, even though it was in line with early European knowledge that the astringency of the fruit was suitable, in the words of John Gerard (1633), to "cooleth the stomacke, and allayeth inflammations." The vitamin C content may have useful in a non-specific way.

Debate exists over the origin of the name bakeapple – sometimes misunderstood as *baked* (that is, cooked) apple. Most students of plant names believe that it is related to the odour reminiscent of baked apples.

NOTES
See: Smallwood and Pitt (1981) 116–7, economics; Chandler et al. (1979), for Micmac usage; Gerard (1633) 1420; Clute (1942) 43, for comments on name.

### BAKING SODA

Baking soda (sodium bicarbonate), sometimes called bread soda, has been one of the best known "kitchen" remedies. In 1936, it was noted to have almost replaced Cooper's chalk or powdered eggshell for heartburn or for a pain in the stomach. The recently recorded Newfoundland oral tradition ascribes many medical uses to baking soda, sometimes employed as "bread soda plaster" – in essence a thick paste – for fly bites, hives, and other skin rashes, and taken internally for indigestion ("heartburn," "acid," and "stomach gas"), all conditions sometimes relieved by alkali. It was also well known for burns and scalds and sometimes promoted for these in newspaper advertisements (for example, for Cow Brand Baking Soda in 1953).

The quantity to be taken internally (dissolved in water) is not generally reported in the oral record, but professional and popular medical writings, some recent, indicate the employment of weak solutions (1% or even less) to relieve the skin irritation of dermatitis and urticaria (see *rashes*) and to treat minor burns.

A teaspoonful of the powder in a large tumblerful of water, suggested as an antacid, is still recommended despite a plethora of over-the-counter medicines.

NOTES

See: Parsons (1936), on Cooper's chalk; Murray (1979) 134, on hives, insect bites.

Representative MUNFLA references: 76-249 (heartburn), 82-122 (acid, rash, burns), 82-158 (burns), 84-320B (fly bites, hives, rashes).


BALDNESS, HAIR PREPARATIONS, STARING HAIR

Male baldness has no doubt long worried some Newfoundlanders, at least if judged by the promotion of hair restorers on the island. The photograph (1910) of the shop front of the pharmacy of Dr. F. Stafford (see p. 19) shows a window display advertising Nyals Hirsutone: "Don't Lose Your Hair."

One baldness treatment recorded a number of times in the oral tradition – its rubefacient (warming) action on the scalp perhaps encouraged this – was Minard's Liniment (q.v.). Its action may not have been as noticeable as the Cantharadine Hair Tonic sold by some Newfoundland druggists, which contained the blistering beetle cantharides, a powerful irritant and rubefacient. In sharp contrast was the application of lanolin, still advertised for baldness in the 1950s, and its association with woolly sheep.

Although commercial preparations advertised in the first half of the twentieth century for falling hair (and for dandruff) did not list ingredients, Salvia presumably contained sage, which has long had a reputation as a hair "tonic." In fact, *The Daily News* (6 August 1910), under the heading "At Last An English Chemist Has Discovered How to Grow Hair," noted that Salvia contained henna that "will positively grow hair;" this, however, is incorrect.

Although the oral tradition suggested that, to avoid hair loss, the hair must not be cut on St. Patrick's Day, some Newfoundlanders probably paid more attention to household and health hints for thinning hair. *The Daily News* (20 March 1894), for example, offered a suitable "hair tonic" containing yellow dock, borax, rum, red onion juice, and lavender.

The failure of hair restorers or "renewers" is perhaps mirrored in the following "tall story" told in Newfoundland: "Rub head with molasses. Go to wood where flies are thick. Flies land on head and stick. When molasses dry pick off flies' bodies leaving legs in molasses. Legs will take root. Wash off molasses after about two weeks and you will have a lovely head of coal black hair."

Whether or not Newfoundlanders used sage washes, sometimes to darken greying hair (and perhaps in the belief that they stopped hair falling out) is not recorded; however, being common elsewhere, it is not unlikely. Certainly available, at least in the early 1900s, was the popular Wyeth's Solution [of] Sage and Sulphur and Lead Acetate for "coloring grey and faded hair." There was, too, some interest in hair colouring aside from the many commercial preparations marketed. In 1964, a Newfoundlander wrote that when this grandmother was in her seventies "she used to use bark in her grey hair to give it a reddish tinge." ("Bark" in Newfoundland referred to the bark and buds of conifers steeped to produce a liquid to preserve fishnets, sails, and so on.)

One particular issue concerning hair in Newfoundland was what physicians called "staring hair." What was this condition, which is no longer recognized? Was it widespread? Was it recognized by Newfoundlanders in general? Staring hair, described as dry, coarse, and lacklustre, was thought to be caused by inadequate nutrition. Perhaps it fostered the application of hair tonics such as the well-known preparations of bay rum. Nowadays, hair tonics, as such, attract little interest, but Newfoundlanders as a whole certainly use more hair preparations (shampoos included) than in the "old days." Lead acetate is still in use in some preparations, but it now prompts health concerns, which encourage some people to use products containing herbs.

NOTES
See: Chase (1862) 260, for sage and falling hair; Adamson *et al.* (1945), for medical view of staring hair.
Representative MUNFLA references: 64-1/96 (bark for grey hair), 69-23/15 (molasses and flies), 84-310B (Minard's).

BALSAM FIR

The resin of the balsam fir (*Abies balsamea*), common throughout Newfoundland, has long been known for treating cuts (see discussion on myrrh under *cuts and wounds*). Usage of the inside of the bark as a poultice for boils or as a plaster for sprains has also been recorded.

The Newfoundland oral record sometimes uses a local name for the fir, namely the "Green Doctor" tree (a fir with the sap running), saying "Find some resin, sap from a Green Doctor tree, and apply it to the cut." Other local vernacular names, "maiden fir" or "she-var," are said to refer to so-called female balsam firs. In fact, since male and female cones are produced on the same tree, female trees do not exist; some consider the name refers to trees with mature cones, but others view it as a way of distinguishing it from spruce which, in places, is considered as male.

"Maiden fir" can also describe the fresh young tops of the fir, or even the fresh juice. As one Newfoundlander reported about an acquaintance, "He called his cure for eczema, maiden-fir. He made it by steeping out fir tree tops. The tree tops had to have seven branches or the maiden-fir wouldn't work. He would boil these tree tops and the substance left was known as maiden-fir."

As perhaps reflected in various common names, the fir has long been an essential part of Newfoundland life. This possibly contributes to the reverence for, and the testimonials to, the usage of various balsam preparations in skin conditions and for coughs. Perhaps, too, it contributed to the reputation of the fir as a blood purifier, thereby rationalizing the use of a decoction for treating boils.

NOTES
See: Introduction to bibliography for general history and background information; Bergen (1899) III, references to fir; Mercer (1991), plaster; *Dictionary Newfoundland English* (1990), green doctor and maiden fir.

Representative MUNFLA references: 66-10/57 (she-var and boils).

BATHING, SPA WATERS, PERSONAL HYGIENE

Bathing in or drinking spa water, and to a lesser extent sea water, has a long history – embracing lay and professional medical care – in Europe and North America for treatment of a wide range of conditions. However, since 1900, with a change in the orientation of medicine, the decline and fall of the spa and water cure, at least in the English-speaking world, is intriguing. Recent studies have confirmed physiological changes when the body is immersed in mineral baths, though apparently no more so than immersion in tap water. The decline of spa treatment was preceded by fading medical interest in sea water. Thus it is not altogether surprising that references in the recent Newfoundland oral record are sparse, even bearing in mind the proximity of sea water to all Newfoundlanders. Some islanders, too, had access to such mineral springs as the one-time chalybeate (iron-containing) spring facilities at Logy Bay, near St. John's; now built over, it once attracted modest interest during the late nineteenth and first half of the twentieth century. There are also magical or holy waters. Micmac Indians have a shrine at Bay du Nord, where a brook is said never to freeze or run dry and the water to have curative properties.

Incidental references to the use of water exist in the Newfoundland record; for instance, warm sea water has been suggested for "flu," perhaps merely intended for tepid bathing to reduce a raised temperature. Warm sea water is also suggested for rickets: "To cure a child of rickets, it is bathed in sea water; the water must not be heated on the stove, but by dropping a hot iron in a pan full." The basis of the recommendation for rickets is unclear, if indeed this "diagnosis" refers to the deficiency disease (lack of vitamin D) of that name. Yet perhaps the suggestion merely echoes past professional medical recommendations for rickets, namely that medicines were generally of little value compared with such bracing and strengthening regimens as cold baths.

*Apollinaris*

"THE QUEEN OF TABLE WATER."

The Carbonate of Soda

which is its natural and chief constituent

is the sworn enemy

of Gout, Rheumatism and Indigestions

1910 advertisement for Apollinaris
from the *Daily News*.

Another aspect of the spa-water story – commercially bottled water as well as artificial spa or table water – affected Newfoundland. Waters advertised to Newfoundlanders in the early 1900s included Apollinaris: "The Queen of Table Water. The carbonate of soda which is its natural chief constituent is the sworn enemy of gout, rheumatism, and indigestion." (It is still available without the promotion.) Kruschen Salts, however, had a greater impact, because of its convenience as well as intensive promotion. Like Apollinaris, the Salts were considered to counteract the presumed deleterious effects of uric acid. According to one advertisement (1940), it dissolved the agony of rheumatism, namely "needle-pointed crystals" of uric acid lodging in the joints.

Uric acid was a major issue in professional medicine toward the end of the 1800s and during the early 1900s. Many physicians, and greater numbers of lay people, accepted a notion – now known to be erroneous – that uric acid was implicated in a myriad of diseases. Much attention was given to the view that lithium, at least lithium carbonate, dissolved uric acid and hence was a valuable medicine. Lithia tablets and lithia spring waters were vigorously promoted, and Newfoundlanders would have been part of this trend if they had acted upon the many advertisements in the St. John's newspapers for Sal Lithofos, recommended for chronic rheumatism, lumbago, neuralgia, and other ailments associated with pain. See also *rheumatism*.

Much spa treatment in general was directed toward rheumatism, and, in fact, the specialty of rheumatologists today is rooted to some extent in the spas of old. But the physiological effects of drinking spa water are much different from bathing, and it is unlikely that Newfoundlanders derived much benefit from Apollinaris water or Kruschen Salts, whatever the theory behind their use. In any case, skin conditions have often been noted to improve with water treatment. In line with this, the Newfoundland record notes salt water for chilblains (q.v.), and fresh water – the foam of a brook – for eczema (q.v.).

Any assessment of sea-water bathing, and so on should be made from within the context of attitudes toward baths in general. Without running water, frequent baths in Newfoundland were generally impossible, even more so for those away logging or at the fishery. The extent to which this was seen by most Newfoundlanders during the first half of the century as a hygiene and health issue – one accentuated by advertisements for soaps (q.v.) – is not clear. A biographer of Wilfred Grenfell writing in 1920 noted, perhaps uncritically and unsympathetically, that "bathtubs are a mystery to some of the patients," who after they have been undressed and led to the water's edge ask plaintively "what do you want me to do now?" Relatively recent changes in attitudes seemingly reflect not only changed hygiene considerations, but also social pressure for a daily shower or bath.

NOTES
See: Porter (1990), for general background; Waldo (1920) 25, on mystery of bath-tubs; O'Hare et al. (1985), for an example of physiological changes in bathing; Parsons (1936), for sea water and rickets; Whorton (1982) 238–69, for background to uric acid; MCG (1993) 2, on Bay du Nord site.

Representative MUNFLA references: 69-28/3 (sea water for "flu").

BEARBERRY, CRANBERRY, MARSHBERRY, AND URINE

Bearberry (*Arctostaphylos uva-ursi*) – commonly called "hardberry" and "Indian hurts" in Newfoundland, and uva-ursi in the medical literature – is well known in professional medi-cine as an astringent tonic and a mild urinary antiseptic. One medical authority in the early twentieth cen-tury indicated various uses, some depending on a "powerful disinfec-tant" action on the "urine and the mucous membrane of the urinary  passages." Since bearberry is found in Newfoundland (even if not especially common), and recent and current herbal writings are again promoting its use – although it is incorrect to suggest its action is "powerful" – perhaps it is surprising that its medical reputation is so little known on the island.

Another "bearberry" – so-called by Newfoundlanders – is *Vaccinium macrocarpus*, better known as the cranberry. This is yet another plant that does not feature in the Newfoundland oral medical tradition, although elsewhere (for instance, in New England, where it is more common) it has long had a reputation for urinary infections, a reputation that has become commercialized in recent years, even if scientific evidence as to its effective-ness is doubtful.

One related *Vaccinium* species – *V. oxycoccos* – commonly known as the marshberry, has been employed occasionally on the island. At least one reference exists to soaking marshberries in water for one week, and drinking a shot glass full every night before bed for fourteen days. It was said this was done to "clean up vaginal infections," a comment that might just cover urinary tract infections.

NOTES
See: Introduction to bibliography for general history and background information, and Potter (1917) 481; Scott (1987), for botanical nomenclature.

Representative MUNFLA references: 89-084 (marshberry).

## BEAR'S GREASE

Bear's "grease" or "fat" has had an extended history of usage in salves and hair pomades. By the early nineteenth century, for instance, James Atkinson was especially well known for promoting bear's grease as a key part of his successful London perfumery business. "Bear's Grease Pomade" became popular during the century, although many brands probably did not contain the expensive grease.

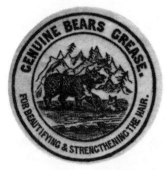

Label for Bear's grease

"Smoochin'" or "smearing down the hair" in Newfoundland could well have employed commercial bear's grease hair dressings. With bears conspicuous in the Newfoundland fauna (at least for hunting), one might expect much local interest; however, few records have been found in the oral tradition, even to the application for "sores on the body" and the use of the "oil" for diaper sores. One hunter remembers that plastering down the hair with fat from a freshly killed bear was supposed to prevent baldness. Although bear's grease (also used as a chest rub) was viewed as an alternative to goose grease (q.v.), the latter has been pre-eminent on the island.

NOTES
See: Jackson (1974), for general background; *Dictionary Newfoundland English* (1990), under smoochin'; Mercer (1991), under tuberculosis; MCG (1993) 2, for Micmac recollection.

Representative MUNFLA references: 69-6/8 (body sores), 84-323B (diaper sores).

## BEAVER-ROOT

In Newfoundland, the common name beaver-root may refer to *Menyanthes trifoliata* (see *bogbean*) or to various water lilies, especially *Nuphar variegatum*, considered here. Although references to beaver-root being employed as a tonic could refer to either *Menyanthes* or a water lily (more likely to be the former), Newfoundland reports of cutting and gathering beaver-root (probably so-called because it is eaten by beavers) from the bottom of a pond (and then boiling the root and using the water to wash eyes) generally refer to the water lily. Micmac usage of beaver-root is reported for both plants, for various conditions from kidney complaints to coughs.

Long-standing professional and domestic medical interest in the water lily in Western medicine – which includes the lotus, *Nelumbo* spp. – relates to the astringent, somewhat bitter taste of the roots. This fits with New-foundlanders' interest in it as both a tonic and an eyewash. A reference exists to "poppy" or water-lily buds being boiled and the steam inhaled for relieving headaches and sinus trouble, but whether there is a pharmacological explanation for this needs study. It should be added that poppies (*Papaver* spp.) are grown in Newfoundland gardens and, as elsewhere, there is sometimes the hope (even belief) that they contain opium; this, however, applies to only one species growing under certain conditions.

NOTES
See: Introduction to bibliography for general history and background information; Cormack (1856) 27, "called by the Indians beaver root"; MCG (1993) 2, Micmac usage.

Representative MUNFLA references: 68-10/8 (eyes), 69-007F (poppy heads, head-ache and sinus trouble).

Personal communication: P.J. Scott (1990), for statement that Ontario water-lily rhizomes were made into a soup and taken for asthma.

BED SORES

Bed sores (pressure sores) are often an intractable problem especially for elderly invalids who must spend considerable time in bed. Nursing care, even by professional nurses, can be difficult, and it is unlikely that New-foundland suggestions to apply "cornstarch" or "flour" accomplished much in severe cases, though clearly such items were intended to dry the sores. Another Newfoundland record – to keep a pan of salt (sea) water under a patient's bed – may be an incomplete recollection.

References to astringent herbal washes for the sores, considered to have a protective if not a healing action, are not found in the recent Newfound-land oral record, in contrast to records elsewhere. This seems to be further evidence of the limited use of plants on the island.

Modern nursing practices to prevent sores embrace far more than appli-cations; they range from regular "turning" of a patient and the employment of special beds and mattresses to the use of specialized dressings.

NOTES
See: Bader (1990), for background; Creighton (1968) 196, for an example of an astringent application of white oak (red oak grows in Newfoundland, but is not common).

Representative MUNFLA reference: 76-249 (flour or cornstarch).

## BEDWETTING

Most older children who suffer from bedwetting "grow out" of the problem by the age of ten, by which time only 5 per cent of those who were bedwetting when they started school (or inappropriately urinating in other situations) still have the problem. Only 1 to 2 per cent of adolescents continue to have difficulties. Such considerations perhaps explain why many remedies tried in the past – within the frameworks of both professional and home medicine – achieved at least some positive reputation.

The history of bedwetting is littered by discarded suggestions, many having been pushed to one side when psychological treatments became more popular during this century. Most folklore collections commonly mention diuretics (or "kidney medicines"), but none have been found in the Newfoundland record. Aside from an infusion of ox-eye daisies (generally known as a tonic or insecticide, but not as a diuretic), only animal remedies are listed in the Newfoundland record: the eating of "rat soup" (catch, kill and skin rat; boil rat in water; and give water to child), "mice soup," or snails for breakfast. Specific directions for the latter regimen involve, as so often with self-care, active patient involvement, which might contribute to a positive outcome. The bedwetter, for instance, had to collect snails each evening for someone to fry for breakfast next morning. This was to be continued indefinitely until a cure was achieved.

At present, the problem of bedwetting is invariably dealt with by a physician and other medical services, but there is anecdotal evidence that, "in desperation," folk practices are tried as well.

NOTES
See: Introductory note to bibliography for general history and information; Brown collection (Hand 1961, vol. 6) 47, for mouse and rat treatment.

Representative MUNFLA references: 68-23/1 (mice soup), 68-24/2 (mice soup), 70-26Ms (rat soup).

## BEECHAM'S PILLS

One of the most persistently advertised commercial medicines in Newfoundland, as in many places, was Beecham's Pills. Readers of the St. John's *Evening Telegram* were told a number of times that the pills were the "most famous home medicine in the world." Another advertising byline, "Worth a Guinea a Box," became even better known, as the pills were said (for example, in 1920) to maintain normal activity of stomach, bowels, liver, skin, and kidney.

Containing soap, ginger, and aloes, Beecham's pills aroused professional medical disquiet in the early twentieth century. Critics such as the editor of Health News in *Exposures of Quackery* (London, c. 1910) protested against the advertising claims and lack of novelty, saying that the

**When You Feel Played Out**

There comes a time when your grip on things weakens. Your nerves are unstrung, the vital forces low, the stomach is weak and the blood impoverished.   You feel old age creeping over you.   Be careful of yourself.   Take

**BEECHAM'S PILLS**

at once; there, is need to renew the life forces.   Weak nerves, wearied brains, sick stomach, feeble blood, torpid liver, sluggish bowels—all feel the quickening effects of Beecham's Pills.  Their use makes all the difference.  The tonic action of these pills upon the vital organs is immediate, thorough and lasting.  They are Nature's own remedy

**For Run-down Conditions**

Prepared only by Thomas Beecham, St. Helens, Lancashire, England. Sold by all Druggists in Canada and U. S. America.  In boxes 35 cents.

Advertisement for Beecham's Pills from the *Daily News* (St. John's), 1920.

active ingredient – the laxative aloes – was present in many other proprietary medicines. Newfoundlanders were also treated to much hyperbolic advertising: "When your brain works like a dog with three legs walks, you need Beecham's Pills. An active brain must have pure blood, not poisoned with products of indigestion – or liver and kidney laziness" (1920). Only slightly less graphic is another 1920s advertisement reproduced below. Notwithstanding, the laxative action has helped to sustain the usage of Beecham's Pills until the present.

NOTES
See Francis (1968), for background.


BERIBERI


In 1914, Dr. John Little wrote about a case of beriberi as follows: "During winter [the patient] lived on dry bread & tea without milk or butter. Had an occasional meal of peas, no beans or potatoes or any other vegetables, no meat. Beginning April 1st felt slight numbness and weakness in legs, later calves of legs swelled and had some pains, symptoms gradually increased until this entrance to Hospital." [in St. Anthony 19 June 1914]

Beriberi – caused by a deficiency of vitamin $B_1$ (thiamin) – was especially significant in drawing attention to nutrition problems in Newfoundland during the early twentieth century; aside from being potentially fatal, the condition was for some time viewed as an Asian problem, certainly not one to be found in North America. Indeed, the disease became very much part of Newfoundland lore. In 1958, Newfoundland's Deputy Minister of Health indicated that in the 1930s beriberi "was rampant." In fact, it is difficult to assess the precise incidence of the disease during the first half of the twentieth century and "rampant" may have been an exaggeration to emphasize, for whatever reason, the progress in public health. Even so, no doubt exists that the shadow of beriberi shaped many health considerations in Newfoundland and became a key plank behind efforts at nutrition reform during the first four decades of the twentieth century.

The issue of nutrition and the general health of Newfoundlanders was raised in Part I. By 1912, physician J.M. Little was linking beriberi with overreliance on white flour; he also indicated that poor diet in general was a problem: "There are many who are well satisfied if they have enough flour, tea, [and] molasses to see them through the winter." Little's comment was but one to imply that Newfoundlanders did not recognize the unhealthiness of an unvaried diet. In 1936, the statement was made that the "relation between beriberi and lack of vegetables and greens seems never to have been appreciated" in Newfoundland, although that ignored much public awareness of the nutritional value of garden food.

But perhaps the basic issue behind the incidence of beriberi was not so much reliance on white flour, or generally bad nutrition, or even "poverty" as emphasized by W. Aykroyd in 1930, but the consequence of lifestyles created by living on fishing boats, as well as by the profound economic difficulties associated with the structure of a Newfoundland outport society based on a merchant-fisherman credit system. All this led beriberi to persist until at least the 1940s, when fortified foods contributed to changing circumstances. In 1944, flour reaching Newfoundland was enriched with thiamine, nicotinic acid, riboflavin, and iron.

General symptoms of beriberi include loss of appetite, lassitude, digestive irregularities, and numbness in the limbs and extremities. Few recommendations for treatment, even of symptoms, are found in the recently recorded Newfoundland oral record – only juniper (q.v.) and wormwood (q.v.). Although neither of these is regarded as a source of thiamin, both were known as tonics. They may have resembled somewhat the "beriberi tonic" provided to patients, such as the one administered by Grenfell physicians, referred to at the beginning of this entry. Other aspects of the hospital treatment included a beriberi diet and electricity and massage to the legs.

It is not known how many Newfoundlanders took heed of nutritional advice, including the value of eating brown flour – which unfortunately acquired the stigma of dole flour. The lack of home remedies in the oral record may reflect the treatment of each symptom as a separate entity, as well as fading memories of a condition no longer extant. Certainly, with such protean symptoms, there is every reason to believe that tonics and blood purifiers other than those noted above were used. No evidence, however, has been found that Newfoundlanders viewed Dr. Chase's Nerve Food as treatment or prevention, even though it was noted to contain vitamin $B_1$.

NOTES
See: R. Knowling for background on lifestyles and Grenfell beriberi tonic. Little (1912); Parsons (1936); Miller (1958).

Representative MUNFLA references: 82-122 (wormwood, juniper).

Personal communications: R. Knowling (1992), for background on lifestyles and Grenfell beriberi tonic; M. Reddy and Grenfell Regional Hospital Service (1993), for hospital record; J. Overton (1990), for brown flour and access to his work on nutrition.

## BIRCH

Birch is almost entirely absent from the recent oral record, despite Philip Tocque's accolade in his *Newfoundland: As it was, and as it is in 1877* (1878). The birch tree, "clothed with its silvery drapery [and] the queen of the Newfoundland forest," had, he noted, a very sweet smell said to be very beneficial in disorders of the lungs. Tocque was undoubtedly referring to *Betula papyrifera* – one of a number of birches in the island – known among Newfoundlanders as "silver birch" or "canoe birch," but commonly called paper birch elsewhere. For yellow birch (*B. lutea*) see *witchhazel*.

Birches have had a minor place in medicine, and textbook accounts have largely focused on the common European birch (*Betula alba*) and the sweet birch (*B. lenta*). It is the latter (which does not grow in Newfoundland) that is especially well known for its aromatic properties and as a source of substitute oil of wintergreen. Other birches are much less aromatic, but the odour of *B. papyrifera* is probably sufficient to account for its reputation vis-à-vis lung disorders. Possibly the aromatic property is also linked to the suggestion that birch be used for frostbite (q.v.), although perhaps the outer layer of the bark (the "vellum") was intended merely as a covering for the damaged area, as was the case in its use for treating burns (q.v.). One Newfoundland record mentions a "famous birch bark medicine" as "mother's cure-all," but this was not a general view.

Because birches have attracted little interest within the regular medical profession, it is difficult to say whether reports that European birch possesses diuretic action relate to a recent Newfoundland record that birch bark can be used for treating obesity (but see comment under *obesity*).

Despite limited medical interest in birch in the past, Newfoundlanders can now (1991) purchase capsules of "Betula alba" by mail order. The promotion of these for a range of conditions, from atherosclerosis to hypercholesterolemia, may be based on its weak reputation as a diuretic, and its even more uncertain claims for stimulant, sweat-producing, and blood-purifying actions. Firm clinical evidence for the claim is totally lacking.

NOTES
See: Introduction to bibliography for general history and information; Tocque (1878) 499, frostbite; Grenfell (1932) 231, for a sense of the general economic importance of birch.

Representative MUNFLA references: 68-26/18 (obesity), 73-51 (mother's cure-all; since it was noted to be bitter, it probably contained other ingredients), 84-296B (burns).

## BIRTHMARKS, MOLES, AGE-SPOTS

The belief that birthmarks can result from a mother's behaviour during pregnancy has been widespread (see also *midwifery* entry.) Treatment recommendations – hardly effective (although some marks fade naturally) – are comparatively limited compared with the many suggested causes. As elsewhere, Newfoundlanders considered a craving for a variety of foods a common culprit: "My sister told me this experience she had when she was pregnant with one of her children. She saw a little boy passing along her window; at the time she noticed he had raspberries and longed to have some. This longing for the raspberries caused a birthmark to be on the child's arm and to prove that was the berries, the mark was shaped like a raspberry." Additionally, if one was upset (for example, by the sight of the blood of a seal), the birthmark was said perhaps to be that of a seal's paw; some felt this mark could also result from desiring seal meat.

Infants with birthmarks might be given food wrapped in cloth to suck on, or some juice from the food. Another Newfoundland reference – rubbing a mark with a piece of afterbirth – echoed that found among the various recommendations of many cultures for removing birthmarks or moles. Nevertheless, in the words of one commenter: "In most cases the midwives admitted that a birthmark was something to be endured for life."

Yet another conspicuous treatment – because it is so foreign to today's world – was to rub the birthmark or mole with the hand of a dead person. The following description of an instance in 1972 is a reminder of the persistence of belief amid disbelief:

My son Joe was born on June 27, 1972 and as time passed the birthmark on this forehead increased in size and was very noticeable. It looked as if he had just falled and bruised his head. When he was nearly two years old I received a call from my mother ... who resides at Pool's Cove. An elderly lady ... had just died and she urged me to come and bring my son. For many years it was the belief of the people of that area that if a child who had a visible birthmark (especially on the face) were to touch a deceased member of the opposite sex (boy-woman, girl-man) that as the body decayed in the grave the birthmark would disappear. So accompanied by my aunt ... (incidently the deceased was her maternal grandmother) we went to the church, MacDermott Memorial United Church, where she laid the hand of the deceased on the forehead of my son and said the words, "in the name of the Father, Son and Holy Ghost, I believe." The birthmark faded with time just as others had in the past.

All this does not mean that professional medical attention was not sought. Wilfred Grenfell felt it noteworthy to record (1932) that "a man came to me once to cure what he firmly believed was a balsam on his baby's nose. The birthmark to him resembled that tree."

   It is no surprise that references have not been found in the oral record to removing age-spots; despite long-standing promotion of beauty products in Newfoundland newspapers, self-consciousness about age-spots probably only emerged during the 1950s, with the availability of preparations such as Esoterica (to "fade age spots.")

NOTES
See: Brown Collection (Hand 1961, vol. 6) 18–22, for many explanations of birthmarks; Grenfell (1932), 95; McNaughton (1989) 119–27, for discussion on birthmarks; Davis (1983b) 83, persistence of concern about birthmarks.

   Representative MUNFLA references: 67-10/59 (rub made on birthmark on hand of dead person), 68-007 (quotation about raspberry), 78-211 (seal mark treatment with placenta, failure of treatment.)

## BITTERS

Over-the-counter medicines known as "bitters," which became increasingly popular in the second half of the nineteenth century, were in reality bitter-tasting tonics (q.v.), commonly recommended (because of their bitterness) as appetite stimulants and whenever liver and bile problems were felt to be present (for example, liverishness q.v.). On the other hand, the high alcohol content – reduced in many cases to around 25 per cent in the early years of the twentieth century – was also a key ingredient. Such "medicines" acquired particular popularity during prohibition times in the United States (1919–33); some evidence exists

MARCH 7, 1930

## At One Time She Didn't Care Whether She Lived or Not

**Biliousness and Constipation Had Her Dragged Down to the Point Where Life Seemed Futile and Useless. Now She's Full of Pep and Enthusiasm**

Nothing will depress a woman more or make her age faster, than a clogged liver and sluggish bowels. The poisons re-absorbed into the system cause a gradual but sure break-down of health. In the train of liver trouble and constipation follow indigestion, headaches, dizzy spells, sallow skin and general listlessness.

**Make Your Liver and Bowels Young Again**

...and you will feel young again! The liver and bowels have everything to do with our general state of health. For ... on them depends the elimination of the poisons that accumulate in the body.

**Take Atwood's Jaundice Bitters**

We of this generation can do no better than take what our great-grand-

fathers took for the liver, stomach and bowels – namely, Atwood's Bitters. No remedy has been more thoroughly proven. Atwood's Jaundice Bitters is unique in that it acts on liver, upper bowel and lower bowel—*all three!* Thus it gives the system a complete cleansing, a thorough cleansing, clearing out the poisons that cause sour gassy stomach, nervousness, sleeplessness, headaches and backaches. A little regular use of this remarkable remedy means full and complete relief from stomach, liver and bowel complaints. It means new vigor and vitality too, for it is a tonic as well as a corrective. Let your own experience convince you.

At All Dealers in Newfoundland
**Gerald S. Doyle, Ltd.,**
Sole Agents

Atwood's Jaundice Bitters advertised in 1930 had the "bonus" of acting not only on the liver but also on the upper and lower bowel.

that this was the case during the Newfoundland liquor prohibition beginning in 1917, although concerns were not so intense as they were in the
United States, partly because of the ready availability of home brew and
smuggled liquor from St. Pierre, and also because alcohol could be obtained
(some say readily) with legal prescriptions from physicians. Some bitters, it
should be said – for example, the well-known Stafford's Mandrake Bitters
and Atwood's Jaundice Bitters (the latter sold with a yellow label) – apparently had a laxative effect, which hardly encouraged their use.

Recently, as part of a re-emergence of interest in herbal medicines,
Newfoundlanders have been offered bitters, albeit non-alcoholic. See under
*tonics*.

NOTES
See: Young (1961) 129–34, for general remarks on bitters; Andrieux (1983), for St.
Pierre.

Personal communication: D. Parsons (1992), regarding concern about bitters
during the Newfoundland prohibition.

BLADDER DISORDERS (SEE KIDNEY AILMENTS)

BLEEDING, BLOOD-LETTING

Aside from the once commonplace applications of myrrh and of substances
acting as styptics (see *cuts, minor wounds*), there are a few other applications
specifically for "bleeding" (generally for relatively minor bleeds) recorded
in the recent Newfoundland oral tradition: a piece of tobacco leaf from
chewing tobacco; the spittle (zap) resulting when tobacco is chewed; and
the Blessed Virgin's leaf "possessing a dark purple spot in the centre of the
leaf or the likeness of a thumbprint" (probably *Polygonum persicaria*).

One Newfoundland recollection of the application of flour to a serious
wound is noteworthy as yet another indication of the perceived lack of
professional sympathy with many elements of self-treatment. A youngster
fell on a "broken bottle and cut off an artery in his hand. To prevent his
bleeding to death his relatives began to pile flour onto his hand and kept
doing this until the plane arrived to take him to St. Anthony. The doctor
had a terrible mess of caked flour to remove before he could treat the
wound, and *was a little sore at the relatives even though the flour had saved
the boy's life*" (author's emphasis).

Folk-medicine records in many places describe charmers, sometimes
called "blood stoppers," who were known for stopping bleeding from
wounds, sores, and gums (including after tooth extraction). This special-
ization has been, and to a lesser extent still is, well known in Newfoundland.
A noteworthy number of reports come from the area of Twillingate, but it

may be that this is linked to a comparatively high incidence of haemophilia in the area. One wonders how many reports of profuse bleeding particularly with tooth extractions were linked to undiagnosed haemophilia: "I used to bleed a lot. It used to bleed right free and then it would clot, but it would clot and fill my mouth out you know. Then the nurse would have to take the clot out, then it would start bleeding free ... I tell you, I just remembered, when my gums were bleeding they went up the Bay and found a junk of ice, iceberg, and got ice and that's what they stopped it with."

Recollections about charmers who could stop bleeding suggest they followed diverse practices: magical, religious, or both. One commonly known procedure was to give the bleeding person (not just from the nose q.v.) a green ribbon. At times words – sometimes said to be prayers or biblical verses, but rarely intelligible to those present – were an essential part of the regimens.

Some charmers were noted to be effective at a distance. "I know what you want, you go on home and Nel will be all right." It is reported that Nel's bleeding stopped. The introduction of the telephone encouraged "telephone treatment" by at least some charmers. Sceptics say success with charming reflects the natural process of haemostasis at work. (See also *charmers, nosebleeds.*)

Part of the story of bleeding involves deliberate letting of blood for treating various conditions, although this had virtually disappeared by 1900. Nevertheless, the benefits of losing blood and "impurities" in the blood remained known to Newfoundlanders (see *tonics.*)

NOTES
See: Creighton (1968) 196, for a "Newfoundland charm" for stopping blood: "The blessed Lord Jesus Christ who was baptized in the River Jordan for us and rose again and commandeth the blood to cease" (Biblical verses are known elsewhere, as well); MCG (1992) 108, for story "I used to bleed a lot."

Representative MUNFLA references: 66-2/77 (charming and tobacco leaf), 66-6/71 (Blessed Virgin's leaf), 67-5/79 (story of Nel), 69-23/33 (flour on serious wound quotation), 76-249 (charmer and green ribbon), 82-215 (charmer).

Personal communication: Troake, (1989), about Twillingate.

## BLOOD, BLOOD PURIFIERS, CLEANSING THE BLOOD, BLOOD POISONING

The role of blood in concepts of health and disease has a long and diverse history. Although centuries-old doctrines of humoralism and vitalism – arguing that blood was a seat of the living qualities, the life-force, of men and women – disappeared almost completely from professional medicine during the nineteenth century, legacies persisted in popular culture. Nevertheless, drinking or applying blood is not commonly reported in twentieth-century North America. It is noted in Newfoundland, as elsewhere, for treating shingles, and it was also rubbed on areas of thrush (q.v.) in the mouth. The application of blood from a black cat was noted in 1899 as a cure for a sty.

Notions of "thick blood," "too much blood," "too little blood," "dirty blood," and "bad blood" have been commonplace and still exist. Home treatment of presumed blood conditions from, say, 1900 to 1950 commonly included tonics (q.v.) and iron, laxatives (q.v.), blood purifiers, diet, and sundry other approaches. Nowadays, doctors are consulted more and more for chronic conditions believed to be associated with the blood, but a renewed interest in tonics and blood purifiers is noted below.

Many so-called blood purifiers recorded in Newfoundland are discussed under specific entries (*alder, burdock, dogberry, elderflower, sarsaparilla, sulphur and molasses*). Of these, sulphur and molasses was possibly the most popular in Newfoundland. The majority of purifiers were bitter or astringent, but certain laxatives, notably senna (made into a tea), were also viewed as possessing cleansing and blood-purifying properties. Many tonics (q.v.) were synonymous with blood purifiers, but the latter were also viewed as a separate category.

Numerous over-the-counter preparations competed with blood purifiers prepared in the home. One, occasionally advertised (for example, in 1920), partly as a blood purifier, was "Dr. Wilson's Herbine," a bitter tonic containing "dandelion," "mandrake," and "burdock." (See also *tonics*).

One factor in the early twentieth century that added to the already long-standing popularity of blood purifiers was the concept of autointoxication, noted in Part I. This was a time when innumerable advertisements for diverse medicines played on the theme of impurities and poisons. Tiz, for instance, was said in one 1915 Newfoundland newspaper to be "the only remedy in the world that draws out all the poisonous exudations which puff up the feet and cause tender, sore, tired, aching feet."

After World War II, however, when the concept of purifiers was fading even from the popular mind, talk of "blood poisoning," albeit not new, kept notions about purification alive. For instance, Newfoundlanders were warned in a 1950 advertisement for Olympene, the Antiseptic Liniment, to "Beware of blood poisoning! The tiniest cut or bruise can be dangerous." At least one Newfoundlander, however, successfully used a soft-bread poultice to deal with a case of "blood poisoning;" this was viewed as a triumph for the claim was that a physician had said regular treatment was "too late" and that amputation of the limb was necessary.

There was continuing worry about red streaks going up the arm or leg. One Newfoundland suggestion to prevent this involved drawing a circle just above the red streak; another idea was to paint iodine above the infected place and along the streak, or around the reddened area. Here the use of iodine, well-known for its antiseptic properties (and a popular remedy in Newfoundland), may well have been reinforced by the magical notion of "ringing" a disease, as implied in the previous suggestion. Self-care, when combining two (or more) concepts or approaches, reflects the widely accepted view that two treatments are better than one.

Concerns about red streaks are still to be found, as are worries about toxins in the blood. In fact, much current popular health promotion is again focusing attention on the need for blood purification and body cleansing in general. Nowadays "toxins" or "poisons" worry many lay people, and the consequent use of laxatives and colonic washouts are often unwisely promoted. After many years of lying relatively fallow, such notions as tired blood are again shaping self-care; and evidence exists of returning interest in "old time" and new purifiers, sometimes for the treatment of such "new" conditions as arteriosclerosis. (See also *tonics*). As an elderly Newfoundlander said recently: "A lot of people used to drink this Wampoles and Brick's Tasteless cod liver oil to build them up after the winter. That was very popular. It's only recently I heard about Barley Green [a newly promoted (1991–92) commercial preparation]. I just heard that it was good to cleanse the blood. My daughter-in-law, she recommended it to me. So Eileen and I, we got a bottle, we took it between us. I didn't see any difference in myself. It was good I suppose, but you got to have faith in those things."

NOTES
See: Bergen (1899) 68, on black cat's blood, also application of heart of black cat to a wound to stop bleeding (see also *animal parts*); Davis (1983b) 133–6, for general comments on too much blood, too little blood; Hand (1980) 188, on blood; MCG (1992) 109, for Barley Green story.

Representative MUNFLA references: 63-1/9 (ring of ink above poisoning), 69-25/5 (soft bread poultice), 69-25/13 (painting ring of iodine), 78-200 (notes on many plants – cherry bark, ground juniper, tansy, blackberry herb, black spruce – as items to clean blood), 79-249 (circle above red streak).

BLOODROOT

Newfoundlanders use the common name "bloodroot" for *Geum macrophyllum*, whereas elsewhere in North America and in the medical literature the name is generally employed for *Sanguinaria canadensis*, a medicinal plant well known primarily as a stimulant and expectorant. *G. rivale* (purple avens, water avens, chocolate root), which grows in Newfoundland, has (unlike *G. macrophyllum*) attracted professional and lay medical interest as an astringent and bitter tonic in the past, although not, as is the case with many herbs, in Newfoundland. No mention has been found in the recently recorded tradition; William Cormack, however, in describing his epic 1822 journey across Newfoundland did report a "strong" Micmac decoction of "Geum vivale [sic *G. rivale*] or chocolate root" for "dysentery, colds and coughs, particularly for children."

Unfortunately, the Newfoundland record offers no clues as to whether the popular name "bloodroot" for *G. macrophyllum* (somewhat different in appearance from *G. rivale*) reflects the view of bitter root – which is not reddish – as a *blood* purifier, or whether there is an analogy to other red roots (for example, of *Potentilla tormentilla* as has been suggested) or even *Sanguinaria canadensis*, although these do not grow in Newfoundland.

NOTES
See: Introduction to bibliography for general history and background information; Cormack (1856), 53; Scott (1987), for the resemblance to *P. tormentilla.*

### BLUEBERRY

The abundance of blueberries (*Vaccinium* spp.) on the island, supporting the traditional activity of berry picking, has spawned a host of Newfoundland recipes, including many for the long-popular blueberry wine. Yet no mention of specific medical usages has been found in the local oral tradition or printed record. This is surprising since elsewhere (in New England, for instance) a medicinal reputation has long existed – seemingly justified on the basis of the astringency of the leaves and roots – as to its ability to control diabetes. Considerable interest followed a 1927 scientific study of blueberry-leaf extract that showed a blood-sugar-lowering action. The study, initiated by reports that blueberry-leaf tea was used for "diabetes among the Alpine peasantry" in Europe, was followed by information that blueberry-leaf tea had some repute as a diabetic remedy in certain rural regions of the United States. This information persists as popular culture and is seemingly well known.

Constituents said to possess hypoglycaemic action have been isolated from *Vaccinium* species, but whether these are present in all species is unclear, as is their clinical significance. Whether the species found in Newfoundland (most commonly *V. angustifolium*) possesses hypoglycaemic activity obviously deserves study.

NOTES
See: Introduction to bibliography for general history and information on the blueberry.

### BOGBEAN (BUCKBEAN)

Bogbean (*Menyanthes trifoliata,* sometimes popularly known in Newfoundland as "beaver-root" [q.v.], but elsewhere as "buckbean") is rarely noted in the Newfoundland oral tradition, although references exist to a decoction of the root being employed as a tonic as well as in treatment of kidney ailments, tuberculosis (and perhaps colds), and worms.

Because the plant is fairly common in Newfoundland and because of professional and lay medical interest in the nineteenth century, one might expect more references than are found in the oral record. The bitterness of the plant accounted for its reputation as a tonic; cathartic (strong laxative) action has also been reported, which may be linked to the suggestion that bogbean be used for worms. The leaves, too, were regarded by some as valuable for intermittent fever, rheumatic and scrofulous diseases, and various skin ailments. However, evidence for the clinical value of these claims, some of which persist among herbalists today, is weak, and it may be that they have arisen from theorizing about reported pharmacological properties.

NOTES
See: Introduction to bibliography for history and general background; MCG (1993) 2, for kidney ailments.

Representative MUNFLA references: 73-19/13 (bobean, apparently bogbean, for colds).

Personal communication: Delberth Smith (1989), for tonic and tuberculosis.

## BORIC ACID, BORAX WATER

Boric acid (also known as boracic acid or boracic powder) has been recommended in Newfoundland and elsewhere for skin conditions, eye infections (q.v.), and snow-blindness (q.v.).

Until recently, boric acid was a frequent recommendation within the framework of professional medicine, particularly as an "antiseptic" dusting power for various wounds, and as a lotion for the eyes and skin. Apart from its employment in treating snow-blindness, its Newfoundland uses are in line with recommendations elsewhere. Professional medical usage of boric acid (and borax, noted below), considered to have feeble antibacterial and antifungal properties, has declined with the realization that, because it is excreted slowly, repeated doses (whether applied externally or taken internally) have a cumulative effect and may be toxic. Particular concern emerged over boric acid in dusting powders for infants.

Borax (a sodium salt of the acid) has been employed in solution for purposes similar to those of boric acid. Its astringency, however, has contributed to its greater popularity as an aid to gargling and in lozenges for sore throats. The recorded Newfoundland reputation of using borax water to treat sties mirrors past, but not present, professional recommendations.

NOTES
Representative MUNFLA references: 63-1/2 (rash with vaseline), 78-205 (borax water for sty; snow-blindness), 82-149 (eye infection).

## BRONCHITIS

Probably all the Newfoundland recommendations for asthma (q.v.) and for colds and cough (q.v.) were tried for "bronchitis." Although the lay diagnosis of this condition is often less precise than that of doctors, the symptoms of painful cough and wheeziness (associated with inflammation of the mucous membrane of the bronchial tubes) suggest bronchitis to all. It is imposible to say whether the condition was exacerbated in Newfoundland by the universal use of wood stoves, but it is likely.

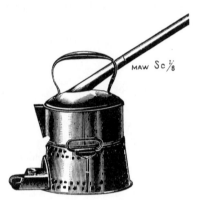

Missing from the Newfoundland recommendations is the advice recorded in home-medicine books – and still offered by doctors – namely, to use "bronchitis" or "steam" kettles (or just steam from an open pan of water) to humidify the air and hence help remove thick catarrh. Although special kettles can no longer be readily purchased, humidification – along with inhalation – is still encouraged. Moreover, such recommendations still occur despite a 1990 double-blind study on treating colds

Late nineteenth-century bronchitis kettle.

that noted "no beneficial effects of steam inhalation on common cold symptoms." The conclusion, in contrast to similar studies in an Israeli population, was based on measurement of nasal resistance, not patient comfort.

For many years, most over-the-counter cough and cold medicines, like catarrhozone (see under *colds*) advertised to Newfoundlanders since the late nineteenth century, have included bronchitis in their list of chest conditions: "colds, cold on chest, asthma and bronchitis, catarrh and deafness." More specifically for bronchitis, Buckley's Bronchitis Mixture became (and remains) a household name.

Nowadays, sufferers from bronchitis usually rely on professional medical advice, although self-care (inhalation, expectorants, and other aids) still play an essential role.

NOTES
See: Macknin et al. (1990), on steam treatment for colds.

Representative MUNFLA references: 76-249 (goose grease), 78-200 (goose grease with red flannel for "wiezed up"), 78-205 (oatmeal and onion poultice), 82-122 (cutout heart of oatmeal paper), 82-218 (kerosene and molasses, Minard's Liniment and molasses, Friar's balsam and sugar).

## BROWN PAPER

Nowadays, a sense of disbelief commonly greets references to the employ-ment of brown paper in folk medicine. In many ways, however, it served as a valuable emergency (or temporary) cover for cuts, perhaps because it was attached to the skin by softened candle wax. Brown paper was also a convenient backing for plasters, both those from home care and those prescribed by doctors.

The use of the paper – soaked in vinegar and applied to the forehead – to relieve headaches (q.v.) has been as well known in Newfoundland as elsewhere. Placing the paper inside the lip for nose bleeds (q.v.) was a common suggestion as well, as was its application to the stomach for seasickness (q.v.).

NOTES
See: Brown Collection (Hand 1961), for various references comparable to New-foundland uses (for example, vinegar and brown paper).

Representative MUNFLA references: 82-218 (nosebleed), 82-238 (headaches) 78-205 (cuts).

## BURDOCK

Burdock has been discussed frequently in domestic medicine books as a blood purifier (q.v.). Perhaps surprisingly, therefore, it was not found in the local oral record, not even for treating the ubiquitous "dirty blood." Burdock was a listed ingredient in a number of the over-the-counter medicines avail-able on the island. Admittedly, the species that has attracted most medical interest, *Arctium lappa*, does not grow in Newfoundland, but the medical reputation of the available lesser burdock, *Arctium minus*, is comparable.

Uncertainty can exist over the botanical identification of burdock, as listed in the oral, or even the printed, record. One Newfoundland reference – to the use of "dock" or "burdock" (steeped and taken as a cure for boils) – is identified by the informant as *Heracleum maximum* (see *wild-parsnip*).

NOTES
See: Introduction to bibliography for introduction and background information; Murray (1979) 132, for dock as wild parsnip, and commercial medicines, including Dandelion and Burdock Bitters.

## BURNS AND SCALDS

A wide range of applications to cover both burns (from dry heat) and scalds (from wet heat) have been suggested in Newfoundland, mostly in line with past recommendations accepted by the medical profession and as much to provide relief as to heal. Those of a greasy or emollient nature include olive oil (also called "sweet oil") perhaps mixed with lime water, butter, cod liver oil, kerosene, vaseline, and soap. Some of the latter were applied alone, but the butter might be churned with cream and mixed with "fine table salt."

In contrast, the "drying" or "cooling" items employed are flour (sometimes "scorched"), baking soda (q.v., in a solution or paste), burned or scorched rags, cold water, white of egg, lime water, milk, and "myrrh and birch rind." Carnation milk, long popular and to hand in Newfoundland, could be included in either category, as could the application of a cabbage leaf softened with boiling water.

The combination of myrrh and birch bark (or "vellum," see *birch*) was considered as a "drying" agent, although it is noteworthy that other commonplace, astringent medicinal plants recommended elsewhere for burns (for example, plantain) have not been found in the Newfoundland record. Mention exists, however, of applications of boiled willow bark and boiled alder roots, both of which provide some astringency. Another Newfoundland suggestion – to cover the burn with any mid-summer flower – is likely to have been viewed as a cooling agent.

Salves, too, are rarely mentioned – another indication that home-made salves have not been as popular as in many places off the island.

Of course, commercial products were available. Astringent preparations of tannic acid were sold, but one wonders whether in Newfoundland, Mecca Ointment, "the household ointment" – already noted for the treatment of boils and promoted for burns – was better known. Druggists made their own over-the-counter preparations as well. A popular one – widely considered to be effective and said to have been found in most Newfoundland homes and in "doctors' boxes" used on fishing and sealing vessels – was Carron oil or lime liniment. It was prepared by shaking together equal parts of lime water and linseed oil.

Overall, Newfoundland burn applications offer nothing unexpected; even applying cod liver oil reflects the ready availability of this well-known product.

Whether a greasy or a so-called drying application was chosen often depended on personal preference and convenience. Home-medicine books and other sources were not consistent in their advice. Medical author G. Black (1927) noted that the "popular idea that every burn or scald should be treated with oil is wrong," though he was concerned more with serious burns or scalds. Even so, for mild cases, "boracic ointment" (a commercial preparation) was suggested.

Additionally, magical approaches to treating burns in Newfoundland existed, although there appears to be little record that charmers (q.v.) blew or talked the fire out of burns as was the case in many other places.

Newfoundlanders, however, did have ways to "transfer" a burn. For instance, if the burn was not too serious, it was held as close as possible to a hot stove. This, it was said, drew out the heat from the burn and lessened the pain. There is some anecdotal evidence that such magical approaches were often combined with an application to the burn. Some commentators, ignoring the possible value of faith in a remedy, suggest that the latter was the only effective component of the regimen.

Although the long-standing approach of cooling is rarely noted in the Newfoundland oral tradition, it was likely well known. Nowadays, cooling under cold running water is viewed as the most effective way of relieving pain for minor burns and scalds. A sterile dressing is also recommended, without any other greasy or local application. On the other hand, current, commercial promotion of burn applications is intense, especially preparations of aloes. Although some of these may be useful, the direct application of aloe gel from a broken aloe leaf may be the most beneficial. It is worth noting that various plant mucilages have long been advocated for burns; it is perhaps surprising, then, that no Newfoundland reference has been found to the use of linseed mucilage, since it was readily available.

NOTES
See: Black (1927) 113; Mercer (1991), for willow and alder, the latter made into a salve; Morton (1990), for mucilages.

Representative MUNFLA references: 66-14/74 (butter), 68-21/21 (baking soda), 68-26/6 (white of egg), 69-25/10 (kerosene), 76-62/63 (cold water), 82-158 (baking soda, lime water, olive oil).

CAMPHORATED OIL
AND CAMPHOR

Camphorated oil (sometimes mixed with butter) has been used in Newfoundland for both rubbing on the chest and – frequently at the same time – imbibing in the case of colds. It has also been employed internally (or as an external application to the front of the neck) to ease sore throats, and as a favoured "rub" for rheumatism.

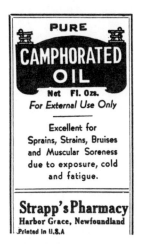

Label for camphorated oil

It is unclear whether most Newfoundlanders generally made camphorated oil in the kitchen or purchased it, though the latter is probably the case. (A common formula was one part camphor to four parts oil).

Camphor – obtained from the wood of *Cinnamomum camphora* by distillation with water – has long attracted usage, both within and outside professional medicine, because of its reputed stimulant, antispasmodic, rubefacient, and analgesic actions; some of these have been linked to effects on the nervous system when camphor is taken internally. Much professional medical interest was sustained by the widely accepted theory that camphor acted as a counterirritant that lessened, by postulated reflex-action, both congestion and inflammation. Camphor has been employed in many conditions aside from colds and rheumatism. Numerous Newfoundlanders best know camphor as an ingredient in Minard's Liniment (q.v.).

NOTES
Representative MUNFLA references: 82-218 (chest cold, earache, sore throat).

### CANCER, CANKER

The fact that cancer was rarely noted in the Newfoundland record of home care is in line with recent comments (1992) among elderly Newfoundlanders that they do not remember hearing much about cancer until the recent decades. Much of this is due to increased publicity, for there is no reason to suppose that the Newfoundland incidence of cancer in the past was any lower than elsewhere. Indeed, some forms such as lip cancer have probably always had a relatively high incidence, as is the case today. One anecdotal account (published 1935) merits quotation, if only to provide a sense of the living conditions sometimes found as well as the heroic stories that are part of the Newfoundland tradition:

They greeted the doctor with cries of 'God bless you, Sir!' and as he unpacked his instruments he was aware of the feeling of honest hospitality which existed even in this small, dirty cabin. After listening to the tale of woe from the old lady he proceeded to unfasten a filthy rag which has been wrapped around her lip. Without any kind of anaesthetic he then began to cut a cancerous growth from the lower lip, which the husband assisted with a dirty thumb and finger. The old lady bore the operation without making a sound, and afterwards busied herself with preparing a steaming cup of tea for the doctor.

A variety of skin cancers and other visible tumours were obviously recognized, for some reached horrendous proportions before eliciting medical intervention. Surgeon John Little, writing from St. Anthony to his parents 14 June 1908, commented on one such large tumour of the face: "I took out the upper jaw and cheek on one side and dissected the whole neck." The warning to be careful of moles because of the belief that an injury to them could lead to cancer can be found in the Newfoundland record, as elsewhere.

Although other widespread ideas (for example, treatment by touching a tumour or swelling with a dead person's hand) have not been found recorded in Newfoundland, they were likely known. (See *birthmarks* for another use of touch from a dead hand). It should be remembered that a principal difficulty of reviewing cancer self-care lies in knowing the correct diagnosis. "Cancer" and "canker" (the latter strictly an aphthous ulcer in the mouth) have been used indiscriminately, although the former can refer to a painful, infected sore. One Newfoundland suggestion for a canker (probably not a cancer) was to take the blood from a rooster's comb, smear it on a rag, and then rub this on the canker. Another recommendation, apparently for a small ulcer on the tongue, was to dip the tongue in molasses. Applying ice, still a known treatment, is also mentioned.

Charmers were certainly consulted on occasions in Newfoundland, sometimes when "growths" were suspected even if not diagnosed by a physician, for the realization that cancer can be "hidden" is long-standing. One regimen, of more than passing interest, suggests animalcules as a cause. The story goes that a certain woman had cancer in her hand and thought she would have to have it amputated. But a woman from Long's Hill in St. John's, recognized for her cures, suggested that a woollen cuff be placed on the hand for fifteen minutes. After that time "the lady took off the cuff and the cuff was full of maggots." The patient was "cured." Aside from reflecting an idea, found elsewhere, that cancer is linked with some form of "beast" or "something" eating away inside, this maggot story is a reminder of the many "blast" stories found in Newfoundland and else-where. These are tales of fairies who by "shooting" at a person produce sores in which hair, stones, sticks, and other bizarre items are found. Speculation (without any firm evidence) as to natural explanations for these stories includes rare tumours known as teratomas (containing tissues for-eign to the site) and infections, say, of the bone. But perhaps more significant is that both the blast stories and the maggot story – responding as they do to widespread social fears of outside agents, illness, and animals – may help some people cope with troubles and fears inasmuch as they find explanations comfortable to them. As well, the stories illustrate a concern with drawing out a cancer (rather than having it cut out, which might leave "roots"), as was done for Newfoundlanders by certain lay cancer "doctors."

The Newfoundland silence on cancer probably resulted from various factors – all of which need study – such as embarrassment (for example, of breast cancer). It should be noted that only in the 1950s did media attention to real and hoped-for breakthroughs from medical science – part of public awareness of the new research explosion – become conspicuous in the Newfoundland press. Almost certainly it encouraged fear. Previously, aside from such breakthroughs as the use of radium, developments in treating cancer often reflected the wishful claims of entrepreneurs promoting a new remedy.

Cancer causes considerable fear and worry nowadays, and one consequence of health-education programs in recent years, as well as more readily available medical services, is that worries are brought into professional care at an earlier stage than in the past. However, this does not mean that many Newfoundlanders do not hold a range of ideas and beliefs about cancer that shape the way they cope; as elsewhere, some express interest in alternative treatment approaches – sometimes sanctioned by professional medicine, sometimes not. Among the many alternative practices attracting attention are offers to restore "balance" and "equilibrium." Despite the current emphasis on new developments and understandings of cancer – Newfoundland is now developing its first building devoted to cancer – the cultural resonances from the past must be continually considered as part of patient care.

NOTES
See: Fitz-Gerald (1935) 75–6, for lip growth surgery (also relevant comments on 164, 170); Little, J.M. papers, for face cancer story; Spitzer et al. (1975), on lip cancer; Hand (1980) 73, on dead man's hand; Couzens (1993) 103, on ice; Bennett (1989) 137–41, on lay cancer doctors; Cassileth et al. (1984, 1991), for introduction to scope of alternative treatments and issues; Patterson, J.T. (1987), for general background to cancer beliefs and attitudes, p. 31 for concept of cancer as a living beast; Rieti (1991a), for blast stories; Arrindell et al. (1991), for range of social fears; CMG (1992), for various references to silence in the past.

Representative MUNFLA references: 67-12/38 (injury to moles), 69-7/2 (blood from rooster's comb), 72/64 (cuff and maggots).

## CAR SICKNESS

So-called traditional self-care, as is evident from many Newfoundland records, is far from static – both for old and "new" conditions. An example of the latter is the extension of the use of blood purifiers to "arteriosclerosis"; another is the management of car sickness. Such suggestions as suspending a bag of salt around the neck and sitting on newspapers or magazines (which, according to one informant "does not work") are apparently analogies to long-standing practices for seasickness. Sitting on the earth is described in the entry on *seasickness*, with carrying amulets considered not uncommon. Promoters of commercial seasickness remedies have extended their products to car (and train) sickness.

The usual recommendation, common everywhere, of suspending a chain from the bumper so that it touches the ground is noted many times in the Newfoundland record.

Current treatments are the same as noted under seasickness.

NOTES
Representative MUNFLA references: 68-10/16 (sit on newspapers), 69-16/5 (bumper chain), 69-22/2A (bag of salt around neck).

## CHAPPED OR CHAFED SKIN

Roughened and cracked skin, sometimes split open because of exposure to the cold and wet, is an obvious occupational hazard of the fishery and logging business. "Sprayed" hands (dry and sore hands) is a term still known today in Newfoundland. Peter Troake, Newfoundland captain of sealing and other boats, has commented: "Carbolic ointment was wonderful when you got bad hands ... We had lysol, too, it's cut-down carbolic and not so powerful. Now in the morning when you get up first, nearly always you had to go somewhere to make your water. Make the water on your hands, nothing no better than that." Urine, as noted elsewhere, was well known for skin problems.

Many other suggestions for applications to chapped and chafed skin can be found, ranging from using a mixture of Sunlight soap and nail polish to rubbing with oakum (q.v.). The latter, at least, is in keeping with professional medical opinion that coal-tar preparations are helpful in certain skin conditions. A number of commercial preparations, aside from the carbolic ointment noted above, were known such as Zam-Buk (see *antiseptic ointment*). All these provided at least some protective action.

NOTES
See: *Dictionary Newfoundland English* (1990), under sprayed; Troake (1989) 37.

Representative MUNFLA references: 69-22/7 (urine for sprayed hands), (cod liver oil for sprayed hands).

## CHARMERS

As noted in Part I, a spectrum of practitioners without professional training provided medical care in many communities. They included "charmers," who offered magical treatment, or what was perceived by some people as a form of faith healing, for a variety of conditions ranging from bleeding to warts. The role of faith on the part of the patient was widely appreciated, perhaps even encouraged, by some physicians who recommended to patients that they try charmers, at least for warts (see below).

The story of charmers is complex because of the considerable differences among them and their various modes of practice. If only because of the influence of different traditions and personal idiosyncrasies, the regimens of one practitioner rarely replicated those of another precisely. Many charmers acquired their so-called gift or endowment and authority in a traditionally accepted way; for example, in the European tradition a seventh son of a seventh son was viewed to have special healing powers, all the more so if born with a caul. (A seventh son [but not of another seventh son] might also have some, albeit lesser, power). Some charmers had authority bestowed upon them by a community, in much the same way elders of native peoples assume that position today; others just acquired it by happenstance or position in a community. Conspicuous in the New-foundland record are charmers with specialized skills to treat bleeding (q.v.), boils (q.v.), cancer (q.v.), toothache (q.v.), and warts (q.v.). Information on charmers with the ability to "blow out" or ease burns – a practice well known elsewhere – is not clearly documented.

How did these Newfoundland charmers see themselves, particularly com-pared to practitioners elsewhere who offered magic free or for sale. Throughout much of North America, the African influence is well known, at least when magical healing power is for hire. In Newfoundland, however, many practitioners have felt that their gift would be lost if payment was received, although it is acceptable through a third party.

Although most Newfoundland charmers had a gift for treating a single ailment, at least some offered help with a spectrum of conditions. Unfor-tunately, few details are known, including whether some charmers used empirical, as well as magical or religious, approaches, at least as part of their treatment. Indeed, a clergyman, recounting a recent case in his congregation, noted that his parishioner, who had had a sore leg and at length had applied to a man possessed of such powers, went through incantations only to be told to "apply some oatmeal and vinegar." Oatmeal and vinegar applications to sore legs were an acceptable part of regular medical treatment at the time.

Women charmers – several of whom are portrayed in the following quotation, probably outnumbered their male counterparts.

There was a lot of, I suppose you could call charmers. I have a sister-in-law, Hannah, people come from all over the shore. Doctors send people to her. She won't tell me what she does. A lady ... passed it on to her. She'd cure warts. There was one boy in particular came from Ferryland. If you want to see hands – they were ugly to look at. And he had gone to a doctor and doctors and doctors. They burnt them off and everything. His mother brought him down to Hannah and in two weeks they were gone.

There was another woman. I was probably eight or nine years old. So I went up to her and she told me to go and get a piece of sheep's wool or sheep's yarn, not washed, with the grease still in it. I went up and when she had finished she gave me it and she said, now you bury that and make sure anyone don't see you burying it. She didn't put the wool on the warts. For every wart she tied a knot on the sheep's wool. That's one of the processes but you're [the visitor] not to tell. And can't release where I buried that wool or what she did otherwise. They went in a week or a week and a half. I never had a wart since.

Now Hannah, she used to come here to Bay Bulls probably two weeks of the summer for her holidays and she'd come three or four times during the year maybe for a weekend. She was my mother's lifelong girlfriend. Every time she came to Bay Bulls there was always three or four people because they'd come and ask Mom, when is ... coming up again? And she'd tell her and friends she told she'd be here Sunday and three or four people come with warts.

Today, charmers have lost their health-care, as well as their social and community, roles.

NOTES
See: Patterson (1895), oatmeal and vinegar; MCG (1992) 011, women charmers and referral by physicians.
   Representative MUNFLA references: 72-249 (boils, warts), 76-249 (toothache), 77-87 (toothache), 82-164 (nosebleed).
   Personal communication: Troake (1990).

CHERRY, PIN, CHOKE (SEE WILD CHERRY)

CHILBLAINS AND COLD FEET

Because of their intractable nature, chilblains (sometimes called "scaldings" in Newfoundland) – those itchy, inflamed areas on the feet or hands (less often on the ears), associated with exposure to draughts and cold and, perhaps, inadequate food and clothing – have prompted many treatment suggestions. Newfoundland recommendations included running barefoot in snow or rubbing snow on the chilblain (probably a well-known practice), applying cold urine or vinegar, rubbing with Sunlight soap, and soaking in cold or salted water (including sea water).
   What many people see as a "common sense" approach – keeping the hands and feet warm, at least out of draughts – is not specifically mentioned. Perhaps, however, this was because many thought chilblains were caused by wearing tight shoes. In fact, some may actually have been sores from shoe trouble:

I'll tell you something now real. When I was in the orphanage, all the boys' boots were made in Harbour Grace; there was a shoe factory. And then up in your toe there was a ridge went along where the leather was joined and I got what they called "chilblains" around the joints of the toes.
   It got watery like a discharge from it, pus from chafing and rubbing. The matron, she'd go to take the bandage she had and she didn't have the patience when it stuck sometimes. It stuck somewhere and it was very painful. She'd tug on it and then your feet were right back to where they were.

Now I'll tell you the cure. When I came home my feet were terrible. Now they weren't pussy all over, but there was so many toes were discharging. I don't think mother has a roll of bandage in the house, but she took a nice clean piece of cotton and scorched it, not burned and put it on.

One treatment that recognized cold feet as a cause involved putting a brown paper bag on the foot under the sock. But chilblains are not only associated with circulatory inadequacies. It is also known that constrictions around the ankles and wrists should be avoided, although this advice generally comes more often from doctors.

The Newfoundland suggestion of applying urine recognizes beliefs in the value of this liquid for skin conditions. No specific mention of salves or ointments, however, has been found in the recently recorded oral tradition – a further indication of the comparative lack of Newfoundland interest in such preparations. On the other hand, a number of commercial preparations were available, such as Mentholatum "for chilblains, chapped skin, burns, bruises, colds." Egyptian Liniment, a cure-all – also promoted around 1920 – was said to be an "all-round remedy that every household should have for prompt treatment of cuts, scalds, burns, frost bites, *chilblains*, sore throats and chest, neuralgia, etc."

NOTES
See: MCG (1992) 108, tight shoes, and 001 for quotation.
    Representative MUNFLA references 67-20/29 (bathing, cold urine), 68-7/3 (cold water), 73-189 (rubbing snow), 76-249 (snow and Sunlight soap).
    Personal communication: N. Rusted (1991), on vinegar.

## CHUCKLEY-PEAR

The sweet, reddish-purple berries of the flowering shrubs (*Amelanchier* spp. – eight in Newfoundland) are commonly known on the island as "chuckley-pears" and, less often, as "wild-pears" or "Indian-pears." (The names Juneberry and serviceberry, well-known in parts of North America, are rarely used in Newfoundland).

Little medical interest (professional or domestic) has been aroused in *Amelanchier* spp. in the past, despite the astringency of the bark and the unripe fruit (hence perhaps, the term "chuckley"). In places where the tree grows, however, tonic properties and usage of the astringency for diarrhoea have been recorded. No evidence has been found to indicate that these properties were recognized in Newfoundland even among the Micmacs, for aboriginal knowledge has been recorded elsewhere. The pleasantness of the ripe fruit sustains interest more than anything else.

NOTES
See: Introduction to bibliography for history and background information; Scott (n.d.) 45.

## COBWEBS

The Newfoundland oral tradition, as elsewhere, refers to the application of cobwebs to cuts (or to the gums following tooth extractions) to stop bleeding. Since cobwebs are rarely at hand when needed (unless stored), it may be that their haemostatic property is best remembered because it captures the imagination, rather than because of its widespread usage.

During the nineteenth century, particular interest emerged, more so in professional than lay medicine, in cobwebs. Recommendation were to take them internally for a panoply of conditions, both as a so-called nerve sedative and as a medicinal agent for tuberculosis and malarial fevers. Much of this interest, however, carried a sense that positive results might be due to placebo action.

NOTES
See: Hartnett (1974), for background, and widespread usage; Brown Collection (Hand 1961), for various references, Green (1990) 222, for uncommon suggestion of use for bleeding at childbirth.

Representative MUNFLA references: 76-249 (cobwebs with myrrh, flour, and ashes), 78-195 (cobwebs).

## COCOMALT AND MALT EXTRACT

A "New Kind of Tonic in Food Form" claimed a 1940 advertisement for Cocomalt. At the time, Cocomalt was undoubtedly one of the best-known health beverages in Newfoundland, for both infants and adults. The advertisement stated: "For years Cocomalt has been the favourite food-drink in millions of homes. It not only furnishes Iron for red blood and strength; it is rich in Carbohydrates for furnishing the food energy needed for the strenuous activities of our high-pressure living. It contains proteins for building solid flesh and muscle, Vitamin D, Calcium and Phosphorus for sound bones and sound teeth." Such claims were part of the promotion of so-called new tonics (q.v.) based on nutritional factors – minerals and vitamins – rather than on bitter or astringent characteristics. Although the latter were often seen as appetite promoters, the newer food tonics were (and are) widely viewed and accepted as food supplements, and hence as "builders" and "strengtheners" for all ages.

A small, but noteworthy, detail about Cocomalt is that it was promoted by a jingle, apparently sung in a number of schools. Gerald Doyle in the 1940 edition of his popular songbook, reproduced "The Cocomalt Song" from the Victoria Cove School Magazine. The chorus went:

Cocomalt! Cocomalt! That's what we all say;
Oh, what fun it is to drink a glass or more each day.
Cocomalt! Cocomalt! We like to drink our fill.
Mixed with water it tastes grand;
With milk it's better still!

The child-welfare movement and teachers who promoted health education were probably a significant backdrop to such practices. Malt extract was promoted in various other products, especially combined with cod liver oil (q.v.), intended primarily for children. Indeed, some Newfoundlanders were pleased to have the taste of cod liver oil disguised! Dee's Malt Extract proclaimed in 1940: "Thousands of mothers give great praise to Dee Brand Malt Extract and Newfoundland Cod Liver Oil. This is a guaranteed tonic for your family." And certainly part of the products' newspaper promotion was directed toward adults. "Bynol [another cod liver oil and malt extract] is a rich tonic food and restorative which gives new strength and energy. When suffering from loss of weight Bynol builds up the body and increases its natural powers of resistance against diseases. Bynol restores vitality and brings good health." (1925) Nowadays, although far from being "new kinds of tonics," malt products still have enthusiastic believers.

NOTES
See: Doyle (1940).

### COD LIVER OIL

Although long established as a self-care product – for many Newfoundlanders synonymous with their island – cod liver oil has been continually and conspicuously promoted by physicians for much of its history. For instance, the value of taking oil by mouth for so-called rheumatism emerged with striking testimonials from respected physicians toward the end of the eighteenth century; tuberculosis received the same play in the nineteenth century.

Early enthusiasm was tempered, however, because cod liver oil was then "raw" (prepared by fermentation of livers in barrels), an extremely unpleasant product said to leave a flavour like that of putrid fish and to give a strong taint to the perspiration of those taking it. This contributed to its decline during the early decades of the nineteenth century, even though physicians said patients accepted the oil. A challenge loomed for producers and entrepreneurs, and countless new commercial products (using different ways of preparation) reached the marketplace from the 1840s onwards. By that time the oil was promoted for a panoply of complaints, including tuberculosis (q.v.), soon to become a scourge in Newfoundland.

The new, ideal oil was fresh, "white" or pale yellow and had no odour of putrefaction. Although considered superior to dark oil (perhaps just as white bread and white sugar were, and are, often preferred to the dark products), some people continued to feel that dark oil was more natural and hence medicinally more effective. Willmott said in 1860 that while many preferred home-made British oil, the Newfoundland oil "assimilates in physical character to the [British] home-made, and is considered by many to be superior in beneficial effect."

In the end, however, commercial preparations of "pure" pale oil pushed interest in, say, crude Newfoundland oil to one side. Only a few references exist in the recently recorded Newfoundland oral tradition to the use of so-called raw cod liver oil made in the outports. One reference is for treating colds and coughs (q.v.); the other for tuberculosis (q.v.). There is, too, one recollection about a refined home-made oil: "Grandfather operated a cod liver factory where the liver was refined into oil. He could drink a ladle full while skimming it into bottles. He never caught the flu or colds, but I've wondered if the oil wasn't a factor contributing to his high blood pressure and finally a paralytic stroke. He died at the age of eighty." Such thoughts about cardiovascular problems, contrary to current views (see below), are typical of many concerns about self-care.

The commercial promotion of preparations of so-called pure cod liver oil was intense. In addition to reinforcing and sustaining widespread interest in the product, it helped to move the perception of cod liver oil from that of a medicinal agent to that of a food, albeit a food for health. As one physician said categorically in 1900, "the oil is a

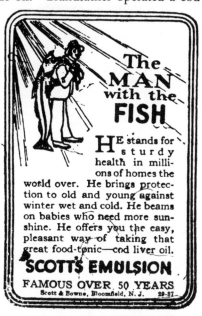

GERALD S. DOYLE, LTD.
Agents for Newfoundland
Newspaper advertisement for cod liver oil,
1930

food and not a medicine." As the Newfoundland advertisements dem-
onstrate, manufacturers capitalized on this belief. Gerald Doyle, who, as
already noted, did so much to distribute over-the-counter medicines to
every outport in the island, had many slogans in promoting his own brand
of "Pure Newfoundland Cod Liver Oil," such as "To build up ... manliness." Many Newfoundlanders saw it as the finest of tonics. Doyle also
promoted Scott's Emulsion and Brick's Tasteless oil, both of which became
household names on the island. The Emulsion was advertised as a pleasant
way of taking that great food-tonic, as was the Tasteless. As one Newfoundlander put it, perhaps overenthusiastically, "Everybody had Brick's Tasteless,
whether you needed it or not."

Another chapter emerges in the cod liver oil story with the recognition
of two constituents, vitamins A and D. Although cod liver oil had been
recommended for rickets during the nineteenth century, it gained greater
acceptance with the recognition of the presence of an "antirachitic vitamin"
(vitamin D) in the early 1920s. The value of its vitamin A content was also
appreciated and promoted, as countless advertisements testify. The precise
significance of this new knowledge for Newfoundlanders, however, was
uncertain. Indeed, although rickets had often been cited as a nutrition problem in Newfoundland, its incidence during the first half of the twentieth century is unclear. W.R. Aykroyd wrote in 1930: "Every grade of severity of rickets may be noted here and there on the coast, but severe types are uncommon. There is a lack of vitamin D in the diet, and the calcium, owing to the relative

**LOOK BETTER-LIVE LONGER**
BY PRESERVING YOUR HEALTH WITH
**VITAMINS A AND D**

See that you and all the members of your family, from infants to grandparents, enjoy the good health that flows from the daily intake of Vitamin-rich Cod Liver Oil. Doyle's Newfoundland Cod Liver Oil—in Golden Capsules or Liquid —is pleasant to take and will help you to enjoy better health. Sold at druggists and dealers all over

**NEWFOUNDLAND**

A 1955 advertisement from
Doyle's Old-time Songbook

absence of milk and vegetables and the large amount of flour and fish eaten,
is low, while the phosphorus is high." Aykroyd, correctly indicating that
"plenty of sunlight" contributed to lowering the incidence of rickets, added
that people "on the Labrador coasts have learnt to prepare cod-liver oil from
the fresh liver during the autumn to use as a general tonic for themselves
and their families during winter and spring."

With regard to vitamin A and night-blindness (see *eyes*), it is not clear
that cod liver oil was commonly employed as a specific treatment, at least
prior to recognition of its vitamin content.

Although memories of daily doses of cod liver oil are commonplace
among many Newfoundlanders today, it seems that not all Newfoundland
families viewed it as preventive therapy, despite intense promotion. In 1949,
in a discussion of nutrition in Newfoundland children, it was said: "Very

few children in the outports received cod liver oil. It appeared on the histories of several young infants, but ordinarily was only used when children were ill."

Cod liver oil has persisted to a greater extent than most other "old time" medicinal products. It remains a tradition in Newfoundland and there is still a significant market for the oil. This is linked to the growing interest in vitamins and, since the 1940s, in fish oils in general, as well as to evidence that oils reduce heart attacks and strokes. All this is justified by the presence of the omega-3 fatty acids, which justify, in turn, cod liver oil's long-standing reputation for treating rheumatism and certain skin conditions. Questions remain, however, about the clinical value and taking large doses. The long-standing issue – whether cod liver oil is to be viewed as a food or medicine – also remains.

NOTES
See: Willmott (1860); Aykroyd (1930); Butler (1900) 138; Piercey (1992) 6, on grandfather and oil; MCG (1992) 110, for quotation on Brick's Tasteless; Scobie et al. (1949), in frequently used in 1949; Davis (1982), for context.

Representative MUNFLA references: 76-249 (lung trouble), 78-200 (raw oil for tuberculosis), 78-205 (cod liver oil and molasses for cough), 82-121 (tonic).

## COLDS AND COUGHS, CATARRH

As in home medicine everywhere, the recently recorded Newfoundland oral tradition contains innumerable recommendations for the management of colds and coughs. These generally imply severe "chest" colds, rather than upper respiratory tract infections, as reflected in the popularity of applying poultices (q.v.) and so-called rubs (see below) to the chest. On the other hand, there seems to have been relatively infrequent use of either expectorant medicines (to bring up catarrh) or diaphoretics (regimens to sweat out a cold).

The most favoured chest rub was almost certainly goose grease (q.v., said to be best if fresh and warm), although other preparations were applied such as kerosene (q.v., perhaps in a "salve" with Sunlight soap and butter), molasses (q.v., perhaps with butter and vinegar, ginger, kerosene, or Minard's Liniment), and bay rum with cod liver oil. Over-the-counter preparations are noted below. Red flannel (q.v.) sometimes covered the rub or was applied alone without medication.

Preparations to be taken by mouth – alone or in combination with other medications – in order to ease a cough included turnip and sugar, and wild-cherry bark (q.v., alone or with dogberry wine or kerosene oil). Other suggestions for internal treatment of cough and other cold symptoms included molasses used in a number of ways. One recommended method was to drink it with kerosene, or heat it with kerosene and let it cool to form a taffy or "cough" drops. The latter might incorporate blackberry root or pepper. Alternative preparations were a decoction of juniper tree roots (see *juniper*), Labrador tea (q.v.), cod liver oil (q.v.), and onion juice (still popular).

The use of turnip for coughs and colds has been well known since at least the seventeenth century. It is noteworthy that William Vaughan – who was associated with early settlement in Newfoundland, although not a visitor himself – mentioned it in one of his writings (1626) on self-care: "The juyce of turneps sodden with sugar candy, or other sugar is good for the cough." Nowadays, turnip is still fairly well regarded for colds in many places outside Newfoundland.

The oral record also underscores that Minard's Liniment (q.v.) – ostensibly an external preparation – was taken internally at times for colds. This was often administered in relatively small doses – for example, about one-half tablespoonful of Minard's Liniment was put in a glass of cold water, stirred and drunk, or taken with a teaspoonful of molasses – but larger quantities were also taken.

Regimens for colds also included "just keeping warm," maybe going to bed with a lemon drink. ("What we did was steep up the lemon, you sliced up the lemon and steeped it out and you drank that and went to bed and covered yourself up warm and sweated it out of you.") Many alternatives (for example, rum) were tried, because lemons, often not readily available, were something of a luxury.

Bathing the feet in a mustard bath (see *mustard*) – or, less popularly, in onion water – was also recommended. Yet another part of treatment, to help one sleep at night, was called "clearing the passages." A drop of eucalyptus oil on a handkerchief or cloth was particularly well known in Newfoundland, at least until World War II, and was in line with strongly smelling applications to the chest that would "catch the breath." Suspending a bag of mothballs around the neck had the same effect, although it was probably less effective than sniffing the camphor in the more volatile Minard's Liniment.

Most of the above regimens were acceptable to physicians at the time, although many would also recommend the expectorant ipecacuanha (available from stores) to help bring up phlegm from the chest.

Another recommendation stands out: namely, to take a well-known laxative – senna, castor oil, or Epsom salts – none of which today have *specific* reputations for treating cold symptoms. Commercial products such as Grove's Laxative Bromo Quinine tablets were also advertised for colds, until the laxative promotion was dropped sometime around the 1960s.

The use of a laxative can be seen partly as a legacy of a long-standing notion in Western medicine that clearing the gastrointestinal tract was necessary in the treatment of all diseases. As one Newfoundland informant, after suggesting Epsom salts, said, it "will drive the cold down through you."

As a postscript to home-prepared treatments, two plants are noteworthy for their uncertain reputations. The first, *Linnaea borealis* (twinflower, q.v.), was reported in 1899, as a Newfoundland remedy for coughs. The second plant – it attracted little interest anywhere, but has a Newfoundland record – is the crowberry or ground blackberries. As one-time midwife, R. Piercey, wrote recently: "A good remedy for coughs was made by steeping the roots of ground blackberries [*Empetrum nigrum*], adding raisins to sweeten and drink[ing] as often as necessary. I often had half a dozen rum bottles full of the mixture ready for my father to take on board the boat when he had bronchitis. It always helped."

Along with home-prepared treatments, many a family kept a commercial cough and cold remedy at hand, aside from those noted above. Dr. Chase's Syrup of Linseed and Turpentine not only became traditional because of the Chase name, but also because of lay familiarity with the two principal ingredients. Linseed was an especially popular item for poultices, and turpentine had a widespread reputation as a domestic remedy for colds. Moreover, the preparation was frequently advertised, as in the 1945 St. John's newspapers: "The combination of linseed and turpentine with some other equally valuable ingredients has made Dr. Chase's Syrup of Linseed and Turpentine the most effective and most popular treatment for coughs, colds, croup and bronchitis not only for children but for adults also." For similar reasons Kay's Compound Essence (containing, in 1925, linseed, aniseed, squill, and tolu) also had popular appeal. But this is not to say that local products such as Stafford's Phoratone and Macs Compound Cherry Bark Cough Syrup (see *wild cherry*) were not in demand.

Many commercial aromatic preparations, some to be applied to the chest, were intended to help clear the passages with or without the aid of steam inhalation. They included the popular Pinex (for coughs, colds, bronchitis, throat tickle, bronchial asthma, spasmodic croup, winter coughs, and hoarseness), camphorated oil (possibly mixed with butter), Vapo-Cresoline (specifically for inhaling) and Vicks VapoRub for the chest, Vapex ("a drop on your handkerchief"), and Penetro ("Rub on throat, chest and back. Outside [it] peps up circulation locally in congested areas. Inside its medicated vapours sweep deep into breathing passages.") Menthol and camphor were principal ingredients in all such preparations.

At times much promotion focused on "catarrh," as if it was the scourge of mankind. Around 1900, for instance, among a number of somewhat similar preparations, Dr. Agnew's Catarrhal Powder proclaimed: "Before it is too late, stop that succession of colds that means nothing more nor less than catarrh ... Don't neglect yourself until consumption makes its fatal appearance. You can be cured – not merely relieved but absolutely and perfectly cured." (See also Catarrhozone in *asthma* entry).

Nowadays, treatment of coughs and colds by over-the-counter medicines, as sanctioned by professional medicine and pharmacy, remains dependent on symptom relief – through expectorants, cough suppressants (for dry not productive coughs), decongestants, and bronchodilators. Many of these medications have side-effects, if not used carefully, and have greater potential than most older regimens to interfere with prescription products.

Some long-standing commercial medications for steam inhalation are still recommended, though this useful approach (with little risk of interaction with other therapy) has declined in popularity. Chicken soup, moreover, still has physician and the lay public believing in its ability to relieve symptoms, although opinion is just as divided as over such regimens as high doses of vitamin C, both for prevention and treatment of colds. As in many other areas, change is more apparent than real.

NOTES
See: Vaughan (1626) 91; Bergen (1899) 113, *Linnaea borealis*; Piercey (1992) 45, 46, for ipecacuanha, ground blackberries; Erichsen-Brown (1979) 338, for reports on *Linnaea borealis*; MCG (1992) 103, on lemon and driving out colds.

Representative MUNFLA references: 68-12/1 (molasses and kerosene), 69-10Ms (turnip juice), 69-27/8 (kerosene), 77-87 (Labrador tea), 78-195 (soak feet in mustard bath, mothballs in bag around neck, tansy poultice), 82-121 (red flannel), 82-164 (juniper tree roots), 82-218 (camphorated oil and butter, goose grease), 82-238 (cod liver oil).

COLD SORES

The use of aftershave lotion (q.v.) for cold sores (sometimes called fever blisters) has been discussed. Other Newfoundland suggestions for sores (most often on the upper lip) – dabbing with lipstick, earwax, very hot water, or peroxide – do not have the drying effect considered to be useful. Peroxide has a mild antiseptic action said to be beneficial, but no evidence exists – as has sometimes been implied – that it attacks the offending virus. Even so, testimonials suggest those approaches may offer some relief. One Newfoundland informant noted that peroxide was more effective than aftershave lotion.

Some doctors consider that ice applied just prior to the eruption of the sore is helpful. In fact, personalized treatments are legion, including the use of local anaesthetics. Although modern prescription antiviral medicine can be especially helpful, the expense is generally not justified. For preventing cold sores linked to exposure to ultraviolet light (sometimes described as sunblisters), a sunscreen is useful.

NOTES
See: Brown Collection (Hand 1961, vol. 6) 192, for ear wax and for various citations, for kissing a redhead (a practice not found in the Newfoundland record).

Representative MUNFLA references: 69-12/4 (lipstick), 66-18/47 (aftershave lotion and peroxide), 84-284A (earwax).

COMPLEXION, FRECKLES, PIMPLES, ACNE

A clear complexion has always been viewed as a sign of good health, particularly in women. No doubt, many blood purifiers (q.v.), considered to be one way to improve the skin and complexion, were tried, as were so-called kidney medicines like Dr. Chase's Kidney and Liver Pills. Local newspaper advertisements (1939) for the latter claimed that "a clear skin tells of healthy kidneys."

Few specific suggestions concerning external applications for the "complexion" have been found in the Newfoundland oral record, apart from soaking in the first snow in May (or "May snow") or wiping the face with a urine-soaked diaper (see *animal parts*). With regard to snow in general, *The Daily News* (20 March 1894) told its Newfoundland readers that "April snow-water bottled and well corked was, as is, used for many a woman for the preservation of her loveliness."

The application of dew is noted for freckles – a practice known elsewhere – along with the first snow in May applied for nine days. Buttermilk was another recommendation for freckles. This, a commonplace practice in many oral traditions, was not so popular in Newfoundland, where buttermilk has been comparatively little used. All these measures were mild, however, compared with many professional medical recommendations offered during the first half of the twentieth century, such as applications of mercury or bismuth, which many doctors hardly regarded as effective.

Although only a few specific suggestions for pimples were found in the recorded oral tradition – for example, to bathe with a solution of Epsom salts or fresh urine – commercial preparations left no doubt that such blemishes needed a commercial product. Although it is difficult to say whether such promotion was solely a marketing strategy, there was at least an emollient (and an alleged antiseptic) action behind the Mecca Ointment's claim (for instance, in a 1955 advertisement) of value for pimples, among other problems. Another ointment, a competitor, Dr. Nixon's Nixoderm – an apparent skin cure-all – also included pimples in its battery of target conditions.

It is unclear just when public worries about acne became widespread. One Newfoundlander, however, does recall: "I had acne after I went away [from the island] and do you know what I took for it, yeast, Fleischmann's yeast, and that cured it up. I went to the States in 1924 and all the Yanks took it."

No twentieth-century account of complexion can ignore the extensive promotion of an unending variety of toiletries and cosmetics. The latter certainly replaced such practices as using the "red paper off a cocoa package for rouge." Newfoundland women were bombarded with advertisements for such soaps as Cuticura to "clear your skin." Further, while Cuticura may have been the most widely advertised toilet soap – that is aside from all-purpose Sunlight soap – Newfoundlanders did have many others to choose from (see *soaps, toiletries*).

NOTES
See: Vinikas (1992), for background.

Representative MUNFLA references: 64-1/96 (cocoa paper for rouge), 66-2/76 (diaper), 69-22M (buttermilk), 76-249 (freckles and May snow and dew), 84-301B (May snow and complexion).

CONSTIPATION AND INNER CLEANLINESS

Constipation, often as much a preoccupation as a problem, has long been assaulted with a legion of treatments, effective and otherwise. In fact, chronic constipation was noted among Newfoundlanders by many writers on nutrition up to around 1950.

Many Newfoundland recommendations for laxatives have been accepted as effective by the medical profession and the public alike. One example, senna tea, was especially well known in the island and, in 1936, reportedly popular and given mostly to children and infants: "The leaves are brought in small packages, and a tea is made from them which is drunk with milk and sugar." The so-called tea was made with either hot or cold water (the latter by steeping overnight.)

Newfoundlanders have also taken much interest in rhubarb. As Rhoda Piercey has said: "Rhubarb roots from the garden were boiled for an hour and strained, a few raisins added, sweetened to taste, boiled and strained again and used for the treatment of constipation. The dose was one or two teaspoons at bedtime. Every mother's child hated it. So did the mothers."

In fact, the famed medical rhubarb used by doctors as a laxative is not the species that grows in Newfoundland; that could only be obtained through a drugstore.

Also widely used were Epsom salts, castor oil, and soap enemas. (Sunlight soap, commonplace in Newfoundland households, was recommended for use as a suppository inserted into the rectum with water). Other recommendations included some which, in contrast, were inconsistent in their actions: blackcurrant roots, squashberry tree (q.v.), and molasses (q.v.).

Non-internal medicine regimens for constipation – such as placing a tobacco poultice on the stomach (reminiscent of the once-popular fomentations), rubbing each side of the stomach (for a child), and sitting on a chamber pot (or over a pail) containing hot water – perhaps encouraged relaxation. Whether another suggestion – to put Epsom salts in shoes – was ever taken seriously is unclear.

A rather striking instance of "first-aid" for severe constipation is reported in Philip Gosse's account of a journey in Newfoundland (1828). On a cross-country walk, constipation was manually dealt with by the use of a "pointed stick."

Laxatives (especially senna tea) were not always used to relieve constipation as such, but to clean "the system" – sometimes as a spring tonic (see *tonics*) or when there was a general state of unwellness, as well as for specific ailments. Their treatment for colds has been mentioned (that is, "for colds they'd give you senna"; or the so-called laxative Bromo Quinine tablets for "colds, grippe, influenza and as a preventative"). And Cascarets (containing cascara sagrada) were to be taken if "dizzy, bilious and constipated." Such roles for laxatives, part of a broad range of "purification" processes, were sometimes rationalized on the basis of autointoxication and the general need for cleanliness noted in Part I.

Laxatives marketed specifically for children had similar roles. Steedman's powders, widely advertised, were promoted for babies when fretful or feverish from constipation; Fletcher's Castoria, also intensively advertised to Newfoundlanders, relieved "constipation, flatulency, wind, colic, diarrhoea." ("Children cry for Castoria" became a well-known byline). Just as popular was California Syrup of Figs: "best and most harmless physic for the little stomach, liver and bowels."

A noteworthy group of commercial laxatives either stressed or implied "liverishness" (q.v.), at least until relatively recently. Two favourites were Beecham's Pills (q.v., "Real relief from Liverishness. The World's Medicine. The Most Famous Home Medicine in the World") and Carter's Little Liver Pills ("Wake up your liver bile without calomel.")

It cannot be said that interest in laxatives has declined in recent years; indeed, the link between laxation and health has been encouraged in past decades by much subtle advertising. For instance, Melcalose was described to Newfoundlanders in 1951 not as a laxative, but as a "bowel regulator." And more recently there has been a resurging interest in inner cleanliness.

Although older laxatives are still used (senna leaves and pods are available in Newfoundland), some of the current interest reflects the recent emphasis on attention to diet (including high-fibre foods) as preferable to medications, certainly to regular use of medications. In fact, Newfoundlanders have been hearing the "natural" message since at least the 1950s, through such products as All-Bran, the "safe, natural way to relieve irregularity."

NOTES
See: Mitchell (1930), Vaughan and Mitchell (1933), on constipation in Newfoundland (Mitchell notes common requests for "opening medicines"); Piercey (1992) 47, on rhubarb roots; Parsons (1936) and Piercey (1992) 46, for senna; Rompkey (1990) 237, for Gosse story; MCG (1992) 013, for colds, worms; Whorton (1993), for background.

Representative MUNFLA references: 76-249 (senna), 78-195 (tobacco poultice on stomach), 78-200 (hot water in chamber pot, Epsom salts, blackcurrant roots), 82-121 (Sunlight soap), 82-122 (molasses, rub each side of stomach).

CORNS

The realization that foot problems receive little attention in the oral record makes one wonder how many Newfoundlanders suffered from bunions, ingrown toenails, and fungal problems such as athlete's foot and nail fungus. After all, fishermen's rubber boots are not considered ideal for continual wear.

Although treatment advice for ingrown toenails was limited to such as cutting a V-shaped notch in the middle of the nail, or softening with hot tallow and cleaning, the ubiquitous corn (localized thickening of the skin) received much comment. The employment of a wad of chewing gum on a corn – mentioned more than once in the Newfoundland oral record – may have reflected desperation when a protective band-aid (also suggested) was not readily available. Covering with squid skin had the same effect, although some felt that certain types of skin had specific effects.

Also described are several more active treatments; for instance, iodine to "burn off" a corn or, as common elsewhere, various ways of softening corns. One Newfoundland suggestion was to make a poultice from white bread, flour, and boiling water and apply it to the corn while hot. When softened, the "core" or "eye" could be pulled out or the corn scraped, or rubbed, with pumice stone (still recommended). Commercial corn applications advertised in Newfoundland were also tried; in the 1920s, Freezone (still available) was said to take the corn "right off without pain." It contained, like most other over-the-counter corn remedies, salicylic acid.

Corns can be as intractable as warts (q.v.). It is therefore perhaps surprising that only one reference to making the sign of the cross over a corn has been found in the Newfoundland record. Moreover, there is no mention of the most appropriate management (applicable to ingrown nails as well): correctly fitting shoes.

NOTES
See: Bergen (1899) 76, for squid skin.
    Representative MUNFLA references: 67-21/53 (sign of cross), 67-1/20 (poultice), 78-195 (cut in nail, tallow, chewing gum, band-aid), 78-200 (iodine).


CRABS

"Crabs" are described in one Newfoundland report as "a sort of lice that can easily be caught from public toilet seats; these crabs go about halfway in through the skin around your privates and are very uncomfortable." Crab lice (*Phthirius pubis*) affect the genital and occasionally other hairy areas, but it is incorrect, albeit commonplace, to blame public toilet seats.

It was obvious to Newfoundlanders – at least until modern chemical treatments became available – that crab lice are difficult to get rid of. One suggestion was to rub the area with tobacco juice, obtained by boiling or steeping tobacco and straining; this undoubtedly had some positive effect owing to the nicotine content. Recommendations noted under the *itch* entry were also tried.

NOTES
Representative MUNFLA references: 68-10/4 (tobacco juice), 69-23/26 (from toilet seats).


CRACKERBERRY

Crackerberry (*Cornus canadensis*, also known in Newfoundland as "crackers" or "bunchberry") is familiar to everyone on the island as a carpet of flowers in the spring and early summer woods and, later, for the striking bright red berries. Surprisingly perhaps, in view of the visual impact, no evidence has been found in the Newfoundland oral record of usages recorded elsewhere.

All that is noted is the actual eating of the berries, despite their lack of flavour. A notion, in an old report (1893) – that in the "Scotch Highlands," it (also known as dwarf cornel) is called the "plant of gluttony," because of its supposed power to increase the appetite – seemingly had little or no recognition in Newfoundland. The statement, however, probably does refer to the closely related *Cornus suecica*, also found on the island, and said to have more flavour. Native North American Indian usage of the root or the whole plant (for example, for coughs, fevers, tuberculosis, infant colic) is likewise unrecorded in Newfoundland.

NOTES
See: Dana (1989 [1893]) 27, for comment on appetite; Scott (n.d.) 59, for note about it being eaten by children; Moerman (1986), for native uses.

CRAMPS IN MUSCLES

Recommended Newfoundland treatments for cramps – mostly leg cramps at night (that is, night cramps) – included the natural response to rub or massage the affected area of muscle contraction, sometimes with "hot kerosene." This was done perhaps seven times, with or without the sign of a cross. In sharp contrast is the suggestion to jump out of bed and put the feet on cold canvas. Two other recommendations also involve movement: 1) place a junk of wood under the "heart of the foot and bear down on it as hard as possible;" and 2) tie a string (a leather belt is also noted) around the arm or leg, twist the string tight, and have someone rub the area before quickly letting go of the string. All this was supposed to get the "blood circulating again."

Yet another practice, probably as well known in Newfoundland as in other places, involved tying an eel skin (preferably skinned from a live eel) around the limb where cramping occurs.

Many charms or amulets were noted, as much for prevention as treatment, including for menstrual cramps (see *female problems*). "Sometimes the stomach of the flounder is found to contain small, flat shells of the shape and size of a quarter. Many old people carried some of those shells as a charm against rheumatism and the cramps. If a cramp was so severe that the shell could not handle it, then the knuckle bone of a beaver was tried. That was even more powerful than a cramp ring of iron. Cramp rings were fairly common when I was a boy. They were made of iron, of course, but not of coffin nails as they were in the old Country." Other suggestions in the recently recorded Newfoundland oral tradition include carrying a haddock bone; suspending a "cramp knot" (a knot cut from a tree or perhaps just a gnarled piece of wood) or a nutmeg in a bag around the neck; wearing eel skin (with knots in it) around the ankle; crossing shoes under the bed toward the feet; and crossing socks on the floor when getting into bed. It is unclear whether such suggestions were also tried at times for menstrual or stomach cramps, for which there were other treatments (see relevant entries).

Physicians have long recommended (as they still do) quinine sulphate as a prophylactic for night cramps. Yet perhaps surprisingly, quinine has apparently not been incorporated into the Newfoundland oral tradition, as it has elsewhere, despite its availability over the counter in drugstores.

Among the countless suggestions in current lay health-literature for managing cramps and the newer advice in professional medicine is the emphasis on first trying non-drug regimens. Massage is sometimes viewed as analogous to the older regimens of rubbing an area a prescribed number of times. Stretching and warmth (bedsocks, and so on) are certainly recommended nowadays by physicians for night cramps under certain circumstances, particularly when such considerations as disturbed sleep patterns have been excluded.

NOTES
See: Brown (Hand 1961, vol. 6) 163–6, for a similar range of suggestions, except pushing against junk wood; Opie and Tatum (1989) 104, on haddock bone against cramp in England; Sparkes (1983) 166, for quote about flounder.

Representative MUNFLA references: 63-6/21 (nutmeg around neck), 66-10/24 (cross shoes), 67-20/30 (junk wood), 68-23/15 (carry haddock bone), 69-7/MS (rubbing area, sign of cross, kerosene, eel skin), 69-13/2 (stone under tongue), 69-23/12 (cramp knot), 69-23/42 (jump out of bed on cold canvas), 76-249 (eel skin).

### CREEPING SNOWBERRY

As noted under *abortion,* the creeping snowberry (*Gaultheria hispidula,* also popularly called "maidenhair," "capillaire," or "magnatea berry") was apparently well regarded in eighteenth-century Newfoundland, in part as an abortifacient. Aside from Aaron Thomas (see *abortion*), Newfoundland visitor Joseph Banks indicated its use as a beverage (1766): "Plant from the Berries of which Syrup of Capillare is made it is call'd here maidenhair & drank by way of substitute for tea." Banks' comment, however, raises some uncertainty about the identity of the plant, since Syrup of Capillaire was at the time prepared from the fern, *Adiantum pedatum.* But in all likelihood, Banks was referring to creeping snowberry. It was certainly fairly well known as a stimulant by the second half of the nineteenth century, and alleged emmenagogue properties were often noted.

One Newfoundland informant seems to have referred to the flowers when calling them "chalices." "They grow on the barrens. They are like a cup, a little white thing, you pick them and they cure the whooping cough." Steeped in milk with a little sugar, they were administered to a baby with whooping cough. ("They thought they were going to lose her [the baby], she used to turn blue. And they cured her right off the bat.")

*Adiantum pedatum,* commonly called "maidenhair fern," which grows in Newfoundland albeit rarely (on mountain tops near Port aux Basques), remained modestly well known to physicians throughout the nineteenth century. The bitterish aromatic fronds were once employed in chest ailments, but no mention of this has been found in the Newfoundland record.

NOTES
See: Introduction to bibliography for history and background; for Banks, see Lysaght (1971) 122, (the editor identifies "maidinair" as *Gaultheria hispidula*); MCG (1992) 002, for whooping-cough story.

CROUP

Parents have long worried about children's croup – with its cough (often described as "barking"), hoarseness, and harsh sounds on inspiration (stridor). One advertisement (1940) in a Newfoundland newspaper recommending Chase's Syrup of Linseed and Turpentine noted that "the croupy cough strikes terror in the mother's heart." The relatively few Newfoundland records about treatment can hardly reflect the countless times it was managed at home.

For croup, non-commercial treatment recommendations in Newfoundland are generally the same as for a cold, although one particular suggestion for croup singled out rubbing the chest with goose grease (sometimes mixed with honey) and covering with red flannel. Other applications are to the throat: rub with camphorated oil or with turnip juice (obtained from covering thin slices of turnip with sugar in a saucer and warming until the juice forms), and then wrap the neck with a sock or flannel. A warm herring, covered with a wool sock, was also suggested as an application to the throat.

No Newfoundland reference has been found to the therapeutic usefulness – noted time and time again in professional and lay medical writings – of humidifying the atmosphere. Although physicians consider this more effective than the suggestions just given, the possibility of benefiting from a rub (perhaps partly psychological as it involved lengthy preparation time such as making turnip juice) or from herring wraps has to be considered.

One commercial preparation frequently promoted for croup, as it was for so-called babies' colds prior to the 1940s, was Vicks Vaporub (q.v.): "When your child has Croup [Vicks Vaporub] rubbed on throat and chest relieves spasmodic croup in two ways. (1) Its medicated vapours, released by body heat reach air passages direct; (2) at the same time it stimulates the skin thus helping the inhaled vapours ease the difficult breathing." It is difficult to overestimate the popularity of this rub, still available today, which contains menthol, camphor, turpentine, eucalyptus, and other oils. Everywhere, Vicks pushed aside home-made remedies.

NOTES
Representative MUNFLA references: 67-14/75 (goose grease and red flannel), 78-200, (flannel, camphorated oil, herring, turnip juice).

## CROWBERRY

*Empetrum nigrum* – commonly known in Newfoundland as "blackberry," and "blackberry heath," as well as "crowberry" – is found all over the island. It has attracted virtually no medical interest (professional or domestic), although the leaf has been noted to act as a purgative. The only recorded uses for Newfoundland, for bronchitis and uterine pains, are considered in the *colds* and *midwives* entries.

NOTES
See: Moerman (1986, vol. 1); Scott (n.d.) 69.

## CUTS, MINOR WOUNDS (SOMETIMES INFECTED)

Suggestions for treating cuts and minor wounds and sores, commonly using ready-to-hand items, are legion in Newfoundland, as elsewhere. The record partly reflects the high incidence of cuts among fishermen, many of which became festered (sometimes called "festers"). Wives had to know how to treat these cuts if the "husband was to have success in the fishing season." As noted elsewhere, recollections exist of frequent sores throughout the Newfoundland population; some people think these were related to nutritional deficiencies.

Initial cleansing of a cut might include bathing with water and salt or just cold water, the latter perhaps also intended to stem bleeding. Myrrh (q.v.), the gummy resin from spruce and balsam fir respectively, was a favoured subsequent application, although sometimes it was applied without initial cleansing. Myrrh bladders (which, some advised, should be kept on hand in case of emergencies) were squeezed out onto the cut. Suggestions included mixing the myrrh with molasses, flour, ashes, or cobwebs (q.v.).

Although myrrh was especially well known, commercially produced turpentine (q.v., a pine product) was probably frequently applied. Alternative applications, utilized alone or in combination (sometimes with myrrh), included: brown paper, cod liver oil, Friar's balsam, iodine, Jeysol (a commercial disinfectant), lanolin, molasses (q.v.), sugar, tansy (q.v.), and tobacco juice. Although scorched flour, ashes, and white puff-balls ("horse's fart") were also specifically recommended, they were really more for styptic action if bleeding was a problem (see *bleeding*). The puff-balls could be shaken over the cut to apply the fungal spores, although in one suggestion the ball was cut into two halves, one of which was placed over the bleeding surface.

A complicated recommendation, perhaps reflecting a favoured family recipe, was the preparation of rosin, sulphur, and cod liver oil mixed together and melted in a glue pot; this was spread on a piece of material (for example, calico or sometimes shirting), left to dry, rolled up, and kept for sores, cuts, and so on.

If a cut or wound was infected (sometimes described as a "rising," a term also used specifically for infected fingers), a poultice (q.v.), a piece of fat pork (q.v.), or an antiseptic (for example, iodine) was the suggested application.

Fairly conspicuous in the record are practices explainable by the concept of sympathy and long viewed as magical or non-natural. Not only was the wound or sore treated, so was the cause. For example, if a nail had caused the injury, the rust might be cleaned away and the nail placed in kerosene or acid, or buried until the wound healed.

Another Newfoundland suggestion, albeit not often recorded, was the application of mould from bread or jam (or mouldy bread) to a cut (or infected area). Although the use of moulds and mouldy substances has a long history, it may be that because the practice has come to be widely known as a folk "antibiotic" treatment, memories are clouded about its actual use.

Compared with records of self-treatments for cuts and so on in other societies, there is nothing especially noteworthy about the Newfoundland recommendations. Many followed professional practices, certainly the employment of iodine and Jeysol, as applications of "antiseptics" to cuts. The compounded Friar's balsam, which like myrrh provided protection for cuts and wounds, has been professionally recommended since at least the seventeenth century.

As home treatments for cuts, cod liver oil and molasses are, in contrast to other suggestions, probably less well known elsewhere. The emollient action can provide ease, however, and some have argued that cod liver oil also had a specific wound-healing property. Probably, the sugary molasses like granulated sugar, has an antimicrobial action on the wound.

If most of the above treatments have faded and the application of myrrh has been replaced by the application of Band-Aids, at least antiseptic ointments (q.v.) persist.

NOTES
See: Butler (1977) 69–71, account of cuts and wounds in 1930s; Hartnett (1974), general account of cobwebs; Wainwright (1989), for general background on moulds.

Representative MUNFLA references: 77-87 (wool, lanolin, tobacco), 78-195 (iodine, cobwebs), 78-200 (mold from bread or jam, cobwebs, "white puffy balls"), 78-205 (brown paper), 82-158 (myrrh, molasses and myrrh), 82-122 (cod liver oil), 85-001 (wives treating husbands).

## DANDELION

The usage of dandelions is still well remembered by many Newfoundlanders. As one said: "Dr. McGrath told us there's more stuff in dandelion for your body like for your blood, whatever kind of chemical is in it, it cleans your blood and everything." Strong memories also exist of making dandelion wine and eating the leaves as a spring green. "Couldn't wait for the spring to break up so we could get the dandelion. We have them then till the greens come, the cabbage and the turnip tops. We have the dandelion first. I like it better than any of it. My God we were strong as bulls from eating that stuff."

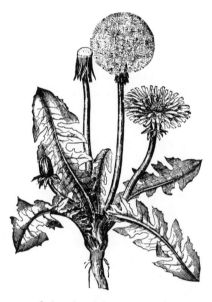

Noteworthy in the Newfoundland story of the dandelion is the general lack of recognition awarded its principal, long-standing reputation as a diuretic. And this despite the common occurrence of this weed.

NOTES
See: Introduction to bibliography for history and background; MCG (1992) 002, for influence of Dr. McGrath and for quotation.

## DEAD-EYES (SEE GALLS)

## DIARRHOEA

Suggestions in the Newfoundland oral tradition for treating diarrhoea (known by a variety of colloquial names such as "runs," "scuts," "summer complaint") include an intriguing variety of approaches: apple (q.v.), arrowroot (q.v.), barley, castor oil followed by milk, dry toast, strong tea, teas of wild cherry (q.v.), juniper berries (q.v.), wild strawberry, and red (not black) spruce. (The latter was also noted for what was called dysentery, evidently referring to severe episodes of diarrhoea). Commercial preparations such as "Certo," "Radway," and "Wild Strawberry" ("You can buy that in a drugstore. I always keep a bottle at hand") are part of the Newfoundland record. Items in the diverse list of treatments are generally well known elsewhere.

Some recommendations – dry toast, arrowroot, and barley, all bland, readily digestible foods – provided supportive care "to keep up your strength." Eating "dough" (or, if that was not available, flour and water or "batter") was, however, considered specific treatment. Moreover, today's still current recommendations – to stop eating during an episode of diarrhoea – are recorded. "For diarrhoea or summer complaint, you'd get the barley and you'd boil it, and strain the barley off, and you had the water and you'd give this to the child with nothing to eat, just drink this, the diarrhoea would stop." Another Newfoundland suggestion, cloves – if given in sufficient amounts to have a physiological effect – might help to ease stomach discomfort rather than stemming the diarrhoea.

Nowadays, the suggestion to use the laxative castor oil (followed by "warm milk to bind") to treat diarrhoea would surprise most people. However, it mirrors the long-standing belief of "cleaning out" the gastrointestinal tract in many disorders, as already noted (for example, see *constipation*). And indeed there is still some belief in this approach, or at least there is a concern that giving an antidiarrhoeal might prevent ready removal of offending pathogens from the bowel. It should be noted that bouts of diarrhoea can accompany chronic constipation, although there is no evidence that any Newfoundland recommendation arose from such a consideration.

The reference to wild cherry bark (q.v.) – also listed in the diarrhoea recommendations as "chuckley-plum" – is not in line with its general recommended uses, although the astringency could be beneficial. Strong tea and strawberry roots were certainly used for their astringency or, in the words of one Newfoundlander, "to dry up your insides."

Of the commercial preparations noted, Certo (a jam thickener [pectin] that could "thicken anything") may not have been a serious suggestion. Radway's refers to the proprietary medicine, Radway's Ready Relief. Although long-standing recommendations from medical professionals for such items as kaolin or codeine are not mentioned in the Newfoundland oral tradition, these products were widely sold.

It is noteworthy that no specific mention is made in the Newfoundland record of the treatment of diarrhoea in infants. In fact, the difference between past recommendations for children or adults has been minimal. Recently, however, professional medicine has paid particular attention to assessing the state of hydration of children – mouth dryness and many other factors, including the nature of the stools – as a guide to treatment.

Oral hydration therapy is recommended, and even long-standing recommendations, such as for kaolin, are considered questionable.

Many Newfoundlanders have started to follow the popular advice of taking yogurt after a bout of diarrhoea, even though convincing scientific evidence of its effectiveness is lacking.

NOTES

See: MCG (1992) 106, for barley; MCG (1992) 111, for Wild Strawberry.

Representative MUNFLA references: 68-8/4 (strawberry roots), 68-10/6 (cherry bark), 69-7Ms (dough, strong tea), 70-14/56 (arrowroot), 78-195 (juniper berries, certo, apple, flour and water, hard bread), 82-146 (castor oil), 82-218 (dry toast, strong tea).

DIPHTHERIA

Diphtheria, once a dreaded scourge of childhood, is characterized by a membranous exudation at the back of the throat and on the tonsils. Symptoms of the disease, which is caused by a bacterial infection, include breathing difficulties – even suffocation – due to the so-called membrane at the back of the throat and effects from absorption of bacterial toxins. Mortality was relatively high in Newfoundland until the late 1940s, when the increased use of immunization against the disease began to have an overall impact. 1959 was the first year in which no deaths were recorded.

It is perhaps surprising that few home treatments are found in the Newfoundland oral tradition, though this may merely mean that knowledge of self-treatment has faded in the absence of the disease. One old-timer has related just one of the many reported lay "triumphs" over doctors. Evidently, the doctor had given the five-year old boy just a few hours to live. The grandmother said:

"Go and get some turnip and peel it and put on two slices."

And I didn't know what she wanted it for, and when 'twas boiled, then I had to mash it up and put kerosene oil into it.

In the meantime she said, "Get some fatback pork and take two slices of it and put one piece in flannel and heat it on a plate on the stove and put it around his throat. One off and one on."

And the poor little thing screeched his life out, you know, 'cause blood was coming from his nose and his ears at the time. So, soon as the turnip was ready, she said "Now get the carrots in."

Now, you know, I didn't know what it was about, and she measured the carrots in the poultice and put that up around his throat. Now that was six o'clock in the night, and he hadn't spoken for three days. Three o'clock that morning he opened his little eyes and he mumbled something. Now, we used to have lime juice a lot then, and I could understand he wanted some lime juice.

And the next morning Old Doctor Macdonald went past the house and I said to mother, "He's comin' down the road, mum. And he's past; he's not comin' in."

He looked up and came back and said "I looked at the house, thought the blinds would be drawn."

Other suggestions such as swabbing the membranous coat with kerosene, salt solution, or vinegar were rarely tried, although they were sometimes suggested by physicians. Drinking "raw kerosene oil" was also noted as a treatment. In 1950, the Newfoundland Deputy Minister of Health, Leonard Miller, still saw diphtheria as a problem: "Only five years ago I visited a village of twelve homes where there had been three fatal cases of diphtheria in the previous week. Without immediate medical aid, parents were using vinegar to remove the membrane from their children's throats." He was probably even more critical of anyone who ate twigs from palm branches, to invoke religious associations of the palm.

Over-the-counter medicines, which were recommended for diphtheria during the early 1900s, included the cure-all, Minard's Liniment. It was applied directly to the throat as well as being rubbed on externally.

The fear generated by the disease is reflected in the preventive measure of washing the clothes of diphtheria patients with Gillett's lye, a recommendation which was extended to other infectious diseases (for example, tuberculosis) and also to children suffering from lice (q.v.). Fumigation of a room or dwelling (to remove "contagion" or "germs") with sulphur was also commonplace.

NOTES
See: Miller (1950); Severs (1975), for background; Fizzard (1987) 174, for quotation on grandmother's treatment.

Representative MUNFLA references: 72-90Ms (palm), 78-200 (kerosene); 82-122 (burning sulphur for fumigation).

DISINFECTANTS (SEE GERMS)

DODD'S KIDNEY PILLS

Intensive newspaper advertising and thousands of copies of Dodd's *Almanac* over many decades helped to make Dodd's Kidney Pills (and other Dodd's preparations) a household name in Newfoundland. In 1900, the *Evening Telegram* ran a typical series of advertisements in which one of a long list of ailments (for treatment by the pills) was noted each day: dropsy, women's weakness, neuralgia, backache, blood disorders, Bright's disease, diabetes, rheumatism, and lumbago. Bright's disease – "one of the deadliest and most feared maladies to which mankind is subject" (1927) – was often singled out in other advertising for the pills. The pattern was followed in the *Almanac's* advertising, two examples of which are shown here:

Testimonials printed in the almanacs often included a local flavour. For instance, from "Princeton, Nfld" (c. 1910), one finds: "I have been subject to a bad back for the last

**Blood Disorders**

are simply kidney disorders. The kidneys filter the blood of all that shouldn't be there. The blood passes through the kidneys every three minutes. If the kidneys do their work no impurity or cause of disorder can remain in the circulation longer than that time. Therefore if your blood is out of order your kidneys have failed in their work. They are in need of stimulation, strengthening or doctoring. One medicine will do all three, the finest and most imitated blood medicine there is, '.

**Dodd's Kidney Pills**

Sold everywhere at 50c.

**The Best Tonic**

The best way to tone up a run-down system is the natural way. The natural way is to remove the cause. The cause is sluggish circulation owing to the blood being filled with waste tissue and other impurities. The way to remove these impurities, is to put the Kidneys in working order by using.

**Dodd's Kidney Pills**

Sold everywhere at 50c.

seven or eight years. I have tried all kinds of medicines but have found them no good. My wife was reading your Almanac and found where lots of people were relieved of complaints like mine, so I got two boxes and now I am feeling much better. I am so thankful that we read your Almanac. I recommend your Dodd's Kidney Pills to all who suffer with backache like I did."

Advertising helped to provide a conceptual framework by linking impurities ("bad blood") with a range of conditions. Many extravagant claims were still being made in the 1930s for what was described as the "standard kidney remedy for fifty years sold all over Newfoundland"; one claim was that the pills stopped "rheumatism at its source." Analyses published early in the century (indicating that the principal ingredients were potassium nitrate, powdered fenugreek seeds along with pine resin, and a very small quantity of oil of juniper) offer no scientific basis for effectiveness. Further, stated constituents are not in line with advertisements, such as in Doyle's celebrated *Old Time Songs and Poetry of Newfoundland* (1927), which still said that the pills were "purely vegetable," a reflection of the concerns about chemical remedies. Nowadays Dodd's Pills contain sodium salicylate.

NOTES

See: Dodd's *Almanac* (c. 1910) 17; *Secret Remedies* (1909) 68, for formula; *Canadian Drug Identification Code* (1993), for current formula.

DOGBERRY, DOGWOOD

Dogberries (the red-berry fruits of *Sorbus americana* or *S. decora,* also commonly known as American service tree, American mountain ash, or the European *Sorbus aucuparia* [mountain ash]) have already been noted in the recently recorded Newfoundland oral record as an appetite restorer (q.v.).

The limited published information on dogberry in professional and domestic medical literature generally refers to the bark, as does a Newfoundland suggestion that recommends a decoction as a tonic and for "bad blood" (see *blood purifiers*). Additionally, dogberry wine (made from the fruits), a popular home-brew in Newfoundland, has, like all wines, been viewed as both a tonic and stimulant, an opinion still current.

C. Millspaugh, in a well-known book *American Medicinal Plants* (1892), made favourable comments insofar as he indicated that *S. americana* was a substitute for wild cherry (q.v.). He noted that the bark of the former had been used as a "tonic in fevers of supposed malarial types," and had been substituted for the well-known cinchona bark, the source of quinine; there is, however, no evidence this practice was widespread. The berries were also reported to be an antiscorbutic, although it is unclear whether this claim was generally accepted. Certainly no Newfoundland reference to such usage has been found.

A tradition well known to students of folklore, "passing through" (q.v.) the limbs of a tree, includes the use of dogberry.

The name dogberry sometimes refers to dogwood, which is generally known in Newfoundland as the red osier or red osier dogwood, *Cornus stolonifera*, rather than to another dogwood, *C. alternifolia*, found in the western part of the island. It is not to be confused with the well-known dogwood in North America *C. florida*, which once attracted professional as well as lay medical interest, but does not grow in Newfoundland. The red osier, in the form of a tea made from the bark, is recorded in Newfoundland as a remedy for colds and coughs. It is also noted as a tonic and perhaps all the more highly regarded for medicinal purposes when mixed with cherry-tree bark: "For my own children I boiled the dogwood and cherry for coughs. It really relieved the coughs that were left after flus."

The medicinal reputations of dogberry and dogwood do overlap; the resulting confusion in some Newfoundland records is, therefore, of little consequence.

NOTES
See: Millspaugh (1974 [1892]) 220–1; Hand (1980) 133–85, passing through; CMG (1992) 013, for dogwood and cherry.

Representative MUNFLA references: 84-217 (dogberry bark for bad stomach), 84-282B (dogwood for colds), 84-296A/B (dogwood for coughs).

DOG BITES

Concern over dog bites – at least from so-called mad dogs – is widely reflected in popular medicine everywhere, largely because of fear of rabies.

A long list of unsuccessful remedies can also be culled from the professional medical literature, all of which were swept to one side when Louis Pasteur introduced rabies vaccination in the 1880s.

In line with many past recommendations found elsewhere, the New-foundland record – albeit with few reports of rabies on the island – notes that the dog in question had to be killed immediately; otherwise the bitten person dies. (Not recorded in Newfoundland is the belief that killing the dog prevents insanity.) Such notions rest on sympathetic magic; one variant was for the bitten person to eat parts of the offending animal. Another Newfoundland suggestion was to rub dog's liver over the wound. Still another – a more modern version – is to shoot the dog, but to clean the wound with an antiseptic such as iodine.

Persistent belief in the apparent effectiveness (no longer accepted) of dog-bite remedies may partly reflect the fact that many bites were from dogs not infected with the disease.

NOTES
Carter (1982), for a wide scope of rabies treatments within professional medicine; Brown collection (Hand 1961, vol. 6) 171–72, for various remedies, but mostly those pertaining to dog hair and use of a madstone (not found in the Newfoundland record).

Representative MUNFLA references: 68-20/14 (kill dog), 69-2/5 (rub liver over wound), 69-17/5 (shoot dog and treat wound with iodine).

DRAGON'S BLOOD

The red resin called "dragon's blood," obtained in the Far East from the fruit of *Daemonorops propinquus* and related species, was commercially available in sticks or lumps. In Newfoundland (where it was sometimes called "ox-blood," possibly adding to the symbolism of the red colour), dragon's blood was employed – after softening lumps (or scrapings taken from the stick) by heat – as a plaster for backache, in a poultice for carbuncles (considered to be especially effective), or as a wrap around the wrist to protect from (and perhaps treat) water pups (q.v.) common among fishermen.

Dragon's blood (for years perhaps best known as a colouring agent in varnishes) has not been especially popular in Europe or North America, at least as a domestic medicine, although it still has magical and religious connotations among some ethnic groups. Although Newfoundland usage appears to be entirely non-magical, this area needs study.

NOTES
See: Greenish (1909) 532.

Representative MUNFLA references: 82-146 (back), 82-218 (carbuncles).
Personal communication: N. Rusted (1991), on dragon's blood.

### DRUNKENNESS, HANGOVERS

The extent of alcoholism in Newfoundland prior to recent times and surveys is not clear, although anecdotal evidence suggests that drinking bouts were commonplace in the lifestyles of fishermen. Nevertheless, advertisements (for example, in the *Evening Telegram*, 23 May 1899) for "Drink habit cured at home" were no different from elsewhere. Furthermore, no indications of widespread problems emerge from the Newfoundland oral tradition – at least few recommendations exist for hangovers. One suggestion, probably generally well known, was to eat butter before drinking. Other treatments – for the hangover itself – included further drinks: "Take another drink the morning after," or a "glass of cold beer first thing next morning."

Worcestershire sauce has been a popular pick-me-up. In 1925, Newfoundland readers of the *Evening Telegram* were told in an advertisement that a good pick-me-up was a raw egg swallowed with a teaspoonful of Lea and Perrins Sauce. A better-known commercial item, even if not always highly regarded, is the still available Bromo-Seltzer.

From time to time certain regimens achieve passing popularity for hangovers, such as tomato juice among Newfoundland university students in the 1960s. At present (1991), there is considerable interest in aspirin (to be taken before drinking), but this has been shown to increase blood-alcohol levels. To date, there is no known way to forestall the effects of drinking too much.

NOTES
See: Zachariah and Morley (1977), for a serious problem in the 1970s.
Representative MUNFLA references: 66-3/29 (butter before drinking), 69-10/5 (tomato juice, a drink morning after).

### DYSPEPSIA, NERVOUS DYSPEPSIA, ULCERS

Professional and domestic medical texts generally indicate or imply that a diagnosis of dyspepsia – abdominal discomfort and bloating, flatulence, and perhaps chest pain – embraces conditions popularly known as "indigestion," "heartburn (q.v.)," or "flatulence." Some Newfoundlanders, however, have viewed (and may still view) all these complaints as distinct entities, each meriting different treatments. As well, heartburn and dyspepsia have been distinguished from "stomach troubles" (q.v.), (hence our separate entries, though the overlap is considerable and confusing). Whatever the appropriate term, many problems existed on the island.

"Indigestion is almost universal," said Dr. J.M. Little in 1908. In fact, the catch-all claims for many over-the-counter remedies hardly clarified; indeed, they confused. Thus Stafford's Prescription A, produced in St. John's, was listed in 1920 and for many years as suitable for "Indigestion, Dyspepsia, Catarrh of Stomach, Gastritis, Nervous Dyspepsia."

The last ailment on this Prescription A list, nervous dyspepsia, was a vague diagnosis not uncommonly made in the early years of the twentieth century. According to one home-medicine book (1903): in nervous indigestion "either the indigestion, in its course, disturbs and involves the nervous system, or the nerves become themselves disordered, and produce the indigestion;" it was also stated that there was "great depression of spirits, amounting at times to complete hopelessness and despondency." Although the textbooks discussing this complicated problem were written for physicians, some of the suggested advice might have seemed appropriate to fatalistic Newfoundlanders: "The conquest of Fate is not by struggling against it, nor by trying to escape from it, but by acquiescence." Unfortunately, the extent to which Newfoundlanders linked dyspepsia with nerves (q.v.) is unclear, as is whether the diagnosis of nervous dyspepsia was even commonly made in Newfoundland.

Dyspepsia was also linked to ulcers. (One Newfoundlander said that "ulcers and indigestion were about the same.") Cod liver oil (q.v.) was recommended as a treatment – perhaps reflecting that, as in the Western popular medical tradition, ulcers on both the inside and outside were commonly considered to merit the same treatment.

Nowadays, dyspepsia and related lay diagnoses are commonly treated with antacids as in the past (see also under *heartburn*, *"stomach trouble"*), although they are now considered to inhibit the action of pepsin – a potentially irritating digestive enzyme – as well as to neutralize acid. Some commercial antacid preparations also include a chemical that some people say reduces flatulence by lowering the surface tension of the gas bubbles. At the same time, cautions are now commonplace, such as the need for some patients to avoid sodium containing antacids. Such concerns encourage a few people, in Newfoundland and elsewhere, to use "natural" peppermint oil, sometimes as sold in capsules.

NOTES
See: Warren et al. (1903) 303, for quote; Little (1908b).
    Representative MUNFLA reference: 76-64 (cod liver oil for ulcers).
    Personal communication: Troake (1989), on differences between terms.


EARS, EARACHE, DEAFNESS

One Newfoundland record states that "if a person's ear is ringing it means someone is talking bad things about them. If it is a woman whose ear is ringing all she has to do is to bite the corner of her apron and the person talking will bite his or her tongue." Ringing in the ear can arise from various causes. If it is due to impacted wax however (as it so often is), biting on the cloth might just help to dislodge the wax.

A considerable number of recommendations exist in the Newfoundland oral tradition (as elsewhere) for treating earache. Especially common were the rise of drops of "Electric Oil" (see *eclectric oil*) or olive oil and the blowing in of tobacco smoke (from a cigarette or a pipe) to produce warmth. Alternatives included using drops of camphorated oil (q.v.) or St. Anne's Oil, perhaps more popular for some because of religious associations with Saint Anne de Beaupré. The suggestion to put raisins (sometimes called "figs" in Newfoundland) – soaked in hot water – in the ear was perhaps problematical, since removal could be difficult. At least little evidence has been found for applying irritating substances aside from camphorated oil.

Onion (the "heart" or core) was also suggested; some indicated it was to be placed in the ear: "The sting from the raw onion would cure it." Others said it was to be placed outside the earhole. Perhaps the latter, on occasions, was more for a so-called mastoid (that is an infection of the mastoid bone behind the ear, once common in Newfoundland) – or worry about its possible existence. Additionally warm applications – including heated salt in a bag – were recommended, as was rubbing with alcohol.

The use of drops in the ear (usually warmed) has been universal, but many of the wide range of substances used – including camphorated oil – have been criticized by physicians as too irritating. Damage has also been done, including among Newfoundlanders, through overenthusiastic use of Q-tips for cleaning ears.

It is unclear from the Newfoundland record whether or not there were many lay attempts to make specific diagnoses, though this seems unlikely. After all, the treatments noted were used, as indicated, to soften wax in the ears – sometimes called "gathered ears" – as much as for earache. And deafness was often helped, since impacted wax is a common cause and softening and removing the wax is useful on many occasions.

Newfoundland recommendations during the first half of the twentieth century generally followed those initially employed by physicians, namely, the application of drops and warmth.

NOTES
See: Creighton (1968) 211, for notes on similar treatments, including tobacco smoke; Brown Collection (Hand 1961, vol. 6) 175–8, for various ways of applying warmth and drops into the ear; Tizzard (1984) 132 and 134, for some sense of concern about mastoiditis; MCG (1992) 002, for onion in the ear.

Representative MUNFLA references: 63-1/303 (buzzing and biting apron), 68-13/7 (hot raisins), 69-7 MS (olive oil), 69-22 MS (smoke in ear), 69-21/8 (molasses), 69-29/8 (heart of onion), 77-87 (Electric oil), 78-200 (gathered ears).

## ECLECTRIC OIL

The recently recorded Newfoundland oral tradition indicates that "Electric" oil was a favoured remedy for earache; it was also recommended as an application to the chest for bronchitis. During the 1940s and '50s, according to recent informants, this Electric oil was the over-the-counter preparation, Dr. Thomas' Eclectric Oil, advertised for coughs, head and chest colds. It was intended as a rub, but like many over-the-counter medicines its use was extended to other ailments. One informant noted that it was found in every store in Sop's Arm during the late 1940s and that "I often drank it raw from the bottle, or two or three drops in a spoonful of sugar, for the sore throat." It was also used as ear drops.

The possibility exists that, in the first two decades of the century, an Electric Liniment (marketed, for instance, by Sears, Roebuck) or Electric Oil was available in Newfoundland. An 1899 advertisement from the McMurdo drugstore in St. John's listed Electric Oil.

NOTES
See: Sears, Roebuck (1969 [1902]) 447, Electric Liniment; Sullivan (1984), for background.

Representative MUNFLA references: 68-10/7 (Sop's Arm, sore throat), 78-200 (chest cold), 78-205 (bronchitis), 82-149 (earache).

## ECZEMA

The term "eczema" has been popularly employed for a range of inflammatory skin conditions, subdivided by physicians into specific forms of eczema and dermatitis according to appearance and cause. Even though skin conditions are common – and in Newfoundland this includes such occupational problems as gum-boot dermatitis – relatively few treatment suggestions exist in the recently recorded Newfoundland oral tradition. Some unidentified salves are noted, and there is the commonplace Newfoundland regimen of applying urine for skin ailments (see *animal parts*). A cod-liver-oil poultice is recorded, a reminder that many physicians and laypeople regarded the oil (q.v.) as useful for skin ailments. Suet was perhaps viewed as an alternative: "I remember mother, I never had it but my sisters did, behind their ears would be sores like cracks, and she would melt mutton suet in the cover of a can and put it on the over, and every morning she'd soften it again and rub it behind the ears."

Another suggestion for eczema, one with magical content, was to bathe in the foam of a brook, before the sun rises, for three mornings, stop for three, and then repeat until cured.

As noted already, the treatment of any skin condition might include blood purifiers (q.v.). Although no such specific reference to this treatment has been found in the Newfoundland eczema record, one treatment that might possibly qualify was the drinking of a decoction of fir-tree tops over time (a tea with seven tops might be specified). One Newfoundland record states: Take the tops of five or six virgin fir trees, sometimes called maiden fir (q.v.); steep over a very hot fire for a full day. Strain into a container and drink. Do not add anything. The informant added: "It's worth all the bloody prescriptions that you can get from all the doctors this side of hell!"

Depending on the severity of the eczema, Newfoundlanders often tried commercial preparations specifically advertised for eczema. During the first half of the century, popular ones were Zylex, Dr. Chase's Ointment, Mecca Ointment, and Nixoderm – emollients, and in some cases, antiseptics – and Cuticura Soap. Most have faded from memory, as have the relatively few locally manufactured items, such as Superb Ointment produced by Allan Morgan of Coley's Point (said to be new in a 1955 advertisement).

Some consider that the claims of the preparations mentioned were as unwarranted as those currently found in the promotion of such "new" self-care skin treatments as evening primrose oil. This item, which has become popular in Newfoundland, as elsewhere, through recent health-food promotion, is considered by many to be useful for numerous conditions, including eczema, premenstrual tension, and psoriasis. It is too early to be certain whether the optimism – some from medical scientists – is overstated. In the meantime, the primrose oil story raises questions about the extent to which lay confidence initially depends on experience, theory, or authority.

NOTES
See: CMG (1992) 013, for mutton suet.
    Representative MUNFLA references: 63-1/8 (cod-liver-oil poultice), 69-23/10 (fir-tree tops), 69-25/15 (bathe in brook), 82-122 (scorched rag, urine).

ELDER (ELDERBERRY), ELDER BLOSSOM

A Newfoundland record of 1899 states: "The inner bark of the elder, boiled until a tar-like decoction is obtained from it, is used for plasters. Elder blossoms are used for inflammations." Only the latter use of elder blossoms has been recorded more recently; generally elder blossoms were made into a poultice or salve for treating sores. It seems likely, too, that teas (made from the bark) were also used occasionally for feverish conditions (see *fevers)*, and perhaps rationalized as a cleansing effect if a laxative response occurred (see below.)

**M. CONNORS, Druggist**

**ELDER BLOSSOMS**

*Water Street West, St. John's, N. F.*

It is uncertain whether the 1899 record refers to *Sambucus pubens* (generally known as elder), or *Heracleum lanatum* (popularly known by many other names besides elder blossom [see *wild-parsnip*]), both of which grow in the island, or even to purchased material. In fact *S. pubens* (also known as catberry and elm-blossom berry) is not one of the *Sambucus* species which have long been popular in medicine, both the professional and lay varieties. Most attention has been given to the European *S. nigra* and, in North America, to *S. canadensis*, both of which are regarded as possessing the same medicinal properties, namely for use in skin conditions (including the flowers) and as a laxative (the inner bark). A rationale for the early Newfoundland reference to the use of the inner bark for plasters is unclear, unless it is merely that it retains heat effectively like other poultice materials.

NOTES
See: Introduction to bibliography for general history and background information; Bergen (1899) III.

Representative MUNFLA references: 63-1/27 (elder blossoms for sores), 82-146 (poultice on sore and for blood poisoning).

EPILEPSY AND FITS

Surprisingly, perhaps, few references to epilepsy exist in the Newfoundland record, given that fits (or convulsions) generally prompt alarm and fear among family and the general populace. The fear of the unknown contributed to the long-standing persistence of a belief in magical/religious causes. One recent Newfoundland record notes that fits were caused by an evil that possessed the body: "These were evil spirits and it was almost impossible to get rid of them. In some cases it was believed that these spirits entered the body because of some wrong the individual had done or because he had 'sold his soul' to the devil for some material possession." Dealing with such beliefs led one to the priest as much as the doctor; for immediate first-aid, however, cold water may have been thrown on the face of the patient.

Fits in young children, commonly in association with fevers, produce particular worry and fear; again, however, few treatment suggestions have been found. One said to immerse the child in cold water, possibly to reduce the high temperature commonly recognized as associated with convulsions. This would undoubtedly be more useful – at least in many circumstances – than another Newfoundland suggestion to take a sweater off, turn it inside out, and put it back on. The latter, however, might at least have kept parents occupied while a single fit passed.

NOTES
Representative MUNFLA references: 64-5/104 (sweater off), 73-150 (evil spirits and fits), 84-300B (cold water).

ERYSIPELAS

Worry always exists with erysipelas – in the past sometimes called St. Anthony's Fire (see *skin diseases*) – a generalized infection of the skin which nowadays demands antibiotic care. Lay diagnosis, however, has never been as precise as that of physicians, and the term at times covers red rashes not linked to infection. Specific recommendations for relieving symptoms are found in the Newfoundland record; they include producing a "cooling" action by applying baking powder, bread and soda water (bread soda), or mashed tansy flowers. Another suggestion was to apply rolled oats soaked in vinegar plus tansy and to cover with a rhubarb leaf; this dressing was to be changed twice a day. The informant added that an ointment had been bought from a druggist, but that "mother-in-law said it would kill him!"

No doubt supportive care was also given, as were blood purifiers (q.v.). Dr. Hamilton's Pills, advertised for erysipelas ("one of mankind's deadliest foes") in 1906, were a laxative. Aside from some relief, it is unlikely that any treatment had specific effects on a condition managed nowadays by antibiotics.

NOTES
Representative MUNFLA references: 78-200 (bread soda), 78-205 (tansy, iodine circle around neck).

EYES

The various recommendations for treating eyes recorded in the Newfoundland oral tradition – aside from snow-blindness (q.v.) – fall into various categories:

*Bad or failing eyesight*   Although in other folk traditions numerous recommendations exist to bathe eyes (for example, with the herb eyebright, generally *Euphrasia* spp.), the Newfoundland record is relatively silent. The only clear recommendation for failing eyesight (aside from night-blindness, see below) is to have one's ears pierced and to wear gold earrings – the importance of gold was stressed. The lack of suggestions is all the more surprising since it seems that cataracts and other eye problems, such as pterygium (a growth of the conjunctiva over the cornea) and perhaps Labrador keratopathy, often went untreated by doctors in rural Newfoundland. Even in 1975 it was reported that in one section of the Newfoundland population there was a considerably higher proportion of persons with uncorrected refraction errors. Whether or not this has some association with illiteracy is unclear.

Glasses, if worn, were commonly purchased by trying them on at "Woolco" or some such place.

*"Sore eyes" and "tired eyes"*   A well-known recommendation was to wash the eyes with "the first snow in May" (or just snow in May), which may have been bottled and saved (May water). One Newfoundland informant thought this practice was linked with May being the month of the Virgin Mary and the need to receive her blessing. Perhaps, too, there was a vague link with a common treatment for sore eyes in Ireland, namely, the water of certain holy wells. The application of fresh urine was also recommended (see *animal parts*), as was getting the ears pierced.

*Sties*   The most common suggestion for treating sties, sometimes called "wests" in the Newfoundland record, was to rub a wedding (or gold) ring on the stye. Specific details vary from rubbing nine times (for nine consecutive mornings or days; sometimes thirteen times was mentioned), to making the sign of the crucifix (sometimes for nine days) or an X on or over the stye. The use of a mother's or widow's ring might be specifically recommended. At least two explanations were used to justify the ring: that it had been blessed at a wedding ceremony, or that it was gold.

Borax washes (q.v.) were also tried, a practice more in keeping with professional medical recommendations.

*Infections, sometimes called "red eye"*   Aside from the general suggestions for sore eyes, specific recommendations for "infections" (conjunctivitis) included eye washes of boric acid solution (q.v.), a decoction of beaver root (q.v. "from the bottom of the pond"), a decoction of maple bark, and the application of wet tea leaves wrapped in cloth.

*Eyelids stuck*   One report notes that stuck eyelids were called "cackies" (seemingly a derivative of caked). Treatment was to bath with cooled, boiled water.

*Foreign body*   The obvious method – to remove the offending body with a cloth or finger – was not recorded, although the less practical (even if relatively safe) suggestion of getting a person to lick the eye was mentioned.

*Night-blindness*    Before the association between night-blindness and vitamin A deficiency was appreciated, Newfoundlanders recognized the value of eating the raw livers of sea birds, rabbits, or codfish (see *animal parts*). Cod liver oil is also noted. In 1921, a report noted that "potatoes roasted in ashes and eaten, skins and all, cod liver oil, and seal livers were said to have been used in a few instances with good results." The reputation of cod liver oil increased after the 1930s with the emerging knowledge about vitamin A content. There is no scientific justification for applying poultices of birds' livers to the eyes, but, like many regimens of the past, this combined internal and external usage of one product was viewed as important.

A noteworthy feature of all the suggested eye treatments is that relatively few medications were mentioned, even for bathing the eyes. As with many other areas of self-care in Newfoundland, herbal preparations are conspicuously few, at least compared with many other places. Yet Newfoundlanders did purchase Murine eye drops, which have been promoted in the island since at least the 1920s; used for "tired" eyes and the other conditions, they are still available.

NOTES
See: Richler (1979) and Gillan (1991), for background on Newfoundland eye conditions; Brown Collection (Hand 1961, vol. 6) 294–5, for a number of examples of rubbing a stye with a gold or wedding ring; Appleton (1921), on bird's liver, potatoes, and so on; Aykroyd (1928), for birds' livers including poultice; MCG (1992) 108, for cackies;

Representative MUNFLA references: 68-10/8 (beaver root), 68-19/7 (snow in May), 68-22/1 (tea leaves for infection), 69-11/3 and 73-142 (pierced ears), 82-149 (boric acid for eye infection), 82-218 (wedding band for stye, lick out foreign body), 84-173 (fresh cod liver for night-blindness), 84-286B (ears pierced).

FAT PORK (FAT BACK)

The ready availability of fat pork (generally salt-cured) partly explains the multiple usages for complaints ranging from seasickness (q.v., with hard bread) to warts (q.v.). When salted meat was suggested for treatment, fat pork was generally used. Long-standing magical and religious associations as well as successful use were all part of its reputation. Newfoundland records indicate that fat pork cooked on Shrove Tuesday (the day before Ash Wednesday) or put away on Good Friday was kept in the home "to ward off sickness" or, specifically, for toothache, sore fingers, and so on.

One commonplace usage – sometimes after soaking in kerosene – was its application to minor infections (a "whitlow," a "gathered finger," or a "rising.") Fat pork was noted, too, for boils (q.v.), and for preventing mosquito and fly bites. Some suggestions (for example, for treating warts) had a magical basis of sympathetic action; the pork was buried or otherwise thrown away after being applied to the lesion.

Testimony that fat back was often effective for other conditions exists, although these rarely reached the Newfoundland record. One Newfoundland report on its value for fevers, however, is in line with a statement in Gunn's once popular *New Family Physician* (1869): "There is great virtue in the simple remedy of Fat Bacon, and the efficacy of this remedy has been generally admitted by physicians who have used it in Scarlet Fever. My plan has been to have the whole body well rubbed, or greased, with the inside rind of fat, uncooked Bacon, during the whole course of the disease. When this simple remedy is applied, it gives instant relief, produces exemption from Fever, and affords instant, refreshing sleep."

Usage had probably become uncommon by the '60s, as much as anything because of the relative unpleasantness of the preparation.

NOTES
See: Gunn (1869) 444.

Representative MUNFLA references: 66-10/28 (mumps), 69-29/10 (infection), 73-189 (cooked on Shrove Tuesday), 78-179/18 (Good Friday), 78-195 (quinsy, warts), 78-200 (fat pork rind for boils), 82-122 (fat pork and hard bread for seasickness).

## FEMALE COMPLAINTS, MENSTRUATION, MENOPAUSE

The expression "female complaints" (or "female diseases"), as used within both lay and professional medicine, refers generally to menstrual irregularities, menopausal discomfort (notably cramps and hot flushes), and vaginal discharges. It is also used, however, for vague symptoms, often viewed as peculiar to the female psyche or body, and carries a negative connotation of weakness. Some see the term, especially when used by male physicians, as fostering stereotypes that women are inherently less suited than men to many situations, that they are not only inferior physically, but also intellectually. Past attitudes (see excerpt below) have also fostered views of women as inherent invalids.

I argue that the system of the *female* is the finer and more complicated, having to perform a double work (child bearing) yet confined to the same or less dimensions than the male. And to perform this *double* function of sustaining her own life, and giving life to her species; it becomes necessary in the wisdom of God to give her such a peculiar formation that, between the ages of fourteen and forty-five, or the child-bearing period, she should have a sanguineous (blood like) monthly discharge from the organs of generation, known under the various names of monthly sickness, menses, catamenia, courses, menstruation &c. Why it should have been so arranged, or necessary, none can tell ...

The female organism is such that, what affects the general system of the male, much more frequently affects the organs peculiar to *her* system only. No reason can be given for it except the wisdom of the Creator, or the necessities of her construction. But this *debility* and *irregularities* are so interwoven together that what causes one must necessarily affect the other. (Dr. Chase's Recipes, 1862)

The Newfoundland oral tradition records are strikingly silent concerning female disorders. That few treatments are listed may reflect reticence when the data was collected, as well as the relative silence in Newfoundland's past regarding many sexual matters. In fact, the only non-commercial treatments noted were for treating menstrual cramps and pain. Warmth (still recommended) was important: "A lot of times they'd have an old hotplate, heat a plate, wrap it in cloth and lay it on the stomach." Hot cloths, also suggested, were perhaps more convenient to use. "Some used to say it was better to put a hot brick to your feet, that the heat to your feet would do better," noted another source. Other recommendations were to keep warm and dry, and to take hot ginger tea (again the heat was considered significant). Amulets are noted under *cramps in muscles*.

No concrete suggestions have been found for managing vaginal discharges, though douching with an astringent tea was perhaps tried. By the 1950s, Lysol was noted for feminine hygiene, a forerunner of the growing commercial interest in vaginal douching. This, plus commercial pads and tampons, is a long way removed from the days when "you had no such pad or anything, just flannelette cut in strips and you had to clean that and boil it in Gillett's Lye and blue it and put them away for the next month."

If the oral record has been relatively silent, the promotion of various commercial female remedies, which also helped to shape attitudes toward women, was just as conspicuous as elsewhere. Although there have always been some health-care practitioners not wedded to stereotype notions of the inferiority of women, the commercial market continually reinforced this idea.

While numerous female remedies focused on regulating menstruation, the implication was that they regulated the timing of the female cycle in general. Well known around the 1900s was Dr. Pierce's Favorite Prescription ("Makes weak women strong," stated one Newfoundland advertisement). At face value this resembled to Lydia Pinkham's Vegetable Compound (see below). However, one published formula in indicating the presence of "savin" and "cinchona" (the latter the source of quinine) suggests Pierce's preparation had more of an emmenagogue action, that is to induce menstruation (and perhaps abortion). DeVans Female Pills and Orange Lily ("a sure relief for women's disorders"), advertised in Newfoundland, also appear to have been primarily emmenagogues.

Preparations indicating painkilling properties were increasingly promoted. There was Dr. Chase's Paradol ("when our first Almanac was published in 1904, we didn't have a product to relieve the pain and suffering of periodic distress" [1966]), as well as Midol ("Dora's down – menstrual pain. Dora's up with Midol [1952]). Other painkillers were undoubtedly used.

The link between nerves (q.v.) and "women's problems," particularly noticeable during the first half of the twentieth century, did as much as anything to underscore the concept of women's limitations. Although associating nerves and women was far from new, commercial preparations expanded and reinforced the notion. By 1900, the intensively promoted Paine's Celery Compound was being advertised (for instance, in the St. John's *Evening Telegram*) for nervous and weary women. (See also *rheumatism*). Attention given to nervous women was in line with the then-current interest in neurasthenia, a diagnosis that became popular during the last decades of the nineteenth century. Often described as due to "nervous exhaustion," neurasthenia was diagnosed as a syndrome of symptoms that included "sick headache, noises in the ear, atonic voice, deficient mental control, bad dreams, insomnia, and nervous dyspepsia." The theme of nervous conditions in women was promoted time and time again in advertisements, sometimes with an amazing lack of credibility, even for the time. Thus in the *Evening Telegram* for 19 November 1900, one could read: "If you are nervous and irritable, you may only need more fat to cushion your nerves – you are probably thin – and Scott's Emulsion of Cod Liver Oil will give you the fat to begin with." Among other intensively advertised products was Chase's Nerve Food. A common promotional theme is reflected in the following 1937 newspaper advertisement: "If there is anyone whose nerves are put to a severe test it is the mother in the home with all the cares and worries of housework and a family of lively, rollicking children to look after ... Once the nerves fail to get their full supply of nutrition from your blood you find yourself worried and sleepless and irritable and headed for a complete nervous collapse." Evidently, Chases's product was the answer.

Nowadays, at least since the early 1980s, such terms as "nerves" and "the blues" have partly been moved into the language of the premenstrual syndrome (PMS, still called by some premenstrual "tension"), even though hormonal imbalance has been viewed as the cause since the 1930s. No evidence is available, however, to indicate that Newfoundland women have responded any differently from other women in North America to the new emphasis on the condition and the ways of dealing with it. Some of these methods, which may be viewed as social (coping through discussion and reading, and not "being alone") contrast with prescription-only drug treatment and with directions to "work through it." Past decades, too, have seen the promotion of many so-called alternative treatments. As elsewhere, at least some Newfoundlanders are purchasing evening primrose oil and vitamins, and paying attention to diet.

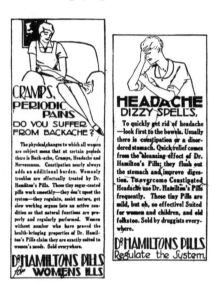

Advertisements for Dr. Hamilton's Pills,
early 1930s.

Tonics (q.v.), well known as a way of improving a general sense of well-being, have constituted another facet of the extensive armamentarium for treating female problems. Laxatives, too, were also encouraged for many vague so-called female symptoms and cramps. This seems to have been the case with Dr. Hamilton's Pills, intensively promoted at times, as in the following advertisements of the early 1930s.

Nowadays, much promotion of self-care for women focuses on urinary tract infections. Some wonder whether this justified the past promotion of Dodd's Kidney Pills (q.v.) for "female weakness" (assuming diuretic action was a property of the pills). One can also wonder if the pills, supported by statements (1927) that the "slightest disorder of the kidneys [that] brings about troubles which are well known and dreaded by most women," offered help with premenstrual tension through diuretic action. At present, besides cranberry juice for urinary tract infections, health-food stores frequently offer bearberry (q.v.) – a herb found in Newfoundland. Other herbs used for so-called kidney troubles include juniper (q.v.). Although this treatment is well established in Newfoundland, prudence is advocated because of possible toxic effects.

One group of herbal remedies (for example, squawvine, black cohosh, blue cohosh), long-known as female remedies, have been widely promoted in North America and elsewhere in recent years as "hormone" or "female" herbs. They have been employed for menopause and menstrual disorders, often with the presumption of restoring "balance." Although some herbs do have oestrogenic activity, this is not necessarily the case for all those now available to Newfoundlanders through health-food stores and other outlets.

Some of these so-called female herbs were once ingredients in such commercial preparations, advertised in the St. John's newspapers, as Lydia Pinkham's Vegetable Compound (at one time containing unicorn root, life root, black cohosh, pleurisy root, and fenugreek). Despite a long pedigree of usage, concerns exist today about the safety of taking some of the hormone herbs regularly – at least black cohosh and blue cohosh, for, say, menopause symptoms.

There is no way of knowing how much self-care is presently employed for menopause in Newfoundland. A recent study in a Newfoundland outport concluded that menopause is commonly viewed as a normal process; certainly many elderly Newfoundland women generally feel it was not talked about much in the "old days." Certainly it was not viewed as a medical event nor a deficiency hormonal disease, as is now implied in various writings on the menopause and by the readiness of many physicians to prescribe hormone-replacement treatment. When various menopausal symptoms are explained by Newfoundlanders in biological terms (linked with nerves or the blood), they are not perceived as unique to the life-change, apart from hot flushes, which may be viewed as a specific way for the body to rid itself of poison, in much the same way as menstruation.

It is possible that with changing times increasing numbers of Newfoundland women will see menopause as more a medical, or at least hormonal, rather than a life, event. Undoubtedly, the hormonal view of hot flushes and the growing professional medical influence in daily lives have encouraged women to try replacement treatment, perhaps with hormonal herbs or such so-called tonics as the increasingly popular ginseng. Further, the notion of retained impurities may encourage the use of blood purifiers.

Although reinforcing female stereotypes is less conspicuous than in former times, self-care remains a major issue in womens' health. This is linked in part to many women's concern that medicalization of numerous health issues – still encouraged by commercial interests – undermines the personal control of their bodies.

NOTES
See: Chase (1862) 189–91; Goodenough (1909) 630, for Pierce formula; Thomas (1982), female remedies and the notion of invalidism; Snow and Johnson (1977), for menstruation beliefs in North America; Davis, D.L. (1983b, 1988), for an outport study of menopause; Stage (1979), on Lydia Pinkham; Apple (1990), Cayleff (1990), Mitchinson (1991), for general background; Bell (1987), on medicalization of menopause; MCG (1992) 108, for hot plate and brick; MCG (1992) 104, on flannelette strips.

Representative MUNFLA references: 67-2/39 (ginger tea), 67-19/4 (keep warm and dry).

### FEVERS

Although feverish conditions were commonplace in all communities, the coverage of associated treatments in the Newfoundland oral record is sparse. For example, while childhood fevers are usually remembered, in general only scarlet and rheumatic fever prompt clear memories. For instance, "One of my sisters had scarlet fever real bad. We used to live on a road, a lane, and it was all barred of from horses, nothing could come around ... My father wasn't allowed in the house ... he had to go to work see. He had to live with his sister." The only herb remedies noted are sarsaparilla (q.v.) wine "made from berries," elder blossom (q.v.), and senna. A possible justification for using the first two was their presumed blood-purifying properties; senna, on the other hand had a laxative action, with a general cleansing action.

The approach of "sweating out a fever" was quite common; that involved taking a hot bath, drinking spirits or possibly Labrador tea (q.v.), piling on blankets, and, perhaps, taking aspirin. When the fever was a symptom of say, a severe cold, chest treatments were also used.

Recommendations based on non-natural approaches are conspicuous in the Newfoundland record, though it is not clear that they were widely used. One suggestion, to "transfer" a fever, is described as follows: kill a hen, pluck it, and place it on the sick person's chest. When the hen is removed it will be black, and inflammation from chest will "come out in the hen." Another suggestion, to put pickled herring on and around the feet, was reported not to work. (See also *measles* and *mumps*.)

NOTES
See: MCG (1992), scarlet fever.
   Representative MUNFLA references: 69-2/7 (sarsaparilla wine), 69-6/3 (pickled herring), 69-25/16 (hen on chest), 77-87 (elder blossom), 82-218 (senna leaves).

### FISH DOCTOR

A fish doctor, a crustacean parasite on cod, is about an inch long and orange in colour. The name is perhaps linked to their being found on wounded fish, although there is also the suggestion that the soft parts were used as a salve for sores. Fish doctors have perhaps been best known as charms to protect against rheumatism and arthritis (q.v.).

NOTES
See: *Dictionary of Newfoundland English* (1990) 178.
   Representative MUNFLA references: 69-7 MS (rheumatism).

FITS (SEE EPILEPSY)

FLANNEL

Wearing flannel – alone or perhaps with an application of goose grease, turpentine, or camphorated oil – for colds, bronchitis, pneumonia, pleurisy (next to the chest), and for rheumatism (over the pain) – has been as well known in Newfoundland as elsewhere. One Newfoundland observer (1936) stated: "A suit of [flannel] is sewn on the body of the person suffering from rheumatism and it is kept on until worn out; or underclothes made from the same material may be worn. A shirt of it is worn all the year round for asthma and bronchitis. It is sewn around the wrists to prevent "sea boils"; it prevents chafing by the sleeves of the oiled jacket." Many Newfoundland reports stressed the use of *red* flannel.

Flannel's long pedigree was recognized by Newfoundlanders. Eighteenth-century medical writers – at a time when "obstructed perspiration" was felt to cause numerous ailments – often recommended flannel to promote perspiration. For instance: "Flannel is warmth without encumbrance, and it acts as a friction to the skin and keeps the pores open; it also creates a uniform atmosphere around the body" (Benjamin Moseley 1787). Innumerable recommendations for the use of flannel appeared in nineteenth-century writings, but these were limited in the first half of the twentieth century to chest ailments and rheumatism, as in the Newfoundland record.

Contributing to the decline in flannel usage, aside from the impact of such newer treatments as antibiotics and other antimicrobials, was the demise of the theory of obstructed perspiration in professional medicine. Nevertheless, the notion persists in popular health literature whenever the state of the pores is considered, as it does vis-à-vis the catching of colds in changeable weather, once rationalized by the notion of closed pores.

Just why *red* flannel became favoured is not clear; nor is the reason for its popularity in Newfoundland. Explanations have included a special power attributed to the red colour, but whether it was this power or merely the red colour (on the basis of the adage that a red colour may cure red conditions) that was believed to help draw out inflammation is uncertain.

NOTES
See: Parsons (1936), for quotation; Renbourn (1957), for general background and Moseley quote.

Representative MUNFLA references: 78-195 (red flannel around the neck for sore throat), 79-189 (grandfather wore a complete set of red flannel underwear), 78-200 (flannel and turpentine for chest cold).

FLIES: BLACK, HOUSE

The scourge of "biting" black flies is known to every Newfoundlander during the summer months. Many preparations to ward them off were tried but with varying success. "One of the biggest things up the Labrador [Captain Troake recorded in 1989] was the black flies, the worst things, and the sand flies you could hardly see. Nobody enjoyed the Labrador. The only thing you could do was to use Stockholm or pine tar, twenty-five percent tar in olive oil – or a mixture of it – and smear it over your face. It was messy, but the flies won't touch it." Pennyroyal, a well-known insect repellent was combined with the tar on occasions, including in a commercial preparation produced by Acme Co. of St. John's. In fact, it was labelled as the "unrivalled preventer of mosquito bites."

Barrier methods for combating flies are also significant in the Newfoundland tradition. Goose grease (q.v.) and various preparations made in pharmacies were used. Newfoundland physician Cluny Macpherson, like many others, may well have favoured "Newfoundland Fly Dope." The formula called for 5 parts of quinine hydrochloride; 70 parts of anhydrous wool fat; 25 parts of cod liver oil; and up to 2 ounces of ionone (a violet scent), according to preference. Kerosene was also tried, but generally considered to be less effective than this Fly Dope. "Black mud" is remembered as part of the Micmac tradition.

Nowadays, barrier methods tend to be forgotten in the face of countless commercial insect repellents, although many Newfoundlanders find them relatively ineffective against the flies.

Various items were tried as relief when barriers failed. As noted under rashes, Calamine lotion, an over-the-counter preparation, was relatively popular for all insect bites. Laundry blue, wrapped in a damp cloth, was also used on occasions for flies, although this had more of a reputation for treating insect stings, as did mud.

Houseflies have probably aroused less concern among Newfoundlanders than black flies, even though the growing twentieth-century fear of house flies as disease-spreaders affected Newfoundland as elsewhere. The "nuisance" season, however, has always been relatively short and somewhat controllable with fly papers and swatters before window screens.

NOTES
See: Troake (1989), 49; Rogers (1989), for general remarks on houseflies; Crellin and O'Mara (1990), on Newfoundland Fly Dope; Saunders (1986) 137, on pennyroyal; MCG (1993) 2, on Micmac tradition.

Representative MUNFLA reference: 73-150.

Personal communication: R. Day (1991), on goose grease.

## FLU (SEE INFLUENZA)

## FRECKLES (SEE COMPLEXION)

## FRIAR'S BALSAM

Among over-the-counter preparations, the compounded Friar's Balsam – an alcoholic preparation of beuzoin, aloes, storax, and balsam of tolu – remains well known for cuts and abrasions (see *cuts*). But it became something of a general purpose medicine: "That's what you'd

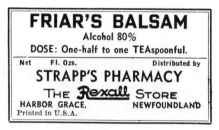

**FRIAR'S BALSAM**
Alcohol 80%
DOSE: One-half to one TEAspoonful.
Net    Fl. Ozs.                    Distributed by
**STRAPP'S PHARMACY**
THE *Rexall* STORE
HARBOR GRACE,                  NEWFOUNDLAND
Printed in U.S.A.

take for a cold if you had a sore throat. You'd take it on a little bit of sugar and partly fill the spoon with Friar's balsam and a bit of sugar and take it to clear the cold out of your throat." It was tried in cases of asthma (q.v.) as well.

NOTES
See: MCG (1992) 3.

## FROSTBITE

References to "frostbite" or "frostburn" in the oral tradition almost certainly include the less severe frostnip; that is local, reversible injury to, for instance, ear lobes, nose, cheeks, fingers, and toes. In professional medicine, the term "frostbite" is generally reserved for cases where permanent injury is produced.

Although gentle rewarming has long been practised by physicians, the notion of applying snow (or cold water) has been widespread in Newfoundland and persists, as elsewhere. ("Rub a bit of snow. Just keep rubbing it, and it comes right back to life.") One Newfoundland informant said it removed the pain. Cold, in fact, has been recommended by some physicians in the past, alongside controversy over the effectiveness of rewarming. A 1927 work on domestic medicine, written by a physician, suggests for frostbite: "Rub with snow or ice-cold water till sensation returns. Artificial warmth applied to a frost bite will cause mortification."

Herb treatment has found little place in the oral tradition, though Bergen (1899) listed "the inside bark of the birch" (q.v.) as an application. It was used with or without cod liver oil. At least two records mention the use of brains of the jay, mixed with either an unidentified herb or with sap from

the inner bark of a fir tree. This was to to be left in place for nine days –
a once commonplace time period in health care that added authority to
the regimen.

Sometimes problems occur with infection in the damaged tissue. A
Newfoundland suggestion to add fresh cow-dung to the affected area might
compound this problem, despite views as to its beneficial action.

NOTES
See: Bergen (1899) 110; Black (1927) 229, and MCG (1992) 002, on snow, and so
on for frostbite; Tyler (1985) 85, who noted applications of beech and oak leaves
and assumed they were applied warm (perhaps this was the case with birch in
Newfoundland).

Representative MUNFLA references 67-20/31 and 67-4/11 (jaybird brains), 66-16/
37 (cow-dung), 68-28/10 (snow).


GALLS

Skin sores (and hard skin) arising from rubbing or chafing are described in
Newfoundland as "galls," a term that also includes blisters and blood
blisters. Galls are also known – particularly by fishermen – as "deadeyes"
when they appear on the palm.

One recommendation found in the recently recorded Newfoundland
tradition for removal of this type of blister was to thread a needle with
homespun wool; pull the needle and wool through the gall; and then cut
off the ends, leaving the wool inside. Evidently, the gall dries up. Another
suggestion was to place oakum (q.v.) between the two surfaces that rubbed
against each other; the impregnated coal tar was probably of some value.
Suggestions to prevent galls included washing the hands often while handling fish and greasing the palms.

NOTES
Representative MUNFLA references: 68-26/5 (threaded needle), 82-122 (oakum).


GERMS, DISINFECTANTS

As indicated in Part I, a close association generally exists between personal
health practices and the effectiveness of public-health education. It is not
easy to assess the early impact of the germ theory in Newfoundland.
Although public fascination and preoccupation with germs was widespread
following the acceptance of the germ theory of disease in the 1880s, the
notion probably emerged more slowly in Newfoundland than in many
other places. There was, for instance, little discussion about prevention
(including disinfection) in newspapers during the 1880s and 1890s, and it

is likely that the lack of a commercial face, along with other communication problems (including illiteracy), made Newfoundlanders comparatively unreceptive to public-health promotion, except during outbreaks of, say, diphtheria. As a postscript to the spittoon story told in Part I, the following comments, written in 1910, are noteworthy: "It is through the fish-hook and the knife that so many septic wounds are caused, and the hospitals and the mission ship, 'Strathcona' are kept looking after their patients. These wounds, through neglect on the part of the fishermen, often become so serious that amputation is necessary. Any form of asepsis is unknown to these people, and attempts to teach them are met with a curious indifference, as they think that the poultice of their forefathers is good enough for them."

Despite these opinions (overly negative since poultices were widely used everywhere at the time for such conditions), concerns in Newfoundland about smallpox, typhoid, diphtheria, and tuberculosis were changing. Indeed, they gave meaning to the announcement by Dicks Company (for example, in 1906) that "germ-proof [writing] slates" were available; unfortunately, it is not known whether such items were taken seriously. Newfoundlanders were also urged to use Dustbane in schools: "Prevents dust rising while sweeping. Dustbane means a saving. Schoolroom dust is unhealthy. It spreads disease and its effect is far reaching" (1925). This is not to say that lay understanding of germs and their roles in disease was comprehensive at the time, or even over the next few decades (see *tuberculosis*).

Disinfectants did much to arouse public awareness of germs. By around 1900, for instance, many carbolic-acid preparations were advertised in Newfoundland – Carbolic Tooth Powder, Carbolic Toilet Soap, Carbolic Ointment, and Carbolic Disinfecting Powder – from the Calvert Company of Manchester, England. In 1925, Stanyl was noted as a safeguard for "germs lurking in cracks and crevices." Later, Jeyes Company products came to the fore.

How much general disinfection was done in and around the home to prevent "house diseases" is unknown. Nor is it known whether all those used were effective. In fact, many Newfoundlanders preferred Gillett's lye as a disinfectant. Also well remembered is the wide acceptance of fumigation – albeit in use long before the germ theory – for disinfecting rooms whenever a contagious disease broke out in the family.

Many over-the-counter "medicines" joined in the "fight" against germs for a wide range of ailments. Around 1905, for instance, Newfoundlanders were told that Liquozone Tonic destroyed the "cause of

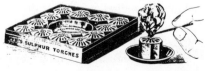

Commercial sulphur candles or torches (1899) used to fumigate rooms.

any germ disease." An offer of $1000 was made for any disease germ it did not kill!

Many preparations were applied to the skin, such as Jeysol, iodine, and Nixoderm (a skin preparation said to kill germs within seven minutes). If by the 1950s, overt concerns about germs had lessened somewhat during the new era of antibiotics and the ever-increasing control of infections, the killing of mouth germs remained a key promotional target. Although Sanitas, as "the all-purpose disinfectant," had long been recommended as a mouth and tooth wash, it was Listerine that gained momentum and remained in the public mind through intensive advertising. (See also *anti-septic ointment*.)

NOTES
See: Musson (1910), for quote on fish-hook and knife wounds.

Representative MUNFLA reference: 78-200 (wash clothes of people cured of TB or diphtheria with Gillette's lye to get rid of germs, smoke dwelling with sulphur.)

GIN PILLS

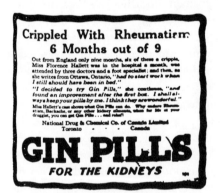

Gin Pills, long advertised "for the kidney" before the above-mentioned promotion of 1930, became one of the best known over-the-counter remedies in Newfoundland during the first half of the twentieth century. The pills are well remembered for changing the colour of urine: "Gin Pills will turn your water green. Well you take a man, an old man, perhaps anywhere he might have to dart and make his water. It could be snow, a bank of snow or something and where he made his water was green, all green. There was no trouble to tell that he was taking Gin Pills."

As with many so-called kidney medicines, Gin Pills were employed for a range of conditions in which some so-called purification seemed appropriate. Although information on the past constituents of the pills has not been found, the colour change was probably due to methylene blue, often included in kidney medicines during the first half of the twentieth century. The term "gin" implied the presence of juniper (q.v.).

Gin Pills – today's contain sodium salicylate – are still being promoted (for example, in Chase's Almanac) but not for kidneys. Instead, the ad says "for prompt pain relief of backache, muscle ache, arthritic and rheumatic pain."

NOTES
See: Troake (1989) 37, urine turning green; Chase's *Almanac* 1993.

## GINGER

Recollections such as the following reflect the popularity of certain notions, among Newfoundlanders for example, that ginger had a long history as a spice and stimulant, as well as a beverage (for instance, ginger beer). "My father put a lot of dependence in ginger wine, about half a teaspoonful in a cup of hot water; it is good relief when he was choked up with asthma, or if he felt a cold coming on." As elsewhere, various ginger essences, to be diluted before use, were sold in stores throughout Newfoundland. Stafford's, perhaps prepared in St. John's, was in demand for many years. Like other ginger preparations (sometimes mixed with molasses), it was recommended for colds and upset stomachs. Its pungency and volatile oil content contributed to relief.

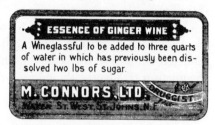

Label for ginger wine

Although ginger has largely disappeared as a home remedy, interest in using the root to relieve seasickness and motion sickness, in general, has recently emerged (See *seasickness*).

NOTES
See: Introduction to bibliography for general history and background information; Piercey (1992), for ginger wine quotation.

Representative MUNFLA references: 67-2/40 (hot ginger tea, menstrual cramps), 67-2/45 (tea made from ground ginger to induce vomiting, perhaps for upset stomach), 67-5/68 (ginger and molasses for colds).

## GOOSE GREASE

Goose grease – a by-product of a goose dinner (keeping grease from a Christmas or New Year's dinner is still remembered by many elderly Newfoundlanders) – has probably been the island's most widely used application (or "rub") "for the chest" and one that has treated "all" respiratory complaints. As one informant said: "Well, when I'd have a cold, mother would listen to this now. She was an expert on preserving goose grease. She had it as clear as amber. She'd have it in a special bottle and heat it in a saucer on the stove. And she'd rub my neck and shoulders if I had a cold or anything."

Mixed with honey, goose grease was also taken internally for croup. In both conditions, aromatic substances (for example, Minard's Liniment q.v.) were sometimes incorporated with the grease. ("My mother, she always treated us herself with goose grease and medicine she would mix up herself ... Nowadays, I don't use the goose grease, but I mix up vinegar and molasses when I have a cold.")

Aside from chest ailments, goose grease was used (with much positive testimony) to rub over aching muscles, sometimes described as rheumatism. It was also (as it still is) used as an application to prevent the flies biting (see *flies*).

Other fats were tried at times. One alternative (probably rarely used) was the fat of a fish called a "pig puffin" (pig fish or sculpin). The fat was rendered out and retained for rubbing on aching backs and limbs, and for rheumatism. Evidently, the odour was obnoxious.

N O T E S
See: MCG (1992) 001, for amber goose grease; MCG (1992) 106, for quotation on mixing goose grease with commercial medicines.

Representative MUNFLA references: 67-14/75 (croup), 73-189 (pig puffin fat), 76-249 (bronchitis), 82-122 (with flannel for colds), 82-238 (colds).

Personal communication: R. Day (1991), for goose grease for flies.

## GUMBOIL

Inflammation or an abscess at the root of a tooth was often associated with bad teeth (see *teeth*). A long-standing professional recommendation – to apply a codeine solution (obtained from a physician or a store) – was presumably tried on occasion prior to the use of antibiotics. Keeping a raisin (sometimes called a "fig" in Newfoundland) in place over the inflamed area was initially more convenient. Stories abounded. In the following, the informant referred to his or her grandfather when talking about the gumboil:

Did you ever hear tell of a gumboil? It comes on your mouth inside, kind of a bubble, something like an abscess. But grandfather had a very big one. He had big feet anyway, he was a big man, one fellow was a little tiny man and the other fellow was a big man. He used to have a lot of trouble with his leg and he used to love to go down to the fishing room, he always used to call that years ago [the waterfront from where the fishery is conducted], that would be way back in the eighties.

Then he would get tired coming up and he would sit down on the bank on the side of the street coming up to the house, there were no cars then, only cars were the merchants and the doctor and the priest. He always wanted salt water and father used to go and he'd always bring him up in the evening a bucket of salt water and he'd put his feet in it. I would wash his legs over and over with the salt water. I don't know what it did to him but it must have been some relief to him.

Preventive dental care and, perhaps, improved nutrition, have reduced the incidence of this painful condition.

NOTES
See: MCG (1992) 008, gumboil story; Tyler (1985), who notes the use of a fig for a gumboil (perhaps a raisin was intended).

HANGOVER (SEE DRUNKENNESS)

HEADACHE

The many treatment recommendations in the Newfoundland oral tradition, as elsewhere, rarely if ever specified usage for particular types of headache. Amid the striking range of general treatments, the suggestions to use aromatic substances were commonplace. They included (for rubbing on the forehead, applying to a headband, or sniffing) Minard's Liniment, Sloan's Liniment, eau-de-Cologne, tansy (perhaps in the form of a poultice kept in place by a band), and vinegar (the last, as commonly noted, should be applied on brown paper). One recent record (1992) is telling: "My remedy for headaches, I suppose it is foolish, but I believe in it. You get vinegar and brown paper and tie it around your head and when the paper got dry, well dip it down in the vinegar again and tie it around again, and after about half-an-hour's time the pain must go. I don't use it nowadays – I don't have headaches very much. But I used it once, I think it was last year." Another account draws attention to the role of women. "There was an old lady down in Blow-me-Down and she always chewed gum and they called her Aunt Ev. If it was bad they'd call her. She'd come up and squeeze this way and that way. I think it was nine mornings she'd come. She'd put a piece of brown paper across the forehead dipped in vinegar, then tie a band on tight." The above approaches, mostly in line with the recommendations of regular medicine (aside from squeezing over nine days), often provided symptomatic relief.

A noteworthy alternative to vinegar was the "vinegar plant" (q.v. "Put vinegar plant in bottle, let stay for a while then put plant on head"). More complicated regimens – perhaps for persistent headaches – could creep into treatment, as reflected in a mixture of pepper, salt, Minard's liniment, and, sometimes, vinegar – all soaked into a cloth and wrapped around the head.

Placing various substances – a cold or wet cloth, wet paper, ice, or cool leaves of alder (q.v.) – on the forehead was probably quite commonly tried, and not just for treating hangover headaches. Cool clothes were also recommended, as was the following suggestion for inhalation. First, one boils in water some poppy buds (said to be water lily, not poppy, though this was grown in some outport homes); then a cloth or towel is placed over the head so the steam can be inhaled.

Perhaps the intractable headaches – the migraines – were the ones that more often attracted magical treatments, such as walking backwards in a circle. Another such suggestion was to stand on the head until dizzy (an idea sometimes rationalized as "sending blood to the head"). In fact, treatments by transference (for instance, cutting and burying hair) have not been found recorded on the island, although they are well known to folklorists.

Severe headaches might also have prompted the use of "penny blisters." According to one informant: "These were the size of a postage stamp. When the white backing was removed the black, sticky surface was applied to the trouble spot, mostly behind my ears. The next morning there were large blisters full of fluid that my mother let off with a sewing needle."

Among other commercial preparations, aspirin (q.v.) was used as soon as it became generally available in the early 1900s. "Headache powders" (see *analgesics*) have also been and are still popular in places. Also successfully marketed in Newfoundland were Nerviline ("corrects stomach trouble and stops the headache"), Dr. Hobson's Headache Wafers, Dr. Hamilton's Pills ("may now be obtained at all general stores [1927]), and Kline's Headache Wafers (in fact these were cachets). Such handy over-the-counter preparations usually contained pain-killing acetanilide, antipyrine, phenacetin, or aspirin. Often perceived to be "strong" medicine, they became dominant in self-treatment.

Today, acetylsalicylic acid – in its various commercial forms including Bayer aspirin (q.v.) – remains prominent in self-care for occasional headaches, except for children under twelve (for fear of Reye's syndrome) and for those with a history of indigestion and ulcers. In fact, the recognition of many potential side-effects from such a long-standing home-remedy contributes to some people's worries over non-natural remedies.

Increasingly, physicians and lay people alike have emphasized various factors considered to precipitate headaches: diet, stress, eye strain, sinus, and so on. Migraine headaches, a special problem, have spawned a considerable range of prescription-only treatments, all of which can have unpleasant effects as well. This has encouraged interest in such "natural" self-care remedies as feverfew.

NOTES
See: Brown Collection (Hand 1961, vol. 6) 205–10, for a long list of treatments including transference; Piercey (1992) 66, on ear blisters; MCG (1992) 105, (brown paper and vinegar); MCG (1992) 109, on Aunt Ev.

Representative MUNFLA references: 68-011E (eau-de-Cologne), 69-007F ("poppy" heads), 76-249 (cool clothes), 77-87 (walking backwards in a circle), 78-195 (vinegar cloth, walking in circle backwards), 78-200 (tansy, Minard's, Sloan's, standing on head), 82-238 (brown paper and vinegar), 89-218 (pepper, salt, Minard's vinegar).

## HEARTBURN

While "heartburn" is commonly viewed as dyspepsia (q.v.), some Newfoundlanders have limited the term to upper chest pain, perhaps associated with reflux. (The expression "stomach trouble" [q.v.], on the other hand, refers to gas and griping without any sensation of burning or reflux.) Newfoundland suggestions for treating heartburn included honey in tea, a solution of baking soda, as well as bread and soda water – all preparations commonly felt "to ease" the stomach. Chewing gum, another suggestion, may have been viewed the same way.

It is difficult to know whether smelling fingers – after they have been rubbed under a sweaty arm or between the toes – played a significant role or, indeed, whether the practice was seriously believed; perhaps the suggestion was nothing more than a personal idiosyncrasy. In addition, the rationale behind eating a "bit of earwax" is uncertain, although the wax was noted to be bitter and, hence, in line with the use of other bitters (q.v.) used for stomach complaints.

By the early years of this century, heartburn (also described as cardialgia) – diagnosed by physicians as pains in the stomach and chest and a generally disturbed appetite – was, as with many ailments at the time, attributed to excess acidity. Recommendations of alkali treatment in popular medical books such as *The New Warren's Household Physician* (1903) suggest swallowing a teaspoonful of soda, magnesia, or chalk in a tumbler of cold or warm water. Newfoundland recommendations for baking soda and soda water are similar.

Until the 1950s, any over-the-counter medicines promoted among Newfoundlanders were generally directed toward all stomach ailments; sometimes, however, heartburn was singled out. Pape's Diapepsin ("Instantly! End indigestion, gas, heartburn, acidity") was one of a number of preparations considered to enhance digestion by increasing enzyme action, rather than counteracting acid. (See also under *stomach trouble*.)

Nowadays, as noted under *dyspepsia*, antacids remain the principal non-prescription treatment, although some specific products for heartburn contain alginates, believed to stop stomach acid from entering the oesophagus. Avoidance of certain foods and attention to eating habits are among other considerations.

NOTES
See: Warren (1903) 309.
    Representative MUNFLA references: 69-21/10 (fingers under sweaty arm), 76-249 (honey, bread soda, baking soda), 84-173 (earwax).

## HAEMORRHOIDS (PILES)

Recorded Newfoundland recommendations for haemorrhoids (distended or varicosed veins around the lower end of the bowel) range widely, as they do in other societies. Applications – also felt to have a general healing action on other skin ailments and sores – include pine tar, oakum (q.v.), and kerosene oil (q.v.). The use of a "maiden fir tree" (q.v.) is also noted, although the directions (to wrap the branch in cloth and apply to rectum, before discarding) make it more of a magical transference treatment, rather than one utilizing the pharmacological properties associated with the fir.

The therapeutic value ascribed to heat for many ailments is reflected in suggestions to sit on a heated object. Sitting on a pork-barrel cover (or head), thoroughly heated in the oven, and then placed on a wooden chair, is one such example. The value of this treatment depended to some extent on the severity of the condition. Another approach using warmth, sometimes recommended by physicians, involved taking a "pile bath" or a regular bath (still recommended); sitting in hot water with the addition of, for instance, Epsom salts can bring ease.

Epsom salts – a laxative – was also suggested for internal administration, thus acknowledging that constipation added to the discomfort of haemorrhoids. Perhaps this is one reason for the Newfoundland suggestion to drink pear juice.

It is noteworthy that astringent preparations, often mentioned in accounts of traditional haemorrhoid treatments elsewhere, have not been found in Newfoundland records. Some commercial preparations – for example, Dr. Bovel's Gum Salve – may possibly have such a property. Pazo Ointment was probably the best known over-the-counter preparation, until superseded by such applications as Preparation H (containing a yeast-cell derivative, shark liver oil, and phenyl mercuric nitrate). Although exceptionally well known, it must still compete with Chase Ointment, advertised in the 1993 Chase's *Almanac*, for "the misery of itching piles."

NOTES
Representative MUNFLA references: 66-21/14 (pear juice), 67-20/32 (heat tub of salt pickle and sit in steam); 69-7 Ms (oakum), 78-195 (pine tar, warmed head of barrel), 82-122 (oakum, vaseline).

## HERNIA

Newfoundland newspaper advertisements for Skull's Patent Okonite Trusses (for example, in the 1890s) and for Brooks Rupture Appliance (in 1918) are one reminder that hernias have long been commonplace in Newfoundland. Indeed, they can be said to be an occupational hazard for fishermen and loggers. If it is surprising that treatment suggestions are not found in the Newfoundland oral record, it may be because trusses remained in common usage long after surgery had become the accepted treatment (unless an operation was contraindicated). In 1951, Newfoundlanders were told to write to Beasley's in Toronto in response to the claim: "Painful trusses abolished. Wonderful new support. Endorsed by the medical profession." (See *Passing through* for children's hernias).

### HICCOUGHS (HICCUPS)

A variety of suggestions are found in the recently recorded Newfoundland oral tradition for what many people (not just Newfoundlanders) have insisted on calling "eggcups". Among the well-remembered "old cures" – none unique to Newfoundland – are holding one's breath, taking deep breaths (sometimes with the head in a brown bag), blowing into a bag, and drinking sips of cold water. In all these, repeating the procedure nine times was commonly suggested. A more vigorous treatment was to take a "spoonful" of pepper with, perhaps, molasses.

Other recommendations included giving the person a fright or surprise, or trying in other ways to take the individual's mind off the situation (for example, spelling first name backwards three times).

Such approaches are still recommended by physicians nowadays. One favoured suggestion for persistent hiccoughs is to breathe from a brown bag; this is justified as a way of inhaling carbon dioxide, an effect also gained by holding one's breath. If the condition is associated with dyspepsia, a long drink of cold water (perhaps with an added carminative or stomach settler like peppermint) is recommended, analogous perhaps to the pepper and molasses noted above. Perhaps underlying these remedies is time: summoning the patience to wait a few minutes can contribute to effective "treatment." If hiccoughs become incapacitating, however, prescription therapy is generally needed.

NOTES
See: Brown (Hand 1961, vol. 6) 212–8, for a range of treatment (holding one's breath and repetition [nine times] are conspicuous).

Representative MUNFLA references: 65-4/80 (deep breaths, holding breaths); 69-6MS (spell name backwards), 69-22MS (give a person a fright), 76-249 (hold breath), 84-323B (pepper and molasses, nine sips of water, head in bag); 84-281B (take mind off hiccough).

### HIVES (SEE RASHES)

### HOPS

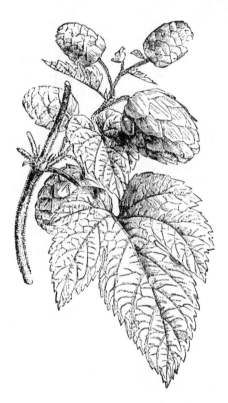

Despite the fact that hops were commonly grown in Newfoundland (hop barm was well known on the island, as elsewhere, as a bread starter) and had a fair reputation in professional and popular medical writings as a tonic, few Newfoundland references attest to their medical usage.

One record refers to the widely known practice of stuffing hops in a pillow to aid sleep, but no evidence has been found that this was popular among Newfoundlanders. In addition, no Newfoundland reference has been found for using hops as a tonic (a reputation justified by its bitterness), or for conditions such as "headache, nervousness, dyspepsia, liver complaints and constipation," although these uses were mentioned in promoting hop pills sold by some druggists around 1900.

NOTES
See: *Dictionary of Newfoundland English* (1990), concering "barm" for hop and other barms; Sparkes (1983) 31, on hop pillows; Helfand (1991) 112, for hop pills.

### INDIAN TEA

"Indian tea" is generally considered to be the often-mentioned Labrador tea (q.v.), although at least one suggestion exists that the former was made from *Rhododendron canadense*.

NOTES
*Dictionary of Newfoundland English* (1990) 267, for *Rhododendron canadense*.

INDIGESTION (SEE DYSPEPSIA)

INFANT CARE, CHILDREN

The story of infant care in twentieth-century Newfoundland is complex. Long-standing practices interacted with commercial influences – as indicated in the mother and baby discussion (Part I). Interaction also occurred between "scientific" infant feeding – often promoted by those in child-welfare movements – and mother's "common sense." Differences of opinion took place against a backdrop of a substantial incidence of infant deaths, although precise numbers are uncertain.

Professional concerns about birthing and care of newborns also faced, and sometimes clashed with, such practices found in the recently recorded Newfoundland tradition as "greasing" or oiling the infant, placing a "belly band" – a two inch wide or so strip of flannel – around the baby, and keeping the infant in an ill-lit room for nine days "to protect" the eyes. The use of the belt was felt by some to protect the cut cord (which was commonly dusted with scorched flour), although a legacy of wearing abdominal belts may have developed to control insensible perspiration and to prevent chills.

The scorched ("browned") flour (or cornstarch) was also used as a talc and was widely known for diaper rashes. Perhaps advice about regular changing of diapers was also heeded; nowadays treatment decisions about diaper rashes can be just as difficult despite a plethora of disposable wear.

Whether the decision dealt with general management of the newborn, infant feeding, medications for such relatively minor complaints as worms (q.v.) and constipation (q.v.), or the seriousness of a fever, there was often (as there still is) much uncertainty about making the actual decision. The question – "Am I doing the right thing?" – must have been commonplace, although midwives who stayed after the birth as well as grandmothers, mothers, and neighbours were often of great help. Uncertainty about what to do was compounded by economic considerations, for commercial preparations such as Cocomalt, for instance, occasioned an expense that might mean sacrifice elsewhere in the home. Even Carnation milk – commonly used for artificial feeding ("Ask your doctor about Carnation milk" for the baby) – had to be bought, although it was used in countless ways in the kitchen as were other condensed and evaporated milks. A 1953 advertisement for Libby's Evaporated Milk stated that it was not only "perfect for infant feeding," but also "for cooking."

The whole topic of infant feeding raised many conflicts. Some elderly Newfoundlanders remember that breast-feeding was "the best" amid such long-standing, artificial feeding practices as giving goat's milk "supposed to be germ free and a safe food for babies." In fact, with women always working – in the home and garden or out on the fish flakes – conditions were not always ideal for regular feeding. When bottles were used in the early decades of this century, they were often glass with rubber tubes leading to the teat. The tubes could not be cleaned properly and the bottles came to be known as "killer" bottles, because of the high incidence of gastrointestinal complaints and deaths associated with their use.

The individual families, ways of reacting to the rapidly changing and often conflicting knowledge concerning infant care were almost certainly inconsistent. Some continued with traditional preventive care for various infant and childrens' diseases, such as "passing through" (q.v.), even after immunizations were introduced.

All in all, relatively little detail remains concerning the bringing up of Newfoundland children, the ways of keeping them well, and the differences among families. Even so, long-standing advice such as "not to stay out in the rain or play in the snow, "not to play too much out in the cold," and to "eat a good breakfast before going to school" was commonplace.

NOTES
See: Campbell et al. (1988), on diaper rashes; Hiebert (1989), on greasing baby; Piercey (1992), on goat's milk, difficulties in mixing work and feeding, and bottles with rubber tubes; MCG (1992) 105, 011, for bringing up children.

Representative MUNFLA references: 84-320B (flour), 84-353B (ill-lit rooms).


INFECTIONS, MINOR; "SPRAINS"

The entry on *germs* indicates that comparatively minor infections (for example, from fish-hook and knife wounds) have been commonplace in Newfoundland. (Various localized infections are considered under *abscesses*, *cuts*, and sties (see *eyes*). These could become a difficult problem if the hand became infected, sometimes called a "sprain." Poultices (q.v.) and commercial antiseptic ointments (q.v.) were commonly employed in treatment. Some people recognized that cleanliness was important: "I had cousins and they didn't use hot soapy water and they were always having infections. With all the pricks from the hooks and your hauling the trawls with the hooks on them there were always cuts."

One noteworthy and entirely different approach – treatment by sympathy – was recorded in twentieth-century Newfoundland, although its usage had generally faded after a period of popularization in Europe during the seventeenth century. For instance, a rusty nail that had caused the initial wound and infection would be dissolved in acid.

NOTES
See: John Little correspondence (letter 12 September 1907), for sprain (on the Labrador); MCG (1992) 013, for soapy water.
    Representative MUNFLA references: 64-5/107 (sympathy).
    Personal communication: Troake (1990).

### INFLUENZA

Newfoundland recommendations for "flu" – meaning influenza characterized by relatively sudden onset of fever and generalized aches and pains – are relatively few. In fact, flu has been (and still is) diagnosed somewhat loosely by lay people and merges into colds and coughs (q.v.). Until around the 1960s (and to a lesser extent to the present), the diagnosis of "la grippe" (or grippe) could refer to either influenza or, according to some textbook writers, to a "variety" of influenza with catarrhal, bronchial, or intestinal symptoms; the latter was perhaps the so-called stomach flu. Doyle was advertising aspirin "for colds and grippe" in 1966, although at this time grippe seems to have also referred to general aches and pains, just one symptom of flu.

Despite few *specific* treatment recommendations in Newfoundland for influenza, a myriad of symptoms were treated according to their severity. Among the recommendations listed under flu was the drinking of Labrador tea (q.v.), which may have been useful as fluid replacement if, as is likely, it had no specific action in breaking a fever or in "sweating out" (aside from the property of being a hot tea). For the latter, hot rum or whisky plus blankets was a better known stand-by, while some saw the same benefits – at least in theory – from bathing in warm sea water.
    Other suggestions for influenza relate to relieving the symptoms of sore throat and cough (molasses and kerosene, or Minard's Liniment) or of a cold (for example, turnip and sugar boiled together, see *coughs and colds.*)
    The laxative senna was advised for accompanying coughs and colds, and also noted specifically for influenza. Commercial preparations made the same point. Grove's Laxative Bromo Quinine was recommended (1920 and later) for "grippe and flu," as were Watkins Laxative Cold and Grippe Tablets. Of particular interest is the little-known "comfort if you lose your taste" practice for the flu: "She'd give you sour jam with no sugar in it and your tastebuds would come back."

Preventive measures were also mentioned by Newfoundlanders, such as the use of moth balls or Minard's Liniment (1930 advertisement). Unquestionably, despite the self-limiting nature of most cases of influenza, many people worried about it, especially those who remembered the horrendous mortality of the 1918 Spanish flu pandemic, which hit Newfoundland as elsewhere. Memories were fostered by a monument erected in 1920 (and still standing opposite the Newfoundland Hotel, St. John's) to the memory of Ethel Dickinson, volunteer nurse, who "gave her life while tending [influenza] patients at King George V Institute, St. John's;" and an advertisement for Minard's Liniment (the *Evening Telegram*, 6 March 1922), which continued to tell readers "Don't wait until you get the Spanish Influenza."

Newfoundlanders, today, are probably assailed by more flu medicines than at any time in the past. Many contain multiple ingredients for relieving cold symptoms, and sometimes in higher doses than recommended for certain patients. Health professionals usually suggest single-ingredient medicines, but the only really effective twentieth-century advance in the armamentarium of professional medicine is vaccination against various strains of influenza.

NOTES
See: Doyle (1966), for aspirin and grippe advertisement; MCG (1992) 005, on taste and jam; Rubia (1980) 197, on turnip and sugar for flu.

Representative MUNFLA references: 69-24/2 (sweat it out), 69-28/3 (bathe in warm sea water), 82-122 (Indian tea, senna tea, moth balls around neck to prevent flu).

ITCH

"Itch" generally refers to scabies, although lice (q.v.) cannot be ruled out. A commonplace Newfoundland recommendation, to rub with sulphur, is in line with past professional medical recommendations for scabies. Other Newfoundland suggestions included sulphur-containing gunpowder (perhaps combined with Minard's Liniment and saltfree butter, or with cod liver oil), as well as gowithy (also known as goldwithy or sheep laurel), actually *Kalmia angustifolia*, which grows widely in Newfoundland. P. Tocque (1878) noted that this plant, when boiled with tobacco and sprinkled over the parts affected, is an infallible remedy for curing dogs of the mange. With well-known toxic properties, sheep laurel also has been recorded in nineteenth-century medical writings as a "cure for itch" of men.

Another recommendation for itch, one not found recorded since 1899 in the Newfoundland tradition, was the use of alder buds (q.v.). Their astringency (when made into a tea), may have provided some temporary relief.

NOTES
See: Introduction to bibliography for history and background information; *Dictionary of Newfoundland English* (1990), under gold-withy; Tocque (1878) 500; Bergen (1899) 110, alder.

Representative MUNFLA references: 82-146 (itch), 82-158 (sulphur), 84-311B (gunpowder).

## JUNIPER

Many references exist in the Newfoundland oral tradition to "juniper," "ground juniper," and "juniper bushes." Difficulty in interpreting the exact plant described in the Newfoundland records (unless the berries are specified) often arises. On the island, the so-called juniper generally refers to what is usually known elsewhere as tamarack or larch (*Larix laricina*), but it also covers "ground juniper" (*Juniperus communis*) and, perhaps, the trailing juniper (*J. horizontalis*).

Most Newfoundland medicinal recommendations for juniper are in line with published information in professional and lay sources on *J. communis*, namely for treating kidney and bladder troubles and stomach disorders, and for use as an abortifacient (q.v.) and emmenagogue (to induce or regulate menstruation.) Both the tops and berries, especially the latter, of *J. communis* have a long history as a diuretic for so-called kidney ailments and as a carminative to settle a stomach. (Teas prepared from the branches were considered less effective.) Backache (q.v.) was associated with kidney ailments; hence such testimonials as: "When my mother would have a backache or she had water problems, she'd send my father off in the woods and pick some juniper berries and she'd steep them and take it and next thing there'd be no more talk about aches."

A measure of the juniper's general popularity is also reflected in the Newfoundland suggestion to use a sugared tea of juniper in a baby's bottle for infant colic. While the carminative action may account for still another suggestion – that the berries (steeped to make a tea) are useful for diarrhoea (q.v.) – an astringent (binding) action is a more likely rationalization. The latter may also account for the recommendation to chew the inner bark of juniper tops for relieving a sore mouth; stimulating the flow of saliva may have contributed.

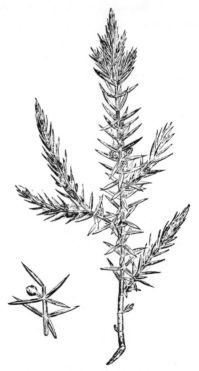

*Juniperus communis*

Some Newfoundland references to juniper branches and "juniper tree roots" for treating coughs and colds refer to tamarack. Although this tree has hardly featured in regular medicine, it was noted in such books as *Dr. Chase's Recipes* (for example, in a Syrup for Consumptives). It is noteworthy that fir, spruce, and pine trees in general (the needles rather than roots) have been widely recommended for coughs and colds (q.v.). A juniper salve (prepared from the inside of the bark of tamarack, and perhaps mixed with vaseline) is said to have been employed for frostbite and sores.

Blood purification (q.v.) also enters the juniper story – *Larix or Juniperus.* Not only does this concept partly justify usage as a tonic (q.v., sometimes specified as a spring tonic), but also employment of roots and branches, inner bark, and, possibly, berries (as a decoction or tea taken internally) for boils or "risings."

An important consideration about juniper – certainly if it is used over considerable periods of time, say for backache or for premenstrual tension as advocated by some modern herbalists – is its toxic effects on the kidney. For those committed to herbal remedies, items safer than juniper, but with similar properties, do exist.

NOTES
See: Chase (1862) 102, for tamarack in syrup for consumptives; MCG (1992) 109, for testimonial.

Representative MUNFLA references: 68-016D (water trouble), 76-249 (juniper bush [not tree] for bladder and kidney), 78-195 (juniper berries for diarrhoea), 78-200 (stomach pain, perhaps with dogberries and alder buds), 78-205 (decoction of branches, roots, or berries for cleaning blood for boils, diarrhoea), 84-321B (salve), 89-217 (infant colic).

KEROSENE

Kerosene – a coal-tar product used in the ordinary kerosene lamps and stoves – is frequently noted in the recent Newfoundland oral tradition. Mention is made of an application to cuts; of a rub for cramps; and of a remedy for coughs and colds, especially sore throats, either rubbed on or taken internally. "The older people put more faith in it [for colds] than the doctor's medicine." It was also tried, primarily as a rub, for influenza and diphtheria.

The Newfoundland story is little different from reports in other places where, in the past, kerosene assumed something of the mantle of a panacea in home medicine. This was undoubtedly encouraged by its inclusion in such popular over-the-counter medicines as Sloan's Liniment.

NOTES
Representative MUNFLA references: 68-7 (quote on faith in kerosene and molasses), 76-249 (sore throat), 77-87 (with molasses for coughs), 78-200 (diphtheria), 82-121

(piles, lice), 82-122 (with molasses for influenza), 82-218 (head lice, with molasses for asthma, bronchitis).

## KIDNEY AND BLADDER AILMENTS

Relatively few specific recommendations exist in the recorded Newfoundland oral tradition for kidney and bladder problems, despite plenty of over-the-counter remedies and concerns about urine. In 1992, one elderly Newfoundlander recollected: "My grandmother told me, make sure you have a clean bladder, mix bread soda and warm milk and take that, and that's the best thing to clean your bladder."

Lay diagnosis of kidney and bladder problems has ranged from backache to changes in urine. Interestingly, Bright's disease is apparently not mentioned, for, although this diagnosis has been replaced by others within regular medicine, it can still be found in many popular traditions as a general term for kidney ailments. Beliefs about causes are rarely recorded, except that a cold or draft might bring on inflammation. Non-specific notions of "kidney-sick" were also sometimes expressed in the promotion of kidney remedies, such as the "great South American Kidney Cure" (1890s).

By and large, kidney (and bladder) medicines were viewed as diuretics to increase urine flow, although in the twentieth century, in the wake of the germ theory, urinary antiseptics also became popular. Although not explicitly stated in the Newfoundland record, increasing the flow of urine was considered not only as a way of dealing with kidney or bladder problems, but also as another way of purifying the blood. A well-known treatment in Newfoundland was concocted from ground juniper (q.v.): made into a tea (or boiled), it might be taken before going to bed for "weak kidneys." Its action, like many other plants, was viewed as diuretic. Just how much information about plant diuretics has been lost to Newfoundlanders is unclear, and some study should be made of W.E. Cormack's (1856) mention of Indian uses of plants for "gravel" (small stones) and as "diuretics." Such plants may merely increase urine flow as a result of increasing volume intake, as reflected in the old adage, "There is nothing better than a good beer that you can drink for your kidneys."

Another more recent record in the Newfoundland oral tradition mentions "mountain fern" as a useful herb for the treatment of kidney ailments. Although the identity of this fern is uncertain, it is probably *Polypodium* spp. Indeed, various ferns (particularly *Dryopteris felix-mas*) have been fairly well known in professional and popular medicine. Among the range of conditions mentioned, however, its action on the kidney has hardly received significant consideration.

It is hard to know whether the Newfoundland recommendation of mouse soup for "bladder disorder" or for kidney trouble was widely recognized on the island, although it did have a reputation in the treatment of bed-wetting (q.v.), as did cooked rat.

One Newfoundland report is of special interest, since it appears to be an unusual alkaline treatment, somewhat in line with a number of eighteenth-century recommendations for the management of bladder stones (see also the bread-soda cleanser noted above). The treatment involved obtaining "small round bone structures" from the heads of "codfish" and browning them on the stove. The "fish's pearls," as they were called, were then ground into a fine powder. Dosage, however, seems problematic, for the suggestion was solely to dip a wet finger in the powder and suck it. Another suggestion for kidney trouble was to roast dry cod's heads until crisp; they were then ground into a powder, mixed with water, and drunk.

A wide variety of commercial preparations for so-called kidney problems and backache have been marketed. Even before 1900, the McMurdo drug-store in St. John's was promoting the South American Kidney Cure already noted. But it was Gin Pills (q.v.) and Dodd's Kidney Pills (q.v.) that became household names.

Another proprietary medicine, once well known albeit not often adver-tised in Newfoundland, was Haarlem Drops. Two ingredients – turpentine (q.v.) and linseed – were well known to Newfoundlanders and also found in cough medicines. Like much commercial promotion for kidney condi-tions, Haalem Drops was also recommended for liver problems. However, this was less obvious a recommendation than Dr. Chase's Kidney and Liver Pills, for which the two organs were viewed as working in conjunction to clean or purify the body. Such concepts, although fading in the 1950s, have not been entirely forgotten, as a visit today to many a health store makes clear. (See also *backache, bearberry.*) Noteworthy, too, were several new claims for kidney and liver medicines, such as "Hardening of Arteries" (for example, in the *Daily News,* 11 January 1930), an instance of the not uncommon "extension" of popular medicines.

NOTES
See: Cormack (1873 [1856]) 53–4; Viseltear (1968), for eighteenth-century treatment of stones; MCG (1992) 1001, for the need to keep the bladder clean, and beer.
   Representative MUNFLA references: 63-1/19 (juniper), 67-4/12 (mouse soup), 69-29/11 (mountain fern), 78-200 (bones from cod's head), 82-122 (ground juniper, senna), 86-254 (browning bones from cod's head).

## LABRADOR TEA (INDIAN TEA)

Newfoundlanders have taken "Indian tea" for many purposes. Philip Tocque, in 1878, mentioned it for "diseases of the lungs, and with good effect;" a later informant went further, saying it would cure anything. Generally, however, it has been limited to treating colds, flu, and stomach upsets (for which "sometimes ginger was added").

Although a precise identification of the plant is rarely given in any of the records, *Ledum groenlandicum* (sometimes, perhaps, *L. palustre* in Labrador) is the usual reference. Occasionally, *Rhododendron canadense* (see *Indian tea*), and perhaps "uva ursi" (see *bearberry*), is indicated.

Labrador tea has long been reported as a beverage rather than a medicine. Aaron Thomas (1794) observed that Newfoundlanders gave their fishing people "Indian tea," which "was put in a Pott with water and Molasses. All was boil'd together and given them with fish and biscuits. This is the common people's breakfast and supper in Newfoundland." Later, Philip Tocque said it was used by some of the "poor of Newfoundland as tea."

In view of its fairly wide reputation as a beverage (including elsewhere, such as throughout Northern Canada, where it is known as Hudson's Bay tea), it is unclear whether the medical recommendations arose from the perceived value of *hot* tea or the specific effects of the herb. The latter can vary from batch to batch; some people have even reported feeling a "high" from drinking the tea (the possibility of adulteration [for example, with *Kalmia angustifolia*] exists.) The adding of a "bit of spruce" to the teapot has been said to enhance healthful properties, a suggestion in line with those who see the tea as supportive care.

Some concerns have been expressed over toxic constituents, especially andromedotoxin – present in higher concentrations when extraction is by boiling (rather than infusing.) Although the precise pharmacological effects require further investigation, prudence is appropriate; it is unwise (certainly for sick people) to take Labrador tea over long periods of time.

NOTES
See: Thomas (1968 [1794]) 71; Tocque (1878) 500; *Audubon Society* (1983) 502, on Hudson's Bay Company; Sparkes (1983), on added spruce (the constituents [in the essential oil as well] are not well characterized); Tattje and Bas (1981), on *L. palustre*.

Representative MUNFLA references: 76-249, 77-87 (colds), 78-205 (bad stomach).

LAXATIVES (SEE CONSTIPATION)

LICE, HEAD AND BODY (SEE ALSO "CRABS"), BED BUGS, FLEAS

Head lice, long a problem, remain an issue in many communities, even though personal hygiene is currently considered to be better than ever before. A common Newfoundland recommendation in the recently recorded oral tradition for treating head lice – often initially diagnosed because of an itching of the scalp, especially behind the ears – was to rub the hair with kerosene. Although this could be effective, by the 1940s DDT had infiltrated everyday use; less toxic substances, in the form of shampoos, available both over-the-counter and on prescription, are now used.

Relevant issues, in Newfoundland as elsewhere, include a general lack of appreciation that head lice produce nits (eggs) that attach so strongly to hair shafts that ordinary washing, combing, and brushing of the hair do not remove them. One Newfoundland record, however, does note the removal of nits with "kerosene oil rubbed over a fine tooth comb." Any oil remaining in the hair was left there for an hour or more and then washed out. The use of fine-toothed combs is noted in other records ("You dreaded to come home every evening with that fine tooth comb going through your hair, I think that's what lost my hair; it took the roots and everything out of my head.") On the other hand, combs employed alone are not entirely effective. Since head lice can survive off the scalp several hours and nits much longer, attention to home hygiene is especially important. One record notes the use of "bitterchips" (quassia chips), boiled to make a tea and used to wash the hair, as a preventive.

Body lice were remembered as a special problem in the Newfoundland fishery, and elsewhere. "Lice always left a dead man as soon as he got cold. You could see them crawling away in all directions." A common treatment was to apply kerosene or a decoction of tobacco. Other suggested treatments were to hang a bag of sulphur under the vest (in part for prevention), or to rub on the sulphur as with itch (q.v.). Clothes might be burned, and pickle water applied. Such treatments (aside from pickle water) were effective, although it is probable that over-the-counter preparations have long been used. Gerald Doyle distributed Kline's Larkspur Lotion ("An effective product for destroying head lice and all parasites that infest the hair on any part of the body"). Powdered Sabadilla (powdered Sabadilla seeds) was also available; like larkspur, it was well known as a parasiticide, although it lacked a particularly strong reputation.

Bed bugs (*Cimex lectularius,* a different species than either head or body lice) hide in cracks in walls and floors and in beds, and, much like fleas, can be difficult to eliminate from households. Although it is unclear how extensive a problem bugs have been in Newfoundland, warnings "to sleep tight to keep the bugs away" suggest they were not uncommon. In a similar vein was the suggestion to wrap a patient in brown paper to keep away bugs. Disinfectants were tried, but "nothing touched DDT." (See *itch*).

For fleas (commonly *Pulex irritans*), one Newfoundland suggestion to keep them "from getting into bed" was to place mint or tansy "between the bottom sheet and the mattress." This is in line with suggestions recorded elsewhere, although pennyroyal is far and away the best-known plant material, wherever it grows.

Head lice, as already mentioned, remain a problem today. That some disagreement exists over the effectiveness of different commercial preparations (including differences between shampoos and lotions) needs to be considered when treatment is instituted.

NOTES
See: Burgess (1990), for background to head-lice preparations; MCG (1992) 104, on quassia chips; MCG (1992) 013, on sabadilla; MCG (1992) 115, for fine comb story.

Representative MUNFLA references: 64-1/91 (mint or tansy; in fact, pansy is listed, apparently meaning tansy), 68-3/51 (bag of sulphur), 69-10/11 (lice crawling from dead body), 69-23/38 (kerosene for head lice), 73-50 (kerosene and comb for nits), 82-121 (kerosene, larkspur).

Personal communication: Troake (1989), on pickle water.

## LIVERISHNESS AND BILIOUSNESS, JAUNDICE

The expression "liverishness" (or "liverish," sometimes "jaundicy") is now rarely heard as a diagnosis in most Western countries (France is an exception). In Britain and North America, until around the 1950s, it commonly referred to a general feeling of unwellness – characterized by nausea, an unpleasant taste in the mouth, and mild dizziness. This was believed to result from a "sluggish" or "congested" liver. Lack of exercise and excessive eating and drinking were thought to contribute to the condition.

"Biliousness" is another loose diagnostic term, viewed by many lay people as merely being liverish, but for some embracing more of a sickly feeling, even vomiting. It was generally associated with blocked bile, but its diverse symptomatology includes neurotic behaviour, at least in the minds of some physicians. By the 1930s, the concept was disappearing from regular medicine, but hardly from lay ideas.

Treatment for liverishness and biliousness, albeit varied, was generally based on purifying the body, particularly on the notion of increasing the flow of bile. For the latter, the celebrated mercury compound, calomel, available from drug and many general stores, was still prescribed by some Newfoundland physicians until the 1930s if not later, although it had long been declining in popularity. A doctor's wife and nurse at the Grenfell Mission in Labrador in 1922 wrote home: "For a week I've been feeling sort of jaundicy and last night got dosed with calomel and salts this morning, as I'm been feeling a bit something like [myself] again."

Calomel had long caused concern because of its side-effects, and, in the 1950s, Newfoundlanders were still being told that Carter's Little Liver Pills were to "wake up your liver bile without calomel." Liverishness had become a major arena for the promotion of commercial preparations, such as bitters (q.v.) and "liver" medicines (generally laxatives), said to increase the flow of bile or to relieve indigestion. Newfoundlanders had various choices besides Carter's: Dr. Chase's Kidney and Liver Pills, Dr. Agnew's Liver Pills, Ripan's Tabules, D & L Pills, Liver Salts, and others. Legislation now prohibits promotion of unsubstantiated claims for action on the liver, a reflection of the fact that the concept of liverishness is now unacceptable to professional medicine. Nevertheless, the concept has not disappeared entirely from popular health beliefs. (See also *constipation*).

Although no reference has been found in the Newfoundland record to the use of "bitters" (q.v.) – even to the readily available dandelion root – to stimulate the flow of bile, it was likely used. After all, Atwood's Jaundice Bitters, with its yellow label, could be purchased with a recommendation of usage for liver complaints.

Jaundice – the yellowing of the skin often, but not always, due to the absorption into the blood stream of bile formed in the liver – is rarely mentioned in the Newfoundland record. Indeed, the only references found to treatment refer to the use of either sheep or chicken manure. The yellow tint is a reminder of past interest in the doctrine of signatures (the notion that medicines carry a sign or "signature" of their potential use). The colour yellow was sometimes thought to indicate its value for treating jaundice. (For sheep manure see *measles*.)

NOTES
See: Yates T.M. correspondence (letter 18 December 1992), for jaundicy and calomel; Bergen (1899) 71, sheep's dung; MCG (1992) 003, liverishness still a concern.
    Representative MUNFLA references: 67-15/51 (hen's dirt), 69-25/17 (sheep's dung).

MAGGOTS

The recently recorded Newfoundland oral tradition, as elsewhere, mentions the use of maggots for wounds and infections. For instance, fish maggots were used to treat "tuberculosis" of the hand (perhaps, in fact, a sore) as well as non-specific infections. In one case, a finger stall containing a few dozen newly hatched fishfly maggots was used. The maggots fed on the pus and "proud flesh" until the wound was "pink and clean."

As unsavoury as maggots sound to most people, maggot therapy attracted considerable interest in professional medicine, especially between 1928 and

1938 in the United States. Much clinical evidence suggested that maggots cured certain localized infections, but interest was pushed to one side by the introduction of sulphonamides and antibiotics.

NOTES
See: Wainwright (1988), for background.

Representative MUNFLA reference: 73-189 ("fish larvae" put on sores to "eat up all the pus"), 78-200 (fish maggots for tuberculosis).

MALE REMEDIES

Female remedies (q.v.) have long been a conspicuous feature of self-care. In contrast, although such "male diseases" as spermatorrhoea (sometimes linked to overindulgence and masturbation at a time when this was felt to be harmful) and enlarged prostate attracted attention on both sides of the Atlantic prior to 1900, commercial considerations (for example, remedies for "male weakness") did little to shape overall attitudes. Nevertheless, male remedies played on individual anxiety by emphasizing traits not part of the stereotype of manliness (strength, self-sufficiency, and so on) that was very much part of Newfoundland culture.

In fact, no clear treatment suggestions for men's diseases have been found in the Newfoundland oral record. Even commercial remedies for lost manhood, male tiredness, and so on were not widely promoted on the island, at least after the early 1900s. The *Daily News* for 31 October 1901, however, did tell "weak" Newfoundland men who wanted to be free, strong, and vigorous for life to write to an address in Detroit. The treatment, said to "enlarge small weak organs to full size and vigour," may have been one of the new organ extracts, probably testicles, promoted at the time.

A widely advertised medicine in Newfoundland newspapers at the end of the nineteenth and in the early twentieth centuries was Dr. Pierce's Golden Medical Discovery. Although this was generally viewed as a female remedy, advertisements sometimes stressed that common problems affect men as much as women. As one newspaper advertisement (1910), in pursuing the popular theme of cleanliness, stated:

A CLEAN MAN    Outside cleanliness is less than half the battle. A man may scrub himself a dozen times a day, and still be unclean. Good health means cleanliness not only outside, but inside. It means a clean stomach, clean bowels, clean blood, a clean liver, and new, clean healthy tissues. The man who is clean in this way will look it and act it. He will work with energy and think clean, clear, healthy thoughts.

He will never be troubled with liver, lung, stomach or blood disorders. Dyspepsia and indigestion originate in unclean stomachs. Blood diseases are found where there is unclean blood. Consumption and bronchitis means unclean image.

DR. PIERCE'S GOLDEN MEDICAL DISCOVERY prevents these diseases. It makes a man's insides clean and healthy. It cleans the digestive organs, makes pure, clean blood, and clean, healthy flesh.

Unlike the Detroit advertisement noted above, there were no apparent overtones of an aphrodisiac property in this promotion. Although little evidence of the use of aphrodisiacs in Newfoundland has been found, one suggestion to restore sexual drive for a sufferer from impotency was noted: to eat shellfish and boiled snails in great quantity. Perhaps more use was made of the cantharides (Spanish fly) – widely known but dangerous to use – available from drugstores.

NOTES
See: Parsons (1977), on nineteenth-century treatments; Hall (1991), on British and general background.
    Representative MUNFLA references: 73-150 (shellfish and snails).
    Personal communication: J. O'Mara (1989), on cantharides.

MEASLES

Worries over long-term effects from measles (albeit uncommon) justifiably persist, although the introduction of measles vaccination in the 1960s dramatically reduced the incidence of the disease. Indeed, the widely held belief that a child with measles should be kept in the dark to protect the eyes is one of the few measles recommendations found in the Newfoundland record. If the eyes did become sore, cold, wet tea leaves were to be applied.
    Another recommendation was to "sweat" the measles out, perhaps by going to bed with hot rum. ("Rum hottens the blood and the measles would all come out;" "When the measles did not come out on your skin it was considered unhealthy.") A particularly well-remembered alternative approach was "to bring out measles" with sheep manure made into a drink. Included in many testimonials throughout the island (for example, "You take this medicine and the measles comes out on you in a few hours."), it was also recently recorded as part of Micmac tradition: "When we had measles there was a crowd in the house. My sister wouldn't drink that and she also died. My brother drank it and me and we was out long before her was up. It looked bad and you had to drink it fast." There were a number of ways of preparing the sheep manure drink. For example, the manure could be placed in a little cloth bag and steeped in milk, which was then drunk. On the other hand, "There was a woman used to mix it. She'd mix it with sugar, steep it, put milk on it and give it to you. Out come the measles. Everybody thought it mutton, but it wasn't mutton!"

Called "saffron," such mixtures, in line with a long-standing notion that manure possessed heating properties, were felt to be suitable for producing sweats. Perhaps at one time an analogy was made to the expensive spice, saffron, either to its colour or its reputation as a stimulant. Another reference to a "yellow" treatment is intriguing: "I remember first they used to go and dig a root out of the ground. I forget what it was called. A yellow root and they steeped that and you'd drink it and they'd be out on you the next morning." Perhaps this refers to the tonic properties of snakeroot (q.v.).

General supportive care for the patient is also reflected in the suggestion to drink Indian tea (q.v.), possibly with the thought of breaking a fever, but perhaps also, as was recommended in many regimens, to replace fluid. Lime juice served this purpose as well. Attention and care had to be given to the scabs: "When we had the measles she'd take the galvanized tub and she would put water and bread soda in it ... put you in that and wash you. And cleaned the scabs." The recommendation of taking senna as a *laxative* in many ailments, other than constipation, is considered under that entry.

NOTES
See: Creighton (1968) 222–3, on sheep tea, nanny tea, or nanny-dung for bringing measles out in Nova Scotia; Brown Collection (Hand 1961, vol. 6) 232–3, on manures (not just from sheep) which are fairly widely reported for measles; Bergen (1899) 71, for comments on general manure usage in Cape Breton, though the term "saffron" is apparently less common; MCG (1992) 002, for manure, milk, and so on; MCG (1992) 104, for bread soda and scabs; MCG (1992) 012, yellowroot; MCG (1993) 2, for Micmac story.

Representative MUNFLA references: 63-1/7 (Indian tea), 69-25/18 (dark room and wet tea leaves), 70-26/MS (rum), 73-142 (measles to come out), 78-195 (senna), 78-200 (sheep manure).

## MENINGITIS

Few recommendations exist in the recently recorded Newfoundland oral tradition for meningitis – infection and inflammation of the membranes (meninges) of the brain – not an easy diagnosis for lay people. Symptoms include headache, vomiting, photophobia, rigidity of the neck, and convulsions. The precise incidence of the disease in Newfoundland during the first half of the twentieth century is uncertain, although tuberculous meningitis was noted as common.

Treatment suggestions included mustard poultices or plasters (applied to the head until "clear water ran out of the nostrils"), or onion compresses or poultices to the forehead or neck (perhaps in response to headache or neck stiffness).

There was, too, a long-standing suggestion to pay attention to the feet, such as to keep them warm with socks, or perhaps to put an onion in the sock. Treating the feet is in line with previous usage of foot baths for flu and headaches (see also *mustard*). It must be assumed that, along with the specific treatments for the head, other symptoms were attended to, even if not recorded.

NOTES
Representative MUNFLA references 82-122 (socks and onions), 82-218 (mustard plasters and poultices).

## MIDWIVES, CHILDBIRTH

During much of the twentieth century many Newfoundland midwives – both those with formal training and those without (sometimes called "lay" or "granny" midwives or "wise women") – have had significant roles, some extending beyond specific childbirth duties to straddle professional medical care and traditional practices: "She was the midwife, an' she was the nurse ... She made her own medicines. The government paid her nothing. She was jus' there for any family. We weren't to bother with the company doctor. I had the midwife, Auntie Elizabeth, for all my babies. There was no limit to the things she used to handle – curing measles and yellow jaundice with a brew made from sheep dung; sour-dick seeds for anybody with hay fever; and yellow root for the cramps."

Although this entry notes only a brief sampling of prenatal care, birth practices, and post-partem care for the mother (for which a midwife might stay in the home for up to nine days) – and does not describe a midwife's general service to the community – it serves to illustrate the scope of practices and concerns over an event that always prompted fear and uncertainty and, on occasion, brought trauma and tragedy. The diversity of recorded practices reflects that, until the advent of general hospitalization for childbirth (the 1960s in Newfoundland), normal deliveries were, in many respects, events for the community and family rather than the professional.

Little information seems to be reported on prenatal care, but one account states: "A lot of them used to have miscarriages but then she [a midwife pre 1940s] would be telling them not to reach up or lift anything heavy. Keep away from salt. But don't sit around. Exercise all the time, do your work and don't worry about it, everything will be alright." Although a tea made from the laxative senna (leaves or pods) was sometimes given at term, it is not always clear whether this was to clean the bowels (as was commonly the intent with castor oil) or to induce or speed labour. It was probably both, depending on circumstances. Enemas were apparently not given as a matter of course unless labour was especially slow. In fact, medications during and after childbirth seem to have been minimal; even ergot, long an important item in regular medicine – to minimize the potentially serious problem of post-partum haemorrhage – and known in popular medicine to speed up labour was apparently not widely used.

Certain non-medication practices to encourage labour – rubbing either the back or the stomach, or nipple stimulation (known elsewhere and attracting some professional interest nowadays) – were apparently not recorded. Another suggestion – to place an axe under the bed to ease labour pains – was found in the Newfoundland record. Infrequent reference to this and similar ideas, which may have aroused more disbelief than belief, supports the view that childbirth in twentieth-century Newfoundland embraced few non-natural practices.

It is perhaps surprising that no reference has been found to the use of raspberry leaves (easily obtainable in Newfoundland); these have long been known to ease childbirth, for which they are still promoted today. In fact, current concerns over caffeine may well be encouraging some pregnant women to use "natural" herbal teas in the belief that they are safe. Raspberry has a stimulant action on the uterus and, in large doses, is a potential abortifacient; although tea made as an infusion is relatively weak, prudence is required when taking the herb during pregnancy, as is the case with many other herbs that have not been fully investigated.

Post-partum birth practices in Newfoundland included blowing into a bottle to help expel the placenta. There is also an intriguing suggestion that the so-called juice from the boiling of berries from "blackberry earths" (also called "blackberry heath") – almost certainly referring to the crowberry, *Empetrum nigrum* – was given to relieve uterine pains (after childbirth and for any pains), as well as to stop bleeding. No known pharmacological explanation exists.

The rationale for another practice – administering juniper tea after the birth – is also unclear. Although it was noted to help "after pains" and to cleanse the body "of any corruption," a suggestion that it has a laxative action seems incorrect. Action on the uterus which minimizes post-partum haemorrhage cannot be ruled out, certainly if the juniper is given over time. (See *abortion*). Many remember that nine days (nine being a popular number in traditional health care) were commonly recommended for post-natal rest. All stimulation was avoided with the intent of reducing the possibility of post-partum haemorrhage: "You got tea with bread and butter the first day. Then no more for three days, dry toast was lived on for three days. They wouldn't give you a drink of cold water." Justifiable worry about haemorrhage is reflected in the suggestion to wear a ribbon around the neck as a preventive, while concern with the mother's lack of strength is further underscored in the following account of "churching" in the Anglican tradition:

We used to be churched after the birth of each child. After I had a baby my husband wouldn't let me set bread until I had gone to church to get more strength. You used to get churched about two weeks after the baby was born or when you were up and around again. You got churched before the baby was christened. On a Friday night you would go to church, come up front, kneel down, and the minister would say a prayer over you. Only regular church-goers bothered with it. It gave you back all the strength you lost at childbirth.

Another aspect of post-natal care was the wearing of abdominal bands for some time after birth, ostensibly to help restore body shape ("till everything went back into place.")

"Milk fever" deserves mention, because it has been elsewhere confused with milk sickness due to drinking milk from cows that had eaten *Eupatorium rugosum*, a substance that does not grow in Newfoundland. On the other hand, milk fever, according to a Newfoundland record, was when milk "gathers in the breast and goes bad." One treatment was to place muskrat fur over the breast. The drying up of milk prompted a number of suggestions, such as greasing breasts ("nowadays use Eversweet margarine instead of grease,"); none, however, included the use of galactagogues, known elsewhere as useful to increase the flow of milk.

Prognostications and beliefs associated with births are not noted here, apart from the long-standing interest in any infant born with a caul (a piece of amniotic sac that sometimes covers a child when he or she is born). In Newfoundland, as elsewhere, good fortune was predicted as a result, as well as the likelihood of the infant becoming a healer (see *charmers*). If the caul was preserved, it was said to prevent drowning or, if hung on a string around the neck, sickness.

If practices described in this entry have to all intents and purposes disappeared, concerns persist over the possibility of birthmarks (q.v.) or deformities arising during pregnancy. Even if frights or unsatisfied cravings during pregnancy – long felt to have adverse effects (especially in producing birthmarks) – are given relatively little attention nowadays, there are new issues creating uncertainty; namely, caffeine (tea and coffee), alcohol, smoking, and many chemical substances. The thalidomide tragedy (1960s) still influences attitudes toward pregnancy.

Considerable interest now exists concerning the demise of traditional midwifery and the emergence of birthing as a hospital, rather than home, event. There are differing views as to how this transition came about in Newfoundland – ranging from a gradual change without confrontation (indeed, that midwives were eager to incorporate medical approaches), to arguments favouring a "take-over" by the medical profession. With the growing authority of medicine (including the role of hospitals) in the twentieth century, an inexorable change was perhaps inevitable in

Newfoundland – even when social changes relevant elsewhere were relatively minimal – because community and other support at birth could only partially allay the many childbirth fears.

NOTES
See: Piercey (1992), for insights on scope of midwives' activities; Creighton (1968) 206, for notes on raspberry-leaf tea for easy delivery in Nova Scotia, and on tansy; Benoit (1983), for quotation about roles of midwife; McNaughton (1989) and Benoit (1989, 1990), for general background and specific detail; Baldwin et al (1987), for prudence over raspberry; Hiebert (1989), on greasing baby; Davis, D.L. (1983b) 68, for churching; Renbourn (1957), on flannel, abdominal belt; Green (1990) 181, on powers of extrasensory perception when born with caul (also Brown Collection [Hand 1961, vol. 7] 146–7, power to see hants, and so on).

Representative MUNFLA references: 69-11 (axe, informant indicated disbelief), 73-60 (caul and drowning), 75-21 (non-stimulant post-partum regimen, binder around mother's abdomen), 76-258 (blowing into bottle), 78-211 (juniper), 82-218 (grease breasts, green ribbon for haemorrhage), 84-281B (for blackberry earths said to be still used in 1984), 89-084 (milk fever.)

## MINARD'S LINIMENT

Of all the proprietary medicines promoted in Newfoundland, the still available Minard's Liniment has been one of the best known. For countless Newfoundlanders it was an essential item in their self-care, and it is no surprise that the recently recorded oral tradition contains many testimonials and recommendations. "My grandfather was a great believer in Minard's Liniment. He thought it was good for everything. If you had a cold you sniffed it. If you had a chest pain you rubbed it on your chest." Recommended uses included arthritis, asthma, bronchitis, influenza, headaches, and sore throats. It was included, too, in compounded homemade medicines such as gunpowder, saltfree butter, and Minard's for itch.

Although the liniment was generally remembered as an external application or rub, taking it internally was not uncommon. As noted under *coughs*, this was given in both small

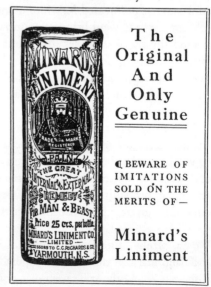

Advertisement 1916

(drops) and large (for example, a teaspoonful every four hours) dosages. The latter, taken over time, would cause concern nowadays, especially with certain patients, because of the toxicity of the camphor present.

Recommendations within the oral tradition mirror decades of intensive newspaper advertising of Minard's for colds, "grippe," (and "flu"), first aid, headache, athlete's foot, neuralgia, sprains, bruises, rheumatism, sore throat, sore feet, and many other ailments. Many advertisements correctly stated that it was "used by physicians."

Advertising claims became less brazen after World War II and today the liniment, with its sharp odour from ammonia and camphor, only claims to provide "relief from stiff, sore muscles, strains, sprains, backache, rheumatic and arthritic pain and chest colds."

The ingredients have mild rubefacient (reddening, warming) and mild analgesic properties, and can provide temporary relief from minor aches and pains. Some people think that these properties may be aided by a psychological component, a result of confidence in the familiar pungent aroma.

NOTES
See: MCG (1992) 004, grandfather testimonial.
    Representative MUNFLA references: 78-200 (headache), 78-205 (arthritis), 82-121 (baldness), 82-218 (asthma, bronchitis).

MOLASSES

Molasses has permeated Newfoundland life for years, and in countless ways. "When the men went into the country hunting or fishing, they always took a good supply of molasses instead of milk and sugar ... It was thought to give them energy." Straddling the kitchen and the sickroom, molasses is still conspicuous in contemporary Newfoundland cookbooks, while many memories exist of switchel tea, that is, the weak so-called tea of molasses without milk.

Numerous other references exist in the Newfoundland oral tradition to the medicinal use of molasses: sometimes warmed ("scalded") for sore throat (q.v., either alone, or eaten or drunker with butter, vinegar, pepper, rum and kerosene, sometimes in combination); for earache; for colds and coughs (q.v.); for bronchitis (q.v.), for constipation; as a blood purifier; and for cuts. One graphic reminiscence exists about the latter:

We was plankin' a boat up there see, and I was spilin' the plank with the drawin' knife and had me hand like that, spilin' and he [his brother] took holt and give it the pluck, and the knife went along and took me finger and sawed 'um down there ... There's the mark there now where I cut it ... And it didn't seem to be gettin' well and this old man, Dicky Tucker, he came in and he done 'n up in molasses and he told me not to open 'n for I believe it was a week without opening 'n. When I opened 'n he was pretty well. Nothing but the pure molasses, plenty of it.

Molasses was sometimes employed in poultices, and scalded molasses was used as an application for minor skin ailments.

The medicinal popularity of molasses is far from limited to Newfoundland, though in many other places it was (and is) known primarily in the form of sulphur and molasses (q.v.), and as a tonic. The latter reputation is not widely noted in Newfoundland, though it is implied when it is said to "give energy," which might have been the intent behind its use in tuberculosis (q.v.). On the other hand, by the 1930s, if not before, the iron content was felt to be a significant nutritional factor for many Newfoundlanders.

NOTES
See: Giovannini (1988) 23, for hunting trips; Murray (1979) 133, for molasses on cuts quotation; *Dictionary of Newfoundland English* (1990) 552, for switchel tea; Mitchell (1930), for iron content of molasses.

Representative MUNFLA references: 66-3/27 28 (molasses, butter and vinegar for cold), 67-5/68 (molasses and ginger for cold), 69-18/1 (molasses candy for sore throat), 69-21/8 (molasses into ear for earache), 69-22 MS (molasses and Minard's for sore throat), 76-249 (sulphur and molasses to cleanse blood in spring; flour and molasses poultice for boils).

MUMPS

Professional medical and nursing treatment recommendations were generally in line with the home management of mumps which, in large families, could cause havoc. The *Daily News* (30 January 1907) felt it newsworthy that Mrs Thomas Tucker of Thorburn Road [St. John's] had ten children with mumps! Treatment regimens included bed rest and hot-water bottles (with protective covering) around the neck. Pain might have been relieved with opium preparations available over-the-counter (for example, laudanum or paregoric) or aspirin (see *analgesics*).

In addition, recently recorded Newfoundland suggestions mention other ways of applying warmth, such as socks filled with warmed coarse salt. Other applications to, or wraps around, the neck included salt herring; fat pork (or salt fat pork, perhaps with added black pepper); or socks filled with coarse salt. (The herring – possibly split into two halves – and the fat pork in strips were covered with cloth first or applied directly and then covered with linen).

These regimens may have given ease in what was a self-limiting condition. Some consider that the distracting discomfort of certain of the treatments was perhaps a more significant psychological factor than faith in the remedies. At the same time, some regimens seemed to be circumscribing the disease within an area, just as tying a silk string around the neck (not found in Newfoundland) is viewed as keeping mumps from "going down."

Vaccination as a preventive measure – introduced into the Newfoundland vaccination program in 1975 – has lessened the incidence of mumps and the occasional complications of orchitis and deafness.

NOTES
See: Brown Collection (Hand 1961, vol. 6) 236, for various ways of keeping the mumps from "going down."

Representative MUNFLA references: 63-1/30 (salt fat pork and pepper), 66-10/28,29 (herring, fat pork), 69-11/6 (salt), 72-64 (warm salt).

## MUSTARD

Recently recorded Newfoundland references to the use of "mustard" generally refer to mustard powder, undoubtedly one of the best-known kitchen remedies from the early nineteenth century to the 1940s. The mustard plaster (sometimes called a poultice, although it was not heated) – made, for example, from one teaspoonful of mustard and six of flour and mixed with water to a suitable consistency – was a commonplace treatment in Newfoundland for colds (q.v.), pneumonia (q.v.), and rheumatism (q.v.). In fact, mustard plasters – once the recommendation of many physicians, rather than poultices – were more likely to be employed for "serious" chest ailments, including asthma, bronchitis, and pleurisy.

Other suggestions for colds were to put the feet in hot mustard-baths and to take internally "mustard, vinegar and molasses." Mustard footbaths, especially popular in Newfoundland from the middle of the nineteenth century until around the

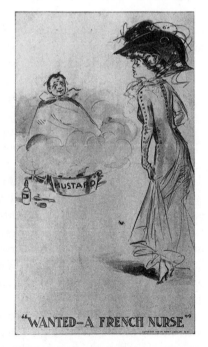

"WANTED—A FRENCH NURSE"

Mustard was "promoted" in many ways, including in this pre-World War I postcard

1950s, were sanctioned by many a domestic medicine book. Thus George Black's *The Doctor at Home and Nurse's Guide* (1927), in giving the theoretical justification held at the time, stated that the foot bath "acts by causing an increased flow of blood to a part remote from the seat of the injury, or from the part where the injury is feared. In order that this derivative action may be efficient, the water should be as hot as can be borne by the patient or, at any rate, sufficiently so to redden the skin. The quantity of water should come up to the patient's knees when the feet are in the bath ... Frequently mustard is added to the water to increase its derivative action." In 1951, Colman's mustard was still being advertised to Newfoundlanders for hot mustard-baths to fight colds "the easy way." A variant noted in the Newfoundland tradition was to add mustard to a baby's bath if a fever was present, although appropriate cooling regimens were probably commonly used. Musterole, a commercially-prepared rub, attracted considerable usage if only because it was less vigorous than mustard plasters.

The long-standing use of mustard (in water) to induce vomiting in poisoning is still well known.

Although mustard baths are generally considered to be a thing of the past, recent promotion (1993) of such preparations as "Dr. Singha's Mustard Bath" has been noted in the province.

NOTES

See: Black (1927) 76, for quotation; *Natural Health* 1993, Jan/Feb 102, for Dr. Singha's mustard bath.

Representative MUNFLA references: 67-15/53 (mustard plaster for rheumatism – mustard rosin and fat), 78-195 (mustard foot bath for common cold, mustard and flour poultice for pleurisy), 82-121 (an emetic for poisoning), 82-149 (mustard in baby's bath), 82-158 (mustard plaster for pneumonia).

MYRRH (MURR, TURPENTINE), FRANKUM

The one-time application of the soft resin, commonly called "myrrh" or "turpentine," obtained from fir or spruce trees as an application to *cuts*, and so on, is noted under that entry. A characteristic testimonial, which notes the resulting ease as much as the cure, was: "If you get a cut the first thing to do, go get a bladder of turpentine, put it right on the cut, heal it up in no time. Kill the soreness and cure it up. A bladder of turpentine just wrap a bit of rag around it that's all. Oh keep it there a day or so, that's all."

Additional uses are recorded for external application (in a preparation with birch) for burns, and for internal use (perhaps taken with sugar or molasses [q.v.]) for the treatment of chest complaints, or placed inside prunes (in place of the "stone") for stomach ailments.

The general confidence placed in myrrh (and in spruce in general) possibly lies behind one report of the value of the solidified resin, frankum, for scurvy (q.v.) – an erroneous belief, or at least vitamin C is not present. Use of frankum as a "chewing gum" is well known in Newfoundland, as it is elsewhere.

NOTES
See: MCG (1992) 002.

Representative MUNFLA references: 68-19/4 (myrrh and sugar for tuberculosis), 82-146 ("kernel" removed from prune and replaced by bladder, with birch for burns), 84-309B (source of vitamin C)

NERVES, STRESS, MENTAL ILLNESS

Everyone living in Newfoundland today knows the expression, "Oh me nerves." It is not always appreciated, however – even by physicians and other health-care workers – that on the island the term covers more than the conditions described by professionals as depression, anxiety, and other mental problems. In fact, so-called nerves is a popular "diagnosis" in many cultures, often covering much more than emotional and social distress. Some of these additional aspects are discussed below, as well as under *female complaints*.

Despite commercial preparations long being available for "nerves" – implying that it is a specific disease (see below) – the term in Newfoundland commonly referred to (and perhaps still does) a self-diagnosis of behaviour as outside the individual's normal pattern, as well as an explanation of various vague symptoms. As in many places elsewhere, nerves was seen primarily, although not exclusively, as a female problem; in some instances, the term referred to the menopause or a "run down" condition, an expression covering tiredness and tension, often referred to in commercial promotions (for example, in 1925, Carnol was advertised as a "nerve remedy and wonderful restorative in all *run down* conditions.")

Another generally acceptable reason for "nerves" or even a "nervous breakdown" was bereavement. "Like I say I tell you if somebody died that belong to you and your nerves would get bad after, they'd think they were still there. They used to believe in ghosts and everything then. So they'd think they were still there. The woman or her daughter or son, her nerves would get so bad, so she'd take Dr. Chase's Nerve Food then and build herself up and she'd be alright again. Her mind would be on the pills then, her mind would be on getting better and forget about the other."

The broad, ill-defined symptomatology of Newfoundland nerves in many ways reflects past concepts of nervous disorders within professional medicine. It has been said that in the eighteenth century almost every disease might be called nervous; later, in the last decades of the nineteenth century, the notion was popularized in neurasthenia, a diagnosis – popular for many decades – based on an ill-defined collection of symptoms. The wide range of symptoms perhaps explains why specific treatment recommendations are rare in the Newfoundland oral tradition, even though advertisements for over-the-counter medicines explicitly focused time and time again on nerves.

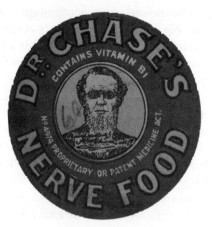

Box of Dr. Chase's Nerve Food

Three examples (composition now unknown) were Dr. Chase's Nerve Food noted above (for "exhausted nerves and palpitating heart" and many other symptoms), Therapion Number 3 (tonic and for nerves), and Asaya-Neurall (for nervous exhaustion – sometimes after childbirth). Even laxatives made the point: Tru-Lax, for instance, was said to be Nature's true laxative for "tense nerves."

An intriguing aspect of the nerve story is undoubtedly the wide range of over-the-counter preparations. Many advertisements implied a specific link between so-called nerves and the character of women, as did the diagnosis of neurasthenia already noted. Further, when advertisements indicated a preparation's usefulness for nerves, they also provided a ready rationalization for diverse symptoms. For instance, Lydia Pinkham's female medicine, mentioned in the Newfoundland oral record for nerves, was one of several that implied a replacement of nervous energy. Examples are Dr. William's Pink Pills, said to contain general tonics often needed by those "who feel old and whose bodies are lacking in certain esssentials vital to energy and vigour." "Kidney" and "liver" medicines (q.v.), too, were sometimes linked to tiredness. In 1952, Carter's Little Liver Pills were promoted for those who were "logy, listless, out of love with life."

Not advertised in Newfoundland newspapers were the standard "sedative" medicines used for treating nerves during much of the first half of the twentieth century, often when tonics were considered inappropriate. The former ranged from the long popular opium to bromides (introduced in the nineteenth century) and barbiturates (from the early twentieth century). Although these sedatives, barbiturates in particular, have long been considered as doctors' medicines, regulatory controls were not in place until recently and opium was still available "over-the-counter" during the 1930s.

The social acceptance of modern psychotropic drugs from the 1950s onwards – in some respects "modernized" versions of tonics and sedatives – has been striking. Whether or not the frequency of the condition of nerves in Newfoundland encouraged the acceptance of the new medicines on the island is unknown. Suggestions exist, however, that some physicians prescribed indiscriminately. One recently published story about a visit to the doctor by a middle-aged woman with nerves (actually a sharp pain in her side), indicates the physician's lack of understanding: "The doctor asks her what is wrong. Ruth hates herself for it but simply replies that her nerves 'are acting-up some awful.' Without further ado (it had been a busy day), the doctor writes her a prescription for nerve pills. Ruth dutifully thanks him and cannot wait to get out of the office."

Nowadays the term "stress," particularly when used by lay people, covers much of the symptomatology once associated with so-called nerves. Careful clarification of the meanings behind the use of the two terms is always needed.

There are many concerns at present about the new "chemical coping" (some say "chemical restraint") because of side-effects, dependence on drugs and doctors, and the fear of becoming "medical victims." Many people wonder if "natural" remedies are safer than chemical ones; some ask if, for example, hops (q.v., commonly found in Newfoundland) as a mild sedative might have something to offer, as do other herbs, like valerian with its mild sedative properties.

The whole subject of nerves and abnormal behaviour raises questions about what Newfoundlanders actually considered as "mental illness," and how it was looked after, for, as indicated, nerves were not viewed as a mental problem. A 1977 study indicated that Newfoundlanders generally correlated mental illness with extremely bizarre or violent behaviour and being out of touch with reality (what popular medical books might have called "dementia" and "mania.")

Although Newfoundland has had a mental hospital since 1854 (in St. John's), it is not clear how it was accepted by outport Newfoundlanders or whether it was used, at times, for social as well as medical reasons. In fact, the history of the asylum tells us nothing about "community psychiatry," much of which fell within home care. Indeed, Newfoundland families (with their extended networks of relatives) and outport communities accepted many people with difficult behaviour, sometimes described as "low-minded" or "dim."

Were there any specific factors that helped Newfoundlanders to accept abnormal behaviours? After all, the often incomprehensible nature of mental conditions has frequently prompted fear and stigma, just as did epilepsy (q.v.). Yet the eclectic nature of so-called nerves may well have allowed some Newfoundlanders to explain and accept conditions physicians diagnosed as "mental." Another factor possibly bringing certain conditions within a socially understood framework was the role of fairies. Although there have always been sceptics about fairy lore, it has had a strong cultural presence in many parts of twentieth-century Newfoundland. Mental and physical disabilities could be blamed on fairies. One record states that people "carried away" by fairies ("little people") were cured by having the priest bless them and talk to them privately. It went on to say that "most times this did not work and the person retained some peculiarity." Records also note that "to prevent oneself from being carried away" it is necessary "to take a piece of bread with you when you go into the woods."

As in fairy lore everywhere, fairies stole infants, replacing them with those deformed or mentally deficient (changelings.) One Newfoundland record describes "dim Pat:"

He is never here when we come around but you see him hiding behind the door or running off up to the woods. Once I told him I had to meet him, I said I was taking a census for the bishop so she brought him in. He's about thirty-two and he's ordinary but he always wears a skirt made out of canvas like you'd make sails with or you'd wear splitting fish. No pants underneath but the big boots and a shirt and this skirt. He's right odd but quite intelligent to speak to and he can fish and make little boats that his brothers sell for him. People say he's a changeling and fairies took the real one away, they're always saying that bout the odd ones.

The extent to which mental problems were seen as a consequence of one's personal behaviour or situation (in the way a tuberculous patient might be stigmatized because of poverty) is a more uncertain issue in trying to understand lay attitudes to mental illness. Indeed, there are few hints in the recorded oral tradition. In one case, dementia associated with syphilis seems to have been accepted without stigma, understood by the community because of the social standing of the individual.

It is impossible to say how "dim Pat" would be managed nowadays, but almost certainly he would have many contacts with, if not continuing care from, professional medicine. At present, powerful psychotropic drugs give a sense that medicine has more answers than ever before. A consequence is that many patients are facing their problems with less cultural support than in the past, if only because rationalizations of the condition do not "connect" with the environment. The consequences need exploration.

NOTES
See: Dinham (1977), for indicators of madness; Davis (1983b), for insights into nerves in Newfoundland, also reference to Chase's and Lydia Pinkham's products; Davis (1984), for details concerning the medical episode of the middle-aged woman;

MCG (1992) 002, on nerves and bereavement; Davis (1989), on Beard, Lydia Pinkham, and legitimacy for nervous complaints, especially for women; O'Brien (1989) 86, for seasonal variations for the year 1860 linked to work and transport patterns; Rieti (1990) 160, for "dim Pat" story; Bennett (1989) 123–4, on fairies and changelings; Helman (1981), for context of acceptance of psychotropic drugs; Thielman (1989), for background to community psychiatry; Gabe et al. (1991), on lay issues concerning psychoactive drugs.

Representative MUNFLA references: 75-150 (little people causing peculiarity).

Personal communication: R. Day (1991), on syphilis and dementia.

### NEWFOUNDLAND STOMACH
### (SEE STOMACH PROBLEMS)

### NIGHT-BLINDNESS (SEE EYES)

### NOSEBLEEDS

Wearing a green ribbon around the neck (sometimes given as a gift, sometimes not) to "prevent" repeated nosebleeds – it perhaps reminded a person not to rub the nose, blow it, and so on until well healed – was a well known practice in Newfoundland. "I had to give him a piece of green ribbon. That's a cure for nosebleed. I went to the store and gave it to Nina to give to him. And he never bleed the nose for years. And one time he went away in the lumberwoods and he forgot the piece of ribbon and his nose would start to bleed after he went away. Said he'd never forget his green ribbon no more." Alternatives included wearing a coloured string or a nutmeg around the neck, or wearing a "lead heart" (a slug from a shell, banged flat) as a necklace. Reciting a verse was also recommended as a preventive measure.

To give a "shock" with a cold object (for example, a key, a spoon or ice) down the neck or on the backbone is still a popular treatment. Another method (albeit noted by one Newfoundland informant as less effective than a cold object) was to place a small pebble or other hard object between the top lip and gum and press as hard as possible with the lips. This may have encouraged breathing through the mouth, a practice still recommended by some people. Perhaps this was done in conjunction with wet cloths on the nose, and pressure. A further suggestion – fairly widely reported in many folk traditions – was to place a piece of brown paper inside the upper lip.

Omitted from the record – even though well-known as a treatment and undoubtedly tried – was keeping quiet and, if necessary, gently packing the nose with a wet cloth, perhaps soaked in tea or a solution of iron for astringent action. Some sufferers ultimately called upon a doctor, who might apply lint swabbed with adrenalin rather than use a conventional styptic. Cauterizing the nose has long been, and still is, a recommended professional treatment for repeated bleeds.

NOTES
See: Murray (1979) 135, for opening quote; Sparkes (1983) 165, on green ribbon; Brown Collection (Hand 1961, vol. 6) 239–47, for many references to the use of brown paper and cold objects, and the wearing of black ribbon; Creighton (1968), on wearing of pierced nutmeg.

Representative MUNFLA references: 76-249 (ice down back), 78-200 (cold object down neck or on backbone), 82-146 (green ribbon, nutmeg, verse), 82-218 (key down back, paper inside upper lip).

## OAKUM

Oakum or tarred fibres of hemp – readily available to anyone who caulks boats, and a reminder for many Newfoundlanders of springtime repairs – was, like many "kitchen" remedies, readily available. It was recommended for chafed skin (q.v.), haemorrhoids (q.v.), galls (q.v.), and infected wounds. A number of skin conditions were (and still can be) helped by coal tar – long employed in one form or another in professional medicine.

What cannot be rationalized on physiological grounds was the use of oakum to stop the flow of mothers' milk: oakum was carried around "in their bosom" for about two weeks. Perhaps the perceived drying action was considered relevant.

NOTES
Representative MUNFLA references: 68-3/52 (stop milk flow), 78-200 (sore breasts), 82-122 (haemorrhoids, galls).

## OBESITY

The extent to which obesity was a concern for Newfoundlanders is uncertain, just as it is unclear whether there was a belief that a "healthy appetite" led to a "healthy body." The notion of strength has also always been a consideration in Newfoundland life.

Although it was apparently felt by some Newfoundland women, until recently, that weight was of little concern after marriage, they might well have been reminded of the sin of gluttony: "When anyone eats a lot of food, I have heard it said, think about the poor man who died eating." Newfoundlanders who were comfortable with the notion that to be plump, or big, is a sign of good health were possibly reassured by advertisements that encouraged putting on weight. Ostrex tonic tablets, for example, were advertised in the 1950s for skinny men and women.

The impact of cosmetics and other advertisements featuring slim women, if any, on Newfoundlanders from 1900 to 1950 is not known. Although little information is in the recorded oral tradition, at least one slimming suggestion exists, namely to drink the juice of steeped birch bark. Although the rationale given – that it would "shrink the stomach" – could be associated with astringency, a slender possibility of a diuretic effect (as noted under *birch*) must be considered. Certainly the reputation of some obesity treatments has rested on initial weight loss through fluid loss.

Few commercial slimming aids were advertised until recent decades. An early one (in the late 1890s), was Professor Compton's Anti-Fat Pellets and, later (1915), Antipon. One characteristic of the slimming promotion, and increasingly so with growing numbers of preparations in recent decades, was the uncertain and contradictory information. An article in the *Evening Telegram* (1951) told Newfoundlanders to "Eat Hearty and Grow Slim." More fat than carbohydrate was the recipe!

NOTES
Representative MUNFLA references: 63-1/379 (saying about poor men), 68-26/18 (birch bark), 69-10Ms (plumpness and good health).
    Personal communication: P. Scott (1991); N. Rusted (1991).

PAIN (SEE ANALGESICS)

PALATE, DROPPED

Concerns about a "dropped palate" (sometimes called "swollen palate" or "falling palate") are rarely found in folk-medicine records. In Newfoundland, the term generally referred to a swollen uvula, which physicians sometimes treated by surgically removing the tip of the uvula. Self-treatments recorded in Newfoundland, as elsewhere, included tying up the hair by pulling it straight up and fixing a bow around it – "to tie in a crown" – or tying it tightly around a stick. It was said that "the palate went up in less than a week," an observation which is compatible with normal recovery of what, for most people, was a self-limiting condition.

Although tying the hair is probably the commonest recommendation remembered, another – to wash out the mouth and gargle with salt and water – may well have encouraged speedier recovery. It is unlikely that adding pepper, as in one suggestion, contributed to the treatment, despite the rationalization that the "heat" from the pepper makes the palate go back.

NOTES
See: Brown Collection (Hand 1961, vol. 6) 184, for tying hair; Fitz-Gerald (1935) 171, for tying around stick.

Representative MUNFLA references: 68-13/15 (tie up hair), 69-30/10 (pepper), 82-149 (salt and pepper on "swollen" palate).

## "PASSING THROUGH"

In 1937, P.K. Devine wrote: "It was quite a common practice to pass a child through limbs of a dogberry tree to secure its future good health and make it immune to measles, smallpox, rickets and other diseases. An old tree standing at Wesleyville, Bonavista Bay, after a hundred years is evidence of this practice. It is to this day known, respected, and uncut as Uncle Joe Tiller's tree." Any "apse" tree (but commonly *Populus tremuloides*) of the right shape was apparently used. Treatment of hernias (q.v.) was a common reason for "passing through," at least for the complaint in children, and in places outside Newfoundland as well. Creighton, quoting a Newfoundland informant, recorded: "My son had the worst hernia as a child and we took him down and passed him under the crotch of the tree three times and he was all cured." Another Newfoundland record notes using a split balsam fir tree for a hernia.

Passing through was used as protection against children's complaints other than hernia, as noted in the opening quotation. In 1955, by which time the practice probably had little following (as had happened to "passing under an animal," see *animal parts),* N.H. Gosse wrote, "I went to go down Bishop's Cove Shore and see if any of the old Apse trees remain that once were split so that children with 'scrofula could be passed through.'" Although prevention of childhood ailments had long changed through immunization, for various reasons it had not brought about complete security.

NOTES
See: Creighton (1968) 216; Devine (1937a) 77, for uncertainty added to observation of passing through dogberry (by including it under dogwood [q.v.]).

Representative MUNFLA references: 84-361B (dogberry).

Personal communication: I. Rusted (1990), for N.H. Jasse information.

## PEBBLES (ROCKS)

A number of references to pebbles exist in the recent Newfoundland oral medical tradition: toothache treated by touching with a pebble taken from a newly dug grave of a good man or woman; seasickness treated with a pebble under the tongue; and warts treated by touching with pebbles that were then wrapped in a piece of rag and dropped on the highway. (Whoever picked up the bundle had the warts transferred to his or her own hands.)

Such suggestions – also commonplace outside Newfoundland, except perhaps the pebble for seasickness – embrace religious and magical concepts. Some people felt that a pebble from a grave was a way of invoking the Trinity in the healing process. The use of a pebble to magically transfer the disease has been an equally long-standing belief.

Nowadays, there is a tendency to perpetuate some of the pebble traditions through modern interest in crystal power for healing. This also invokes the once widespread professional medical use of minerals, some of which were based on empirical observation, as is well illustrated in early lapidary writings. But, as with animal parts and preparations (q.v.), professional medical interest faded in the sixteenth and seventeenth centuries.

NOTES
See: Riddle (1970), for background.
    Representative MUNFLA references: 69-23/36 (seasickness), 78-200 (toothache, warts), 84-361B (pebbles and the Trinity).


PITCHER PLANT

Newfoundland's provincial flower, *Sarracenia purpurea*, the pitcher plant, attracted limited professional and lay medical interest in the 1800s. In 1822, when Newfoundland explorer W.E. Cormack indicated that a decoction of

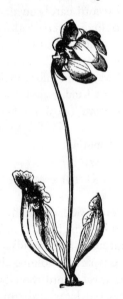

the root (also known as "Indian cup") was known to the Micmac for treating "spitting of blood, and other pulmonary complaints," professional medical interest had already been caught by its growing reputation for treating stomach ailments. More intense interest, however, emerged – at least for a while – concerning the value of the root in treating smallpox. C. Millspaugh, in his influential *American Medicinal Plants* (1892), referred to American Indian use of an infusion of the root for smallpox (as had P. Tocque when writing on Newfoundland in 1878). Millspaugh, however, reminded readers that participants at an 1861 meeting of the Medical Society of Nova Scotia had stated that there was no "reliable data upon which to ground any opinion in favour of its value as a remedial agent" against smallpox.

Medical opinions commonly differ over therapy. Standard medical texts of the 1890s still mentioned the plant, although one stated that it is "now but little used in medicine" as a diaphoretic, diuretic, and stomachic, as well as for atonic dyspepsia. Employment for venereal disease by the "Indians of Nova Scotia" was also noted, as was usage of an alcoholic, rather than aqueous, extract. Further, an account of Newfoundland in 1888 promoted the plant, particularly as an excellent remedy against the "gout."

It is unclear whether twentieth-century references to Micmac and other Indian usage for treating smallpox, "consumption" (tuberculosis), and blood-spitting – also noted in the recently recorded oral tradition – reflect persisting active interest or are simply a memory. In 1993, the only recorded recollection of the pitcher plant being used on the Micmac reserve, Conne River, was the use of its water trapped in the plant as an eye wash.

The astringency of the pitcher-plant root possibly contributed to the belief that it could stop bleeding from the lungs or the upper gastrointestinal tract, although no current scientific basis for this action exists. The frequent association of spitting of blood with tuberculosis (q.v.) possibly explains suggestions that the pitcher plant might be helpful in treating that disease. Astringency also rationalized the plant's usage for stomach complaints and perhaps, too, it was linked to fevers and, hence, smallpox.

Although modern chemical and pharmacological studies might offer alternative explanations for past usages – including the plant's reputation as a diuretic and strong laxative – the historical record hardly suggests that the pitcher plant is a wonder drug waiting to be rediscovered.

NOTES
See: Introduction to bibliography for history and background information; Cormack (1856) 53; Tocque (1878) 502; Denis (1888) 17–9; Chandler et al. (1979) and Green (1990) 863, for twentieth-century references; CMG (1993) 2, Micmacs at Conne River.

Representative MUNFLA references: 76-249 (blood spitting).

PLEURISY AND STITCH ("PAIN IN THE SIDE")

"Mild" or "dry" pleurisy is highlighted by pain in the side, especially during breathing when the pleura or membrane surrounding the lungs is inflamed. Although so-called standard home treatments for chest ailments were tried, the common Newfoundland recommendation for pleurisy among the various poultices (q.v.) seems to have been linseed meal. Until the advent of antibiotics, this was also a commonplace professional medical treatment. Mustard (q.v.) was also recommended.

Another and different type of pain in the side exists in the oral record, although sometimes the distinction was not made sufficiently clear. Known as a "stitch" and acquired on fast walking or running, it has prompted a number of treatment suggestions: placing a pebble under the tongue or a rock in the pocket; or finding a flat rock, spitting on it, throwing it over the left shoulder, and walking away without looking back. The self-limiting nature of a stitch might account, in part, for the belief that these practices can be helpful.

NOTES
Representative MUNFLA references: 69-6/7 (pebble in pocket), 69-23/24 (pebble under tongue), 69-25/20 (mustard "poultice"), 69-29/12 (linseed meal), 76-249 (pleurisy), 78-195 (linseed meal, mustard), 84-281B (under tongue), 78-195 (linseed meal, mustard).


PNEUMONIA

The entries under *poultices, colds* and *coughs* indicate that mustard plaster was sometimes used for treating all manner of chest complaints, at least before the advent of antibiotics. Such "strong" treatment (which could produce blisters on the chest) was once a common first approach used by physicians and lay people for the worrisome pneumonia, or at times if this disease was even suspected. Generally, a patient was kept warm in bed with a warming regimen (maybe dill tea) hoping for what was known as the crisis to come, after which the fever would break. The failure of a crisis to occur signalled a bad prognosis.

Milder acting poultices were preferred by some people and initially tried. One elderly Newfoundlander said recently: "I don't remember too many people dying [in the old days]. I remember my mother had pneumonia when I was young. My two aunts came to look after her. She was upstairs in the bed and they got a pot and they boiled oatmeal. They made oatmeal poultice. They put it between two pieces of cheesecloth and they went upstairs and put it on her chest. And then when that was cooled they had another one ready and they put that on. She was nearly scalded, the poor woman, but she got over it." Onion, when mixed with oatmeal (scalded first), was also specifically noted for pneumonia. That practice mirrors the high regard in which onion – either applied externally or taken internally – has been held for chest conditions. Additionally, placing raw onion in a sock was noted. Another Newfoundland suggestion for pneumonia – the application of linseed meal with raw cod liver oil – serves as a reminder of the adage "The worse the smell the better the medicine."

A further recommendation – ice bags (or tepid water) – mirrored one-time professional advice that cold could relieve pain by modifying the inflammatory process. Little evidence exists, however, that this was a wide-spread lay practice.

When penicillin became generally available after World War II, its success in treating pneumonia, perhaps more than its value for other infections, had considerable public impact and encouraged lay demand for antibiotic treatment as a cure-all beyond the medical evidence of its effectiveness. Indeed, it was one factor that led to the suggestion that faith in treatment had become less important. Hugh MacDermott made some interesting comments in 1938 when discussing a house call for pneumonia: "I went into the house. The bed had been brought down into the kitchen. It is the custom in small houses, when the family think that the end of a sick member is near, to bring the bed downstairs. This is done because of the difficulty of turning with a coffin on a narrow 'stairhead.' It may not be a wise procedure; for it is too easily forgotten that the sick person was well once, and had probably taken part in this act and knew its significance. It may well destroy the patient's hope of recovery."

NOTES
See: Bennett (1989) 96, dill tea; MCG (1992) 004, oatmeal poultice; MacDermott (1938) 265.

Representative MUNFLA references: 68-21/15 (linseed and olive or cod liver oil), 69-9/6 (Sloan's Liniment and goose grease on chest; swallow goose grease), 76-249 (tansy poultice, mustard plaster, onion in sock), 78-195 (linseed poultice), 78-200 (ice bags), 78-205 (oatmeal and chopped onion), 82-122 (linseed meal and old cod liver oil).

## POTATO

The potato is a good example of a widely employed item from the kitchen. Usage is noted under various entries: *burns and scalds, frostbite, poultices, rheumatism,* and *warts.*

## POULTICES

The use of innumerable poultices, a way to apply local heat, has been a popular practice among Newfoundlanders. Lay usage has often been in line with past professional medical usage (see *abscesses.*) Dr. J.M. Olds, the prominent Newfoundland physician and surgeon, once remarked that a physician must discover each family's favourite poultice and prescribe it if the family is to accept him as a good physician. In fact, by the 1930s poultices were becoming less popular in professional practice; even by 1900, medical thought was questioning "the time-honoured poultices" of bread and milk, flax-seed (linseed) meal, or elm bark since they "undoubtedly furnished culture media for the propagation of innumerable hosts of bacteria" and might cause infection through broken skin.

Newfoundlanders used poultices mostly for abscesses, boils, and carbuncles (q.v.); infections arising from splinters (gatherings, festerings, "risings"); colds and coughs (q.v.); pneumonia (q.v.); and sore throats (q.v.).

The bread poultice was probably the most popular treatment for boils and carbuncles. A "basic" form – described in medical textbooks – was prepared by adding boiling water to a thick slice (say three-quarters inch) of bread. This preparation, without overly mushing the bread, was applied to the sore area, which may have been coated with a layer of oil. Occasional Newfoundland recommendations exist for the use of stale or hard bread, softened by milk. Various items – from salt to vinegar – might be added. Sometimes, it seems, these was not used solely as medication, but to help prevent the poultice from becoming offensive in a short time. Perhaps this was also an intention of the "tansy poultice," for which the directions were: "Pick bunch of tansy on Lady Day (August 15), crumble some bread and tansy in boiling water. Add scraping of sunlight soap and boil together. Put poultice on gauze then on boil." If the poultice was employed for chest conditions, the aromatic ingredient may have helped "clear the passages" or the congestion.

A few other poultices containing plants are noted in the Newfoundland record. One was based on chickweed, sometimes called "chicken weed" (perhaps mixed with flour and water). Another – "macerated inner bark of the larch [juniper] mixed with castor oil" – was described, in 1936, as a "favourite poultice" possessed of great "drawing power."

Another favoured poultice for boils was made from soap (the widely used Sunlight soap was often specified), plus molasses and flour. Sugar might be substituted for the molasses and the flour omitted. It is easy to appreciate that some Newfoundlanders preferred such poultices to those prepared from fat pork (q.v.) or fatty meat, obviously more unpleasant to use.

Possibly the commonest poultice recommended for chest conditions in general was made from linseed meal, a poultice also widely recommended by physicians for pneumonia. A St. John's surgeon remembers barrels of linseed meal in the General Hospital during the 1930s. Linseed poultice, a popular treatment everywhere, "retains its heat and moisture for a long time; the oil it contains keeps it soft and prevents it from sticking." It was also easy to make: "Mix ground flax seed with boiling water until a smooth cohesive mass is formed."

---

**M. CONNORS, Druggist,**

## LINSEED.

*Water Street, West, St. John's, N.F.*

Label for linseed

---

Although the use of poultices in Newfoundland homes has been pushed to one side since the introduction of antibiotics, a few commercially made poultices (for example, from kaolin, magnesium sulphate) are still available. There remains, moreover, some appreciation that the application of local heat contributes to treating acute and chronic inflammations, though it tends to be forgotten. One noteworthy point in the Newfoundland record involves dealing with "ploughed flesh," a side-effect of a poultice that results from keeping the poultice in position for too long. Suggested treatment was to add a pinch of sugar to the next poultice. Some undoubtedly tried to avoid another poultice.

A postscript to any story of Newfoundland poultices should deal with the question of whether substitute ingredients, not recorded, were tried, because of availability and perhaps their usage elsewhere. One likely candidate is the plant, toadflax (*Linaria* spp., of which the yellowed-flowered species is popularly known as "butter and eggs"). The medical reputation of this plant has not been strong, at least since the time of John Gerard, who described, in his influential *Herball* (1597), a number of toadflaxes as diuretic and laxative (or at least possessing what was called a "deobstruent" effect on the liver and spleen.) A positive effect on jaundice was also noted. Of more interest is the mention of its beneficial effect on the "deformity" of the skin. Perhaps this information persisted, for, although few subsequent writers on herbs mentioned toadflax, a reputation for its use in "dropsy, jaundice and various cutaneous eruptions" continued. The application of the whole plant as a poultice or fomentation to haemorrhoids and other skin ailments was also reported in 1847. Although this was recorded elsewhere at times, by 1892 an influential writer was stating that the herb had dropped out of professional use entirely, except among homeopathic physicians. Whether it remained in popular Newfoundland culture is unclear.

NOTES
See: Introduction to bibliography for history and background information; Bergen (1899) III, for chickweed; Parsons (1936), on juniper.

Representative MUNFLA references: 68-22/3 (bread poultice for infected cut, also with salt), 68-10 MS (linseed meal), 69-25/1 (with salt and butter), 69-25/2 (with kerosene), 69-27/14, 69-22/1 (tansy poultice, boils), 82–158 (soap, flour, and molasses), 82 218 (Sunlight soap and vinegar).

Personal communication: F. Woodruff (1990), concerning Dr. Olds.

RASHES

Depending on their severity, rashes may or may not demand relief by medication. Whereas measles and german measles (rubella) generally do not need specific applications or treatments, the spots of chickenpox are itchy and Newfoundlanders, like sufferers elsewhere, have long applied calamine lotion purchased over the counter.

One of the commonest self-limiting (even transient) conditions is urticaria (commonly known as "nettle rash" or "hives"). Frequent in children, although possible at any age, urticaria is generally an allergic reaction. Despite current medical opinion that topical treatments have little place in management (nowadays oral antihistamines are commonly recommended), many traditional applications persist, often involving astringent washes (for example, tea) or sodium bicarbonate. Calamine lotion was (and still is) commonly used. In fact, simple procedures are rarely listed in the Newfoundland oral record, aside from the first-aid application of rolled oats soaked in water, the use of baking soda (perhaps made into paste with bread and water), and leaves such as "dock" and rhubarb.

A sulphur and molasses preparation, mentioned as a blood purifier (q.v.), was often employed in skin conditions. Listed, too, are the practices of rubbing animal blood over the rash; and crossing the hives with the sign of a cross, using the thumb nail.

Diaper rashes are noted under *infant care.*

NOTES
Representative MUNFLA references: 82-218 (paste of bread, soda and water, dandelion, rhubarb, and dock leaves).

RHEUMATISM (AND ARTHRITIS)

As in Western cultures, the Newfoundland oral tradition contains innumerable suggestions – external applications, internal treatment, and other practices (charms, bracelets, and so on) – for treating "rheumatism" and "arthritis." Lay usage of these two diagnoses has been generally loose and interchangeable; even mild muscle aches have been called rheumatism or arthritis.

The Newfoundland suggestions listed below are very much a "shopping list;" but as with sufferers elsewhere, more than one approach was (and is) often simultaneously taken. Some people say this is prudent. "I walked the floors night time cause my arthritis was so bad. Now I uses a number of things (copper bracelet, and a potato and a hazelnut in the pocket) I'm not sure which one works, but as long as I don't get it again I don't care." Attitudes that indicate that "doctors pills did not help," were commonplace as well.

*Suggestions from the recently Newfoundland recorded oral tradition:*
• External applications to affected area.
  1  Mixture of vinegar, turpentine, and eggs. Put ½ pt. vinegar, ½ pt. turpentine, and 2 eggs in shell into large wide-mouthed jar. Leave 48 hours until eggshells dissolved. Shake to make liniment.
  2  Mustard plaster. Mix mustard, rosin, and fat. Spread on muslin and apply to affected part. Leave on for three to four days.

3 Other applications: liniments and grease rubs. These include such popular commercial products as Sloan's and Minard's Liniments, as well as goose grease, and such less well-known applications as a dissolved jellyfish in water, or a white gin and vinegar preparation in which a pack of razor blades were said to have been dissolved.

4 Eel skin or eel. Well known for "cramps," the use of eel skins, or the eel itself, has also been recorded for "rheumatics"; for example, an "eel skinned alive for her rheumatics on her leg." It was thought that the oil of the skin might draw out the pain.

5 Covering with red flannel (even red flannel underwear).

- Internal medicines

1 Teas of sarsaparilla berries and roots, alder buds, or celery seeds

2 Cod liver oil

3 Mixture of sulphur and gin. Mix ¼ cup of sulphur in 26-oz bottle of white gin. Drink a few tablespoons each day.

- Other treatments

1 Copper bracelets. The most common cure for rheumatism among the old fishermen was to wear seven strands of copper wire around the ankle or wrist or both. This was kept on as long as the illness remained. Also suggested were copper rings and copper plates.

2 Aluminum rings

3 Fish parts. Carry haddock bone in pocket or suspended as necklace around the neck. Suspend a fish doctor (q.v.) around the neck.

4 Steal a potato. Carry the potato in a pocket until it has dried up or gone hard. Keep as close to afflicted area as possible. Some suggestions do not require that the potato be stolen.

5 Carry a lodestone.

If relief is obtained from at least some items in the first group, it may be linked to the presence of a rubefacient (a mild reddening and warming) action. The suggestion that dissolved razor blades might work is probably associated with notions of transferring or absorbing the disease (as is the use of eel skin.) Flannel (q.v.) was generally applied to the painful area alone or used with the other remedies, although flannel underwear also had a reputation as a preventive agent.

The second group, internal remedies, includes so-called blood purifiers (sarsaparilla [q.v.], and alder [q.v.]). Cod liver oil (q.v.), long been recommended for "rheumatism," is still promoted for "joint pain and stiffness." A sense has existed that the oil is a *specific* treatment for rheumatism; this notion has received support – although further investigations are needed – from recent scientific and medical studies.

Celery seed (in fact the fruit) has been known as a remedy for rheumatism since the nineteenth century, although the historical pedigree is not particularly strong and positive scientific support is unavailable. The interest of many Newfoundlanders in celery may well have been encouraged by the intensive advertising campaign – often appearing in newspaper column after column – for Paine's Celery Compound in the late 1800s and early 1900s. The preparation was promoted as a cure-all with striking claims for nervous troubles, melancholia, Bright's disease, liver complaints, neuralgia, dyspepsia, as well as rheumatism. One eye-catching advertisement (1894), having noted that "The future of Newfoundland depends upon strong and robust women," claimed that Paine's Celery Compound was the answer. Although celery for rheumatism was seemingly buried among other claims, its reputation strengthened in the first half of the twentieth century for reasons not entirely clear.

Of the items in the third group, the use of copper bracelets (and the use of copper in inflammatory disorders in general) has recently attracted scientific interest. Although the clinical value of bracelets remains to be evaluated through therapeutic trials, some positive data exists. Lay interest in copper was given a boost in recent years with its promotion in the nutrition and health literature. Indeed, an astonishing list of problems has been attributed, on questionable evidence, to copper deficiency. Included are anaemia, skeletal defects, degeneration of the nervous system, reproductive failure, elevated blood cholesterol, cardiovascular problems, impaired immunity, and defects in the pigmentation and structure of hair.

The charms mentioned in the third group (for example, haddock bone or fin, and lodestone) have reputations outside Newfoundland for counteracting both cramps and rheumatism. Perhaps Wilfred Grenfell added a local slant, however, when recording that the "peculiarity of the fin [as a charm] consists of the fact that the fish must be taken from the water and the fin cut out before the animal touches anything whatever, especially the boat. Anyone who has seen a trawl hauled knows how difficult a task this would be, with the jumping, squirming fish to cope with, and a host of naked hooks tossing around."

The potato has been widely employed in many places. Mostly it was to be carried in the pocket, but one Newfoundland recommendation referred to wearing potato as a ring around the finger. In fact, there seems to be an extension of these notions into a belief that eating potatoes is good for you: "If anybody ate an awful lot of potatoes they'll never have arthritis. I have no arthritis and I'm an awful potato eater: potato cakes, mashed potato, potato in soups, potatoes in stews and I can eat them raw." One rationalization – "it's the starch in potatoes" – is not acceptable nowadays: "Arthritis is in the bones and this starch gets in the bones."

As in other areas of self-care, over-the-counter medicines are a conspicuous part of the rheumatism story. Aside from the preparations noted above –

Minard's Liniment, Sloan's Liniment, and Paine's Celery Compound – numerous other commercial medicines were promoted among Newfoundlanders. In the early nineteen hundreds, Kickapoo Indian Sagwa was advertised in Newfoundland, one of a line of preparations widely promoted in North America by invoking a "pedigree" of native Indian medicine. But much longer lasting – to become a household name in Newfoundland – was Dodd's Kidney Pills (q.v.), a preparation said to clean or purify the system. Cystex ("end rheumatism while you sleep") was another example.

Throughout the early decades of the twentieth century much "purification" was aimed at removing or allegedly removing uric acid. This was based on an erroneous theory that disease was caused by an excess of the acid. The concept, emerging for a while in the early 1900s, tended to persist in popular explanations for rheumatism after it faded for other conditions. (See also *bathing*). Kruschen Salts was an over-the-counter medicine promoted in Newfoundland and elsewhere on this basis. Numerous advertisements indicated its role in relieving the agony of rheumatism.

The use of painkillers has long been part of the therapeutic armamentarium against rheumatism, especially substances which also have anti-inflammatory activity. Among those consistently promoted in Newfoundland ("at any outport store" it was said in 1927) were TRC's (known also as Templeton's Rheumatic Capsules), which, like aspirin, were listed for rheumatism, lumbago, neuritis, neuralgia, and sciatica.

Self-care for rheumatism has rarely provided anything but temporary relief. Although professional medicine has claimed greater success in recent years because of steroids and other potent drugs, the resulting side-effects have caused many concerns. Indeed, in many ways, self-treatment of rheumatism today is as vexing an issue as it was in the past. Many physicians are frustrated when contemplating the wide range of contemporary self-treatment practices. The following treatments and practices, recorded in the United States during the 1980s, are also representative of information from Australia, Ireland, and the United Kingdom: diets, copper bracelets, vitamins, acupuncture, cod liver oil, vinegar and honey, alfalfa, yucca, sea water, laying on of hands, Mexican border clinics, vaccine therapy, uranium clinics, osteopathy, faithhealing, and embrocation.

NOTES
See: Introduction to bibliography for general history and background information; Bergen (1899) 100, for potato as ring; Walker and Keats (1976), for suggestive evidence concerning value of copper bracelets; Grenfell (1932) 95, for haddock fin; Puckett Collection (Hand 1981) for extensive and analogous collection of suggestions including fish bones, and so on; MCG (1992) 002, for eating potatoes; Brown et al. (1980), Cassidy et al. (1983), Gray (1983), Kestin et al. (1985), Podgorski and

Edwards (1985), Puller et al. (1982), Struthers et al. (1983), for recent rheumatism treatments and concerns.

Representative MUNFLA references: 76-249 (copper bracelet, carry potato, carry lodestone), 77-78 (dissolved jellyfish), 78-195 (carry hazelnut), 78-200 (carry haddock bone), 78-205 (Minard's), 82-122 (Sloan's).

### SAFFRON (SEE MEASLES)

### SALT AND SALTED PRODUCTS

A noteworthy feature of recently recorded Newfoundland health care beliefs is the frequent reference to salt – long viewed as an essential food and readily available in Newfoundland as salt fish and other salted products. Many specific references to usage exist, aside from such warnings that if beef is too "fresh" – not salty enough – it can cause disease. Apart from the widespread symbolism of salt, there are beliefs that it has a general protective function, including against fairies.

Salt (often described as "coarse salt"), packed in small bags and heated, was employed for various ailments: earache (q.v.), toothache (q.v.), mumps (q.v.), and general aches and pains (for example, backache). Again, belief in the therapeutic value of warmth was one factor at play. Salt was also employed – perhaps commonly as it is still – in the form of a gargle for a sore throat (q.v.).

Sea water (or salt water) was well known, although there is no evidence it was widely used. Apparent reflections of the once widespread promotion of salt water within professional medicine (either to be taken internally or for bathing [q.v.]) are found in Newfoundland recommendations for using sea water to treat a swollen palate (q.v.), sore throat (q.v.), bed sores (q.v.), chilblains (q.v.), headaches (q.v.), cuts and welps, and freckles. Pickle water may have been viewed as a substitute or alternative.

Additionally, salted products were suggested. Salted herring has been commonly reported for sore throats as well as for croup and mumps. An alternative treatment for the "chest" or for colds was rubbing in salted butter.

NOTES
See: Toussaint-Samat (1992) 457–78, for background; Brown Collection (Hand 1961, vol. 6) 305, concerning bags of heated salt for toothache; Green (1990) 966, for little bag of heated salt for aches and pains; Rieti (1991b) 76, on salt and fairies.

Representative MUNFLA references: 64-1/82 (protection against fairies), 76-249 (gargle for sore throat), 78-195 (wormwood and salt, salt herring for sore throat), 78-200 (salt butter, salt herring for croup, hot course salt for toothache), 82-149 (earache, swollen palate).

## SARSAPARILLA

One of the most popular blood purifiers (q.v.) during the nineteenth century and well into the twentieth was "sarsaparilla," the principal commercial sources of which were *Smilax* spp. from Central America and the West Indies. Around 1900, Ayer's Sarsaparilla was a prominent over-the-counter preparation helping to sustain – through much newspaper advertising in Newfoundland – the long popularity of the root. ("The Sarsaparilla that makes rich red blood, strengthens the nerves, builds up the whole system.") Competing preparations that were to have an influence included Nyals Sarsaparilla and the local Macs Extract of Sarsaparilla Compound with Iodide of Potassium, "The Great Blood Purifier."

In North America, substitute sarsaparillas were employed, especially in home medicine. Locally available *Smilax* species (for example, *S. bona-nox*) have been reported for general "blood purifying" action, as well as specific diaphoretic (sweat-producing) and alterative, as well as stimulating, properties; reputations, however, were uneven.

In Newfoundland, mention of sarsaparilla sometimes refered to *Aralia hispida* as well as *A. nudicaulis* (yet another sarsaparilla, called American sarsaparilla or wild sarsaparilla); these (the roots, but perhaps more the berries) have a Newfoundland reputation as a "tonic" – similar to that throughout North America. Sarsaparilla wine (from berries) has been known on the island, although hardly as well as blueberry and dogberry. It was considered to be of value for fevers and, as with the berries, for colds and rheumatism.

Unlike sassafras, another "blood purifier," sarsaparilla is still viewed as a relatively safe beverage.

NOTES
See: Introduction to bibliography for general history and background to sarsaparillas.

Representative MUNFLA references: 68-21/16 (rheumatism), 69-2/7 (sarsaparilla wine for fever), 76-249 (tonic), 78-195 (berries for cold).

## SCURVY

Although scurvy is another deficiency disease that caused much concern in Newfoundland, it never aroused the same negative response, with respect to Newfoundland's image, as did beriberi (q.v.). In fact, early reports (for example, by Lind 1753) indicated that the disease was, somewhat surprisingly, absent in Newfoundland. But, as with beriberi (q.v.), it is difficult to assess the incidence of scurvy. In fact, full-blown cases may not have been common. Promotion of the value of Newfoundland's abundant berry crops, including how to store them for winter use, was possibly one factor at play; further, body stores of vitamin C last longer than thiamin for beriberi.

The recently recorded Newfoundland oral tradition contains scant reference to scurvy, although the need for vitamin C during World War II accounts for a reference to the value of rose hips. The use of spruce beer (q.v.) was noted until the 1950s, although as indicated in the entry it contained no vitamin C. A tea made from spruce tops, on the other hand, was helpful as a vitamin source. Perhaps it was the various uses of spruce in daily life that encouraged medical confidence in it; this is perhaps reflected in the following report of a practice that, despite lay opinions, had no value as a source of vitamin C: "Many years ago in Harbour Grace there was a lack of vitamin C. Newfoundlanders had trouble getting fresh fruit and vegetables. Therefore they chewed frankum off the spruce trees. It was said that this would supply them with their vitamin C." Certainly at the time there was concern over subclinical cases of vitamin C deficiency and infantile scurvy. The latter led to vitamin fortification of milk, another factor that removed elements of self-responsibility from self-care.

NOTES
See: Lind 1753 (1772 ed.) 146; Severs (1964).
    Representative MUNFLA references: 84-309B (frankum).

### SEAL FINGER

A well-known hazard of sealing, "seal finger" (and "seal hand") – generally considered to be caused by infection from a micro-organism carried by the seal – was not treated successfully until the advent of antibiotics, although the earlier sulphonamide treatment (emerging in the 1930s) was sometimes of benefit. Until then, as Newfoundland physician J.M. Olds once said, "heat, splinting and amputation were the only procedures available." In 1957, Olds indicated that some amputations were done in order to allow the fisherman to work without the handicap of a stiff and incapacitated finger (which was at least straight if it had been splinted.) "Seal finger is usually contracted in late April or early May. The patient wanted to go fishing in late May or June, as soon as the ice conditions permitted. He knew that if the finger ever did get well it would be stiff and cold. Therefore, he demanded amputation in order to be able to do his work and there was nothing to be gained by refusing him this relief." Other medical practitioners, less sensitive to the social limitations of handicap or ill-health, may have been more reluctant to amputate.

That few treatment recommendations exist in the recently recorded oral tradition may partly reflect a recognition of the intractable nature of seal finger. Even so, symptoms such as redness, painful swelling, and stiffness were treated with various poultices and skin preparations. One specific Newfoundland suggestion for seal finger was cow-dung poultices. If these offered temporary relief, they did not prevent the development of stiffness. Perhaps other treatments were tried, as described in a general review (1952) of practices employed by sealing captains:

1. A covering bandage was saturated with camphor oil and kept in place for one or two days at a time according to the severity of the infection. A partial destruction of the tissue took place followed by healing.
2. White wheat flour was made into a paste with alcohol and spread on the infected finger. This treatment was less radical and less effective.
3. A thick layer of soft soap (sometimes mixed with ordinary washing soda) was spread on the infected hand. The covering bandage was saturated with hot water, and the whole hand or finger was from time to time placed in very hot water. Naturally, this treatment was extremely painful, but apparently quite effective.

NOTES
See: Rodahl (1952), for general review; Olds (1957); also Troake (1989) 49, for differing views of contracting seal finger.
    Representative MUNFLA references: 69-23/40 (protect hands while sealing), 78-200 (cow dung).


SEASICKNESS

Seasickness, an especially frustrating problem for many Newfoundland fishermen, has a long history of often ingenious, albeit failed, treatments recommended by fishermen, sailors, and doctors. A Newfoundlander said recently:

I must tell you. When I was young at home I couldn't go out, the end of the Narrows, you get into the motion of the water, it's all motion. I always get seasick. When I joined the Navy I had weeks of it, vomiting out food. I was told by an old sailor to get a cup of the bilge water. Bilge water is what's down under the floor in the hole of the ships. This is loose water going between the flooring and the timber. But I wouldn't attempt to do that because I know what sort of a taste it would have. There was oil and everything into it. That was senseless.
    I was told to take that and I was put cook for one trip and I was still sick. The captain picked on me. The man's place I took he was a fireman and the Spanish influenza was on the go and he had died. So he said, "Young King, you're going to have to cook on the way down till we get to Halifax," he said to me. Now I had no knowledge of cooking, none whatsoever. He came down, got out of the wheelhouse, a small boat about a hundred feet long. He got out of the wheelhouse and he came to me and he told me when to put the vegetables on and when to

take them off and all that. And he said, "You listen to me, you'll overcome this, don't stop eating. If you stop eating and you have this seasickness, you're going to bring up blood after a time straining. But when you vomit food you're relieving yourself." But I got over it and it could get rough and it made no difference.

Whether or not Newfoundland physicians knew such writings as Herman Partsch's *Sea-Sickness. A Comprehensive Treatise for Practical Use* (Boston 1890), with its notions of cerebral anaemia produced by the sickness, is unknown, but the book's recommendations are not found in the Newfoundland oral record. They include:

1   Sit on a handful of earth in the boat.
2   Sit or stand on mud in the boat.
3   Take the aromatic cow-parsnip (wild-parsnip, q.v.).
4   Eat one of the following:
    a. buckshot; b. turnip; c. hard bread alone, or with fat pork softened in sea water, or molasses.
5   Drink bilge water or sea water.
6   Place a piece of brown shopping paper inside shirt next to chest.
7   Start smoking before you leave the wharf, then smoke at regular intervals (15–20 mins.) while at sea.

Nowadays, most people view these beliefs as mere "superstition" and of no value whatsoever, or at best as having some slight psychological benefit, often called a "placebo response." Certainly, in one sense, the story of seasickness as a whole suggests uncritical acceptance of treatments by physicians and lay people alike, based on flimsy, often anecdotal evidence. Yet apparently bizarre items such as bilge water should not be dismissed out of hand. Any consideration of past treatments must assess the combined factors of empirical observation, the role of theory (some found within professional medicine, such as settling the stomach or strengthening it), as well as sociocultural factors.

Sitting on earth or mud may have provided a relatively fixed position, albeit not the one recommended by many physicians of fixing the eye on the unmoving horizon, or staying in a hammock. As well, there were "seasick chairs," though they probably did not reach Newfoundland. Readers of the *Daily News* (21 February 1906) were told that the Hamburg-American Steamship Co. was testing a chair, powered by electricity, which kept the chair in constant motion.

Herbal remedies such as wild-parsnip (a recommendation not found in the Newfoundland record since 1899) might be rationalized in the context of many stomach remedies – at least those which have carminative properties – to settle the stomach. Over time, various writings (including *The*

*Newlanders Cure* [1630] by William Vaughan, of special interest to New-foundlanders,) recommended other aromatic preparations, as well as bitter ones such as wormwood (q.v.) intended to "strengthen" the stomach. However, there is no evidence that such stomach remedies were any more effective for seasickness than the use of turnip, fat pork, hard bread, bilge, or sea water; some felt the latter two were more effective on a full stomach.

The idea of applying brown paper to the chest or pit of the stomach was probably well known for treating seasickness; it is certainly recorded outside Newfoundland. The origin of the practice is uncertain, but it may be a variant of wearing an abdominal belt or scarf, or applying something warming to the stomach, perhaps along the lines of the carminative substances discussed earlier. Belts were attracting some interest in the early 1900s. One was described in the *Daily News* (1901) as having a buckle and screw to give extra pressure, while McMurdo's drugstore advertised Anti Mal de Mer Belts in 1906.

A practice like smoking, through its associations with growing up, acquired a special aura that may have encouraged a greater placebo response than occurred with many other treatments noted above. Newfoundlanders certainly clearly remember their early experiences, and how they got over seasickness. All in all, the "shopping list" of items reflects a trial-and-error approach for many. Lack of success meant some men were unable to continue in the fishery.

In the past fifty years or so, commercial medicines have crowded out home approaches. A considerable change came about with the accidental discovery (1947) of the value of antihistamines. The story is that dramamine was administered to a pregnant woman for urticaria and, unexpectedly, her car sickness was relieved. Antihistamines and scopolamine have been core treatments during the past forty or so years, but side-effects still remain an issue. Recommendations receiving current attention include ginger and acupressure. Wrist bands can be purchased that put pressure on a point found on the inside of the wrist.

NOTES
See: Vaughan (1630) 74; Partsch (1890); Money (1970), for medical context and treatments such as eyes on the horizon; Brown Collection (Hand 1961, vol. 6) 271, for brown paper *Onlooker* (1991), for current interest in Britain concerning motion sickness and brown paper; Wake (1991), for blotting paper as an alternative; Graedon and Graedon (1991) 407, for a popular health book promoting acupressure; MCG (1992) 001, for opening quotation.

Representative MUNFLA references: 67-5/71 (buckshot), 67-5/72 (bilge water), 67-14/77 (sit on earth), 68-3/219 (smoking), 69-21/16 (brown paper), 73-189 (sea water), 76-200 (bilge water), 82-121 (turnip, hard bread), 82-122 (eating pork, hard bread, molasses).

## SKIN DISEASES (SEE ALSO COMPLEXION, ECZEMA, ITCH, RASHES; SOAPS, TOILETRIES)

Many treatments for skin conditions are widely reported in popular medicine everywhere. Aside from specific recommendations (dealt with in the entries listed above), some "cure-all" remedies were tried. Cod liver oil and olive oil were well-known emollients and more widely used than urine, another general purpose treatment. Cure-alls were promoted at times by commercial preparations such as Dr. Agnew's Ointment: "Will eradicate almost every kind of skin disease" (1900). Even "cure-alls" specified specific conditions. D.D.D. Lotion was noted (15 March 1922) for "salt rheum" of the face, reflecting winter conditions of the skin of many Newfoundlanders. The expression, although not widely used, is still remembered.

Two other ailments merit comment. One is the occupational condition, squid hand – that is, inflamed hands arising from using squid as bait. Protective gloves and salt water are recommended.

The second ailment, not discussed in other entries dealing with the skin, is "shingles," which in at least one Newfoundland record was seemingly described as "St. Anthony's fire," a term more usually employed for erysipelas (q.v.). Shingles, a very painful condition, is recognized as difficult to treat. Among Newfoundland treatments was one with religious overtones – an application of blood (for example, blood from a finger prick) from someone named Cahill.

### NOTES

See: *Dictionary of Newfoundland English* (1990) 523, on squid hand.

Representative MUNFLA references: 67-8/22 (called St. Anthony's Fire, treatment by Cahill), 68-3/218 (squid hand), 68-13/14 (no treatment), 72-90Ms (shingles).

Personal communication: Troake (1991), concerning squid hand, salt rheum.

## SNAKEROOT

Innumerable plants (mostly native to North America) are popularly known as "snakeroots." An example found in Newfoundland is *Coptis groenlandica* (also known as "golden-root," "gold thread," "yellow snakeroot," or "yellow-mores"). The name is appropriate because of the thin, snaking rhizomes, although the name sometimes refers to a plant's reputation for treating snakebites.

A Newfoundland recommendation for treating mouth ulcers with the rhizome (made into a tea, sometimes called juice) is in line with practices elsewhere in North America. Newfoundland Micmac informants see it as very much part of their tradition: "You take it right out of the ground and you're ready to chew them up for a sore mouth, cold sores like that." Some consider it valuable to chew on the rhizome for sore lips.

The bitter taste and astringency of the plant (and other *Coptis* species) accounts for its reputation in Newfoundland and elsewhere as a tonic. In turn, this probably justifies a suggestion that "snakeroot be used for a bad stomach," although some have suggested that the presence of the alkaloid berberine may have a specific action in providing relief.

NOTES
See: Introduction to bibliography for general history and background information.

Representative MUNFLA references 69-6/13 (ulcers on tongue), 82-121 (for worms); MCG (1993) 2, Micmac usage.

SNOW-BLINDNESS (ICE-BLINDNESS)

Many treatment recommendations in the Newfoundland oral tradition testify to the frequency of snow-blindness, an acute inflammatory reaction to bright light especially when reinforced by the high-reflection factor of snow.

One of the worst experiences of my life with regards to health I suppose was the experience of being snowblind. This happened during the winter of 1934. It was caused by the brightness of the sun during the month of March. The eyes being exposed to the sun's rays caused the eyes to be very sore and for several days you would stay in a dark room, usually the bedroom, with the blinds closed. The remedy, including staying in the darkroom, was tansy boiled and a poultice made and put on the eyes. The cure took about a week to ten days. It was a cruel sickness with burning, smarting eyes all the time.

Suggestions, other than those in the opening quotation, include moist tea leaves. One regimen of this common recommendation was to place "leaves on the closed eyelids. After 24 hours the eyes will be cured." Testimony that this took the burning out of the eyes or "eases it" is strong, as it was for the recommendation to apply mother's milk. Only rarely tried, if at all, was "a rabbit's intestine" in place of the tea-leaves.

Another suggestion, drops of pickle water (salt and water) placed in the eyes for a day or so, is another example of self-treatment that employs ready-to-hand items. This was said to work (speeding normal recovery time), although the brine was hardly the normal saline which physicians might recommend to provide a little comfort.

Professional treatment (see Grenfell's comments in Part I) has probably been little better than lay care. That might include solutions of zinc sulphate and boric acid (q.v.). The best care – prevention by dark glasses – has long been recognized by Newfoundlanders. Micmac informants remember the use of birch bark with slits, a reminder of the slitted "spectacles" associated, in the past, with Inuit people. Nor has recent mention been found of looking at a black object or cloth held in the hand, as suggested in William Vaughan's *The Newlanders Cure* (1630).

Cold compresses (for example, with tea-leaves as noted above) are considered by physicians to give some relief, but many feel that the "success" of most remedies is a consequence of the self-limiting nature of the condition. It would be seen as a coincidence if the snow-blindness disappeared after twenty-four hours of tea-leaf treatment, as in the recommendation noted above. Nowadays, if antibiotics are given, it is done with the intention of preventing secondary infection.

NOTES
See: Tizzard (1984) 83, for opening quotation; MCG (1993) 2, Micmac birch bark; Roberts (1986), snow spectacles with slits; Gillan (1991) 52, for discussion that depicts snow or stenopaeic spectacles made from hollowed-out caribou antlers, "they protect the eyes from snowblindness and damage from ice crystals"; Vaughan (1630) 76.

Representative MUNFLA references 76-249 (dark glasses), 78-200 (tea-leaves, raw potato, onion mixed), 78-205 (boric acid), 82-122 (breast milk), 82-164 (tea-leaves), 84-323B (potato), 84-371 A/B (pickle-water).

## SOAPS, TOILETRIES

The commercial promotion of certain soaps (for example, Cuticura) to improve the complexion (q.v.) – "clear the skin" – has already been noted. The "all-purpose" Sunlight soap has acquired many accolades in Newfoundland. "No soap can beat it ... for washing the babies, and men used it for shaving." No wonder it was popular for poultices, helped as it was by intensive marketing.

Newfoundlanders were also bombarded, during the first half of the twentieth century, with information on medicated, germicidal, and other soaps, all part of the intensive British and North American promotion of outer and inner cleanliness. However, as already indicated, the lack of running water and baths probably minimized the impact. Even so, the promotion served as a constant reminder to Newfoundlanders, perhaps a public sensitizer, of many public-health issues.

Even before 1900, Newfoundlanders were told about Sulpholine soap (and Sulpholine lotion to cure skin diseases), a reflection of the general promotion of medicated soaps. Later, as with disinfectants, there was a sustained attack on germs on the skin. Calvert's Carbolic Soap was available by 1900, and later, in the 1930s, Neko Germicidal Soap was vigorously promoted as a destroyer of disease germs, preventer of infection, destroyer of body odours, and remover of dandruff. Lifebuoy Soap became better known. (One 1940 advertisement went: "Handyman! Your hands are germ carriers. Before you eat hands need a Lifebuoy wash to purify ... Lifebuoy lather is antiseptic for personal freshness.")

Subsequently, advertising strategies expanded on the "beautifying" properties of soap, as well as the dreaded complaint of body odour ("Play safe! Don't let friends whisper 'B.O.' about you!" went a lifebuoy advertisement in 1951, a theme the company had been using for many years.) That is not to say household soaps like Proctor and Gamble's White Naphtha Soap were forgotten; indeed, that was the subject of a promotional song in Doyle's songbook, "Song of the P. & G. White Naphtha Soap"

Oh! This soap it is so popular,
'Tis used in every bay;
Some call it the White Naphtha,
And I'm sure it's come to stay.
Now the merchants who stock this soap,
They say it's selling well,
And the men who manufacture it,
Are Proctor and Gamble.

Since the 1950s, with the promotion of an expanding range of products (including deodorants like Arrid – "new cream deodorant" and Old Spice stick deodorant [1950s]) – and, more recently, with stores opening in Newfoundland, such as the Body Shop, which limit their stock to toiletries and related items, the influence of toiletries on images of the body has become both more overt and subtle.

NOTES
See: Vinikas (1992), background; Doyle (1927); MCG (1992) 002, for Sunlight soap.

SORE THROAT, QUINSY

A striking range of suggestions exist for sore throat (some for "laryngitis") in the recently recorded Newfoundland oral tradition. Some were for "glutch" or swallowing: "My throat is so sore that I cannot glutch anything." The suggestions also cover a quinsy, a peritonsillar abscess or collection of pus that would generally be lanced and drained by a physician.

A commonplace suggestion was to tie a sock (perhaps dirty, perhaps red wool or red flannel) around the neck, although informants remember soaked fat pork, salted herring, or other fish as well. Such "wrappings" were (and are) sometimes seen as ways of providing therapeutic warmth or drawing out the soreness. In fact, one record indicated that the salted fish was to be warmed and that it was "the steam from it, the vapour from the salt" that was effective.

Additionally, preparations to be swallowed slowly included molasses, possibly mixed with lemon, kerosene, "liniments," vinegar, cod liver oil warmed or mixed with raisins and sulphur, as well as blackcurrant jam (perhaps dissolved in water). The latter, or at least "blackcurrant," has been widely promoted commercially in the form of blackcurrant lozenges since at least the early nineteenth century.

One informant related a somewhat alarming experience, but one which suggests the empirical tradition at work:

I had a quinsy throat and I nearly choked in bed, and I got out four o'clock in the morning, come down in the dark and I was going for the Listerine bottle and what did I do only take the peroxide. And my gosh, the foam in my mouth. The throat was so sore I thought I was going to choke. But anyway the peroxide did the trick. After I had it done, I didn't know if I was poisoned or no, I felt so queer. But I wouldn't be afraid to use the peroxide, it did me so good then. Thank God I never had a sore throat like that since.

It is unclear whether Listerine was to be used as a gargle. In fact, aside from salt- or pickle-water gargles, gargling is not often mentioned. Home-made candies (as noted under *colds and coughs*) were perhaps more popular. A "grandmother's" recipe for laryngitis was to mix molasses with vinegar and lemon juice, and boil. The mixture was then dipped in cold water to make taffy candy and sucked for twenty-four hours.

Another sore throat recommendation from the Newfoundland oral tradition again illustrates the pervasiveness of Minard's Liniment (q.v.): "Ten drops or more were mixed with cold water or molasses." The rise of eclectric oil (q.v.) was also noted, as was chewing raw onion.

As with so many other areas of home care in Newfoundland, there has been a seeming lack of recent interest in herbal medicines. Elsewhere, however, many astringent herbs have been commonly used to ease sore throats. In fact, popular and professional medical writings indicate that astringency was probably more beneficial than many of the above Newfoundland suggestions. Many over-the-counter preparations – gargles, sprays, paints, and lozenges containing astringent and antiseptic substances – were once prescribed by physicians.

From the 1960s, a more cautious approach to treating sore throats emerged, because of fears of streptococcal infections affecting the kidney. In consequence, overuse or misuse of antibiotics for sore throats has become something of a concern, especially as many cases result from viral infection.

A place remains for non-antimicrobial treatment. Although salt-water gargles are still advised, gargling with two to three soluble aspirin tablets is probably a more frequent suggestion. It is commonly recommended that professional advice be sought if the sore throat persists for more than two days.

NOTES

See: *Dictionary of Newfoundland English* (1990) 217, for glutch; Bergen (1899) 78, for salt herring; Creighton (1968) 229–30, on salt herring as a well-known remedy in Nova Scotia; MCG (1992) 109, peroxide story; MCG (1992) 002, for warming fish.

   Representative MUNFLA references: 76-249 (blackcurrant jam, honey, salt gargle, onion, Vicks), 78-195 (dirty sock, red flannel, salt herring, pickle-water), 78-200 (Eclectic oil and sugar), 82-164 (kerosene and molasses), 82-218 (camphorated oil, stocking), 84-281B (liniments and molasses), 84-309B (for laryngitis), 84-320B (warm cod liver oil).

## SORES (SEE CUTS)

## SPITTING OF BLOOD

With so much tuberculosis (q.v.) in Newfoundland during the first six decades of the twentieth century, it is a little surprising that few treatment recommendations for spitting blood have been found (other possible causes include lung cancer and damage to the blood vessels of the lungs due to coughing.) Only the use of the root of the pitcher plant (q.v.) and, from an older record (1899), *Lycopodium lucidulum* and the application of ice to the chest (see *tuberculosis*) are noted. Although the spores of *Lycopodium* spp. have been employed as a haemostat for cuts, and so on, that hardly explains its internal usage. A possible justification for the use of the pitcher plant is its astringency, but no scientific data supports its value.

NOTES

See: Bergen (1899), 113, for lycopodium.
   Representative MUNFLA references: 76-249 (pitcher plant).

## SPRAINS

Sprained wrists (not referring to infections, q.v.) were common among fishermen, especially during the early part of the fishing season. As a precaution many wore strands of yarn (perhaps nine, perhaps red) around the wrist. Bearing in mind that sprains were common, there are surprisingly few treatment suggestions in the recently recorded Newfoundland oral tradition. Presumably most sufferers merely bound a sprained wrist or ankle with a tight bandage, as universally recommended. Oakum (q.v.) may have been applied first. Cow-dung was also known as an application, as was comfrey (scrapings from roots as well as leaves); the latter has long had a striking reputation on both sides of the Atlantic for managing sprains. Although comfrey is not found growing wild in Newfoundland, it was (and is) cultivated in some gardens.

Red flannel (q.v.) was noted to help relieve pain.

NOTES
See: Introduction to bibliography, for history of and background to comfrey.

Representative MUNFLA references: 68-7/19 (tie nine knots in piece of fishing line and put round wrist; keep on for nine days), 68-11/M1 (comfrey root), 69-13/01 (flannel), 79-24 (tarry oakum), 84-287B (red yarn around wrist).

SPRUCE AND SPRUCE BEER

Teas made from spruce tops and spruce buds (from white and black spruce [*Picea glauca* and *P. mariana*], respectively) are recognized in the Newfoundland oral record as a tonic (q.v., sometimes a spring tonic) and as a beverage. The name of one over-the-counter medicine, Sprucine, marketed in the early twentieth century, drew on and encouraged this interest; containing "spruce gum, wild cherry, hoarhound, and tar," it was recommended for coughs and promoted as invaluable for the first stages of consumption (tuberculosis) if taken with cod liver oil.

A significant item in sustaining Newfoundland interest in spruce has been spruce beer. This had become popular in Newfoundland by the second half of the eighteenth century as a beverage possessing antiscorbutic (antiscurvy) properties. Joseph Banks, in his account of a visit to Newfoundland in 1766, claimed that spruce beer was the "common liquor of the country," a sentiment echoed thirty years or so later by another visitor, Aaron Thomas, who referred to that "grand and important article, not only in Newfoundland, but in the habitable world! It is Spruce Beer! In the Country it is the principal beverage of the people." Thomas, in extolling the many virtues of the spruce tree in the economy of the island, perhaps added testimony to the confidence placed in a drink made from it.

In Thomas' time, spruce beer was prepared either by fermenting an extract of spruce (black spruce was generally noted) or adding such an extract to beer.

Subsequently, references to spruce beer, usually fermented (or occasionally to "taking essence of spruce directly"), were erratic in the nineteenth-century medical literature. Rare is the enthusiasm of Napheys' *The Prevention and Cure of Disease* (1875): "Spruce beer is an admirable remedy in scurvy, and a wholesome, agreeable drink for those exposed to the disease.

It was used successfully by Captain Cook – to preserve the health of his crew." In fact, by that time – toward the end of the nineteenth century – fermented spruce beer, with its pedigree of tradition, was viewed as a dietetic preparation in the same context as ginger beer or molasses beer. This underscored a wholesome reputation, even without the addition of egg and sugar as described in one preparation noted by Banks in 1766, which recalls the earlier popularity of diet drinks.

The vitamin C content of spruce beer depends, in part, on the method of preparation, and it has recently become clear that, despite the vitamin's long-standing reputation as an antiscorbutic, the amount of vitamin is insufficient – certainly if prepared by fermention – to treat scurvy. In fact, Newfoundland usage of spruce beer (including the unfermented product) during this century lost any medical associations, except as a tonic. Even so, at least one recollection exists of the beer still being employed in the 1950s for home treatment of what was thought to be scurvy in children. In terms of vitamin C content, teas made of spruce tops are more beneficial. A question recently raised, but as yet unanswered, is whether an antiscorbutic constituent (not vitamin C) is present in the spruce beer.

Although commercial spruce beer is not easy to find nowadays, Chafe's Spruce Beer (Goulds, Newfoundland) is available (1993) and helps to keep alive a tradition.

NOTES

See: Thomas (1968 [1794]) 59–62; Naphys (1875) 804; Carpenter (1986) 226, for information on vitamin C content; for Banks (1766), see Lysaght (1971) 39–40.

Representative MUNFLA references: 76-249 (spruce beer as tonic), 78-195 (spruce buds and beer as tonic).

Personal communication: R. Day (1992), on spruce beer for scurvy in 1950s.

SQUASHBERRY AND WITHEROD

In Newfoundland, squashberry refers to *Viburnum edule* and perhaps, on occasion, to *V. trilobum*. One record from the recent oral tradition indicates its reputation as an emetic to produce vomiting: bark was taken from the middle of the tree, steeped to make a tea, and used to produce vomiting. Vomiting may be linked to another recommendation that squashberry (the fruit, not the root) be used for stomach trouble, but a more likely rationalization is the bitter and sour taste of the fruit. Some people have felt that squashberry jelly and wine can help settle a stomach.

Another *Viburnum* species, *V. cassinoides*, popularly known in Newfoundland as witherod, has been noted (1899) for preparing plasters. This – presumably another means of retaining heat rather than for any specific medicinal effect – was recommended for colds, muscle aches, and so on.

The *Viburnum* species have not had a major place in professional or domestic medicine, apart from perhaps *V. opulus*, introduced into Newfoundland, and *V. prunifolium* – both regarded as useful for female disorders because of a reputed effect on the uterus. While it seems clear that not all *Viburnum* species possess these actions, studies are merited on squashberry.

NOTES
Bergen (1899) 116, for *V. cassinoides*.
Representative MUNFLA reference: 68-1/68 (as emetic).

## "STOMACH TROUBLE"; NEWFOUNDLAND STOMACH; STOMACH FLU (SEE ALSO DYSPEPSIA, HEARTBURN)

"Stomach trouble," as it was often called, has been commonplace in Newfoundland. In fact, in 1941 two physicians, D. Steven and G. Wald, commented on what was then known locally as "Newfoundland Stomach," a name for diverse symptoms: prolonged constipation and some non-specific complaints, such as irritability, dyspepsia, itching and burning sensations, and lassitude. At the time, some suggested that a vitamin $B_1$ deficiency caused this syndrome. "Stomach sick" is also noted in the record: "If you were sick, I don't know if you heard tell of it, but it you were stomach sick and have a sort of a headache, my mother always would have senna tea [see *constipation*] she would call it and that was for an upset stomach if you felt sick."

Recommendations in the Newfoundland oral tradition for treating stomach trouble – commonly referred to as "gas," "griping," or "cramps" (not menstrual cramps sometimes meant by the term) – include the inner bark of the "squashberry tree" (q.v.) and teas from juniper (q.v.), alder buds (q.v.), and dogberry (q.v.).

Well-known kitchen remedies also noted – especially when "indigestion" was specified – were antacid, baking soda (q.v.) and aromatics, such as nutmeg and peppermint, acting as carminatives or "settlers." Another suggestion for stomach ailments (including cramps, "flu," stomach flu, and "sick to your stomach") was ginger tea (which could be made from crystallized ginger, or more commonly from ginger essence purchased from almost any store.) One notion – at least for stomach flu, although the idea probably extended to other ailments – was that a *hot* beverage, no matter what it was made from, was the important consideration. Whisky in hot water was suggested for gas.

Non-medicine treatment included placing a pebble under the tongue, or kneeling down with the "rear end" up as far as possible, and putting the head to the floor in order to break wind.

Because stomach trouble was apparently widespread in Newfoundland (some came to see it as ulcers), the treatment recommendations in the recently recorded oral tradition are surprisingly limited. On the other hand, numerous proprietary remedies were always available. "Radway's" was, in fact, mentioned in the oral record for "gas," though just as well known was Alka-Seltzer.

Much stomach indigestion was treated in the early decades of the twentieth century by preparations purported to aid digestion by supplementing enzyme action. Pape's Diapepsin was one example frequently advertised in Newfoundland (see under *heartburn*).

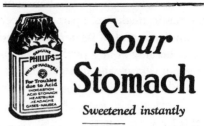

*Sour* **Stomach** *Sweetened instantly*

Just a tasteless dose of Phillip's Milk of Magnesia in water. That is an alkali, effective, yet harmless. It has been the standard antacid for 50 years among physicians everywhere. One such one and only time it once many times it volume in acid. It is 'he rich way the acid pleasant and efficient way to kill the excess acid. The stomach becomes sweet, the pain departs. You are happy again in five minutes. Don't depend on crude methods. Employ the best way yet evolved in all the years of searching. That is Phillips' Milk of Magnesia.

Be sure to get the genuine Phillips' Milk of Magnesia prescribed by physicians for 50 years in correcting excess acids. Each bottle contains full directions—any drugstore.

GERALD S. DOYLE, LTD.,
Sole Agents for Newfoundland.

Newspaper advertisement, January 1930

In general, other over-the-counter medicines, many already long-standing, overtook such enzyme preparations in popularity. Gallons galore of Phillips' Milk of Magnesia have been swallowed by Newfoundlanders who were probably swayed by advertising that stressed sour or acid stomachs; this was part of the widening medical interest in acidity throughout the body as the cause of various ailments. "The whole world, it would seem, is suffering from too much acid" was one comment in 1935, and in Newfoundland at the time, the well-known physician Cluny Macpherson was prescribing alkaline treatment for various medical conditions. Such professional practices probably helped to reinforce the popular preoccupation with antacids. Certainly Newfoundlanders had a considerable choice: Ki-moids, Alka-Seltzer, Eno's Fruit Salt ("neutralize gastric acidity"), other effervescent salts, and Milk of Magnesia.

Antacids, as noted under dyspepsia, remain a principal over-the-counter treatment for relieving stomach ailments.

NOTES

See: Steven and Wald (1941); MCG (1992) 106, for stomach sick; Whorton (1989), for quotation on world and acid (outlines the interests in United States in acidosis and alkaline diets).

Representative MUNFLA references: 68-1/68 (squashberry); 69-22 MS (juniper to relieve cramps in infants), 69-23/20 (kneeling down), 76-249 (whisky in hot water, and baking soda for gas), 78-195 (juniper, alder, dogberry), 85-001 (hot beverages).

Personal communication: I. Rusted (1991), on Macpherson.

### STRAWBERRY

That Extract of Wild Strawberry is still available in Newfoundland drug-stores is a reminder of the one-time popularity of Kline's Extract of Wild Strawberry "for the treatment of diarrhoea, dysentery, pain in the stomach and cramps." When "bottled for Gerald S. Doyle," it contained strawberry leaf, blackberry root, rhubarb, logwood, ginger, and chloroform. Most people remember this extract for relief of "summer complaint," the diarrhoea of summertime.

### SULPHUR AND MOLASSES

Sulphur and molasses has been described as a "standard" springtime purgative in Newfoundland, although some viewed it more as a blood purifier (q.v.) or as a tonic (q.v.) with mild purgative action. With perhaps two cups of molasses to one and a half teaspoonfuls of sulphur, the preparation was used in various spring regimens, which included taking a teaspoonful for nine consecutive days (or perhaps for three days), followed by three without and three with. Single doses were also used: "In the spring, according to my grandmother, everyone in the family, from the oldest grandparent to the youngest grandchild would be given a few tablespoons, or even a glass, of a mixture of sulphur and molasses to purify the blood after the winter."

Until well into the twentieth century sulphur was widely recommended by physicians for internal use, sometimes with the idea that it had a specific action on rheumatism. (External usage of sulphur is considered elsewhere; see *itch* and fumigation under *germs*).

Although the molasses (q.v.) served primarily as a vehicle to administer the unpalatable sulphur, it was also viewed as having its own health-giving properties. Treacle is a loose synonym for molasses; in Britain, sulphur and molasses is commonly known as "brimstone and treacle."

NOTES
See: Murray (1979) 133, and Saunders (1986) 137, for regimens of sulphur and molasses.

Representative MUNFLA references: 64-4/5 (quotation on sulphur and molasses).

### SYPHILIS

The incidence of syphilis and other venereal diseases in Newfoundland during the first half of the twentieth century is uncertain. A feeling exists that the relative isolation of the outports kept it at bay. However, an Act for the Prevention of Venereal Disease (1921) recognized the existence of the disease, and, in the 1930s, congenital syphilis emerged as an issue. In

1943, some physicians viewed it as a significant problem in small outports outside St. John's. The Deputy Minister of Health, Leonard Miller, noted (1950) that the disease had "been present in some localities for many years." Times were changing, however. The 1940s saw the emergence of penicillin, soon to transform the treatment of the disease away from the relatively painful, and hardly popular, arsenical drugs introduced in 1910. Some physicians supplemented this with unpleasant mercurial preparations.

Newfoundland records of the oral tradition, as elsewhere, offer relatively few suggestions for venereal diseases (perhaps a reflection of reticence on the part of informants). Nevertheless, a genital discharge was probably treated symptomatically with salves and astringent teas.

One "treatment" suggestion, not unique to Newfoundland, was that syphilis could be cured by intercourse with seven different girls, an idea not far removed from having intercourse with a virgin, possibly as a way of "transferring" the disease. If taken seriously, these notions, sustained in part in the male subculture by public secrecy and shrouding of information about venereal disease, had public health implications; at the least, they prompt questions for health education.

NOTES
See: Smallwood and Pitt (1981) 420, congenital syphilis; *Northern Medical Review* 1943:1,17, comment on problem in outports; Miller (1950); Hall (1991) 44, for persistence of idea of intercourse with a virgin.

Representative MUNFLA reference: 68-7/12 (intercourse seven times).

TANSY

Entries on abortion (q.v.) and female remedies (q.v.) indicate tansy's best-known uses and widespread reputation. But tansy is also regarded as a tonic. Some Newfoundlanders recognized this latter reputation – attributed to its bitterness – as well as its presumed action as a blood purifier; for these properties the expressed "juice" was perhaps considered most effective.

Additionally, tansy (*Tanacetum vulgare* and *T. huronense*, sometimes called "golden buttons" because of the small, yellow flowering heads) has been popular in Newfoundland

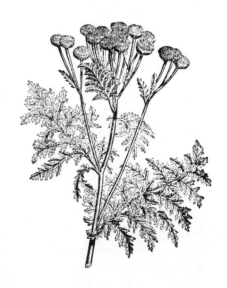

as, or in, poultices for colds, pneumonia, and other chest conditions. Whether this was more for its odour – to clear the passages or to improve the odour of the poultice – is unclear. But at least the tansy in a "poultice" placed around the forehead for headache was felt to have specific benefit.

Tansy was also noted for toothache and for erysipelas (as an application of the flowers), although these were not well-established recommendations. A usage – rubbing the tansy on the skin – for warding off fleas was also recorded.

Undoubtedly, a 1936 comment was apt: "Tansy is used for a great number of ills and is thought so highly of that in some homes it is gathered for winter use." Perhaps it was collected from a tansy patch planted in gardens, rather than from wild plants. One record speaks of a relevant experience. The informant had a "swollen kneecap" as a result of a fall. A local woman, who had a reputation for her medical skill, offered advice: "Go up in Henneburry's garden up there and pick a bit of tansy and steep it and put it in poultice [the tansy alone] on her leg five or six times and she will lose all that." (See *yarrow* for possible confusion of the two plants).

NOTES
See: Introduction to bibliography for general history and background information; Parsons (1936), for quote; Creighton (1968) 198, for the notion of tansy as a blood purifier; Rubia (1980) 201, for tansy as a poultice (identified as yellow flower); Sparkes (1983) 30, for tansy patch; MCG (1992) 104, for tansy and knee.

Representative MUNFLA references: 67-2/38 (chest congestion), 76-249 (poultice side of face for toothache; on chest for pneumonia, pleurisy, abortion), 78-195 (cold), 78-200 (tansy around head for headache), 78-205 (erysipelas), 82-122 (tansy or linseed meal mixed with cod liver oil for pneumonia), 89-084 (value of tansy juice).

THRUSH (THRASH, WHITE MOUTH)

Thrush – an oral candida infection – is common in infants from a very early age. A sign of the problem is when feeding (by bottle or breast) becomes difficult and a white coating on the tongue, the inside of the cheeks, and the tonsils appears – hence the term "white mouth." Thrush also occurs in adults, particularly in circumstances involving antimicrobial therapy, pregnancy, or diabetes.

Surprisingly few treatment recommendations appear in the Newfoundland record, which may partly reflect that physicians have long been more readily consulted for children's ailments than adult complaints. Alum (q.v.), as noted in the entry, has not been reported as a Newfoundland remedy, although it is commonly used elsewhere. It is far from clear whether suggestions to wipe the inside of the mouth with molasses or pickle water were helpful.

The use of blood has not been widely reported. Nevertheless, the recommendations to drip blood from a cock's comb into the mouth or to rub blood from a rooster's comb with a white rag may have been fairly well known practices for this condition.

Nowadays, thrush is invariably treated by antifungal medicines prescribed by physicians.

NOTES

See: Bergen (1899) 69, blood from comb.

Representative MUNFLA references: 82-122 (roosters blood and pickle-water).

## TONICS, SPRING TONICS

Advertisements in Newfoundland newspapers rarely had a local touch, but in the *Evening Telegram* of 6 March 1925, the McMurdo Drugstore in St. John's advertised in its Store News:

### Spring Tonics

Now that to all appearances we are to have an early spring, and it is the time when one does not feel quite alright a bottle of any of the following will pick you up very quickly

| | |
|---|---|
| Wampole's Extract of C.L.O. | $1.20 |
| Compound Sarsaparilla | $1.00 |
| Quinine Iron Tonic | .50 |
| Compound Hypophosphites | 50c and $1.00 |

Another advertisement of the time proclaimed the locally produced Stafford's Mandrake Bitters as a spring tonic and blood purifier. Like other "bitters" (q.v.), it probably contained alcohol, a reminder that beer and other alcoholic beverages were also promoted at times as tonics. Earlier promotions of spring tonics in Newfoundland included Paine's Celery Compound and Dr. William's Pink Pills.

Much Newfoundland interest in spring tonics during the first few decades of the twentieth century was reflected in home-made preparations: "Everyone needed a tonic in the spring. The man of the house cut branches from pine, dogwood, juniper and cherry trees. He peeled the rind from the trees and boiled and strained it and then added sugar. The daily dosage was two or more teaspoonfuls." This quotation implies "polypharmacy," but many Newfoundlanders relied on a single spring tonic, of which juniper (q.v.) was probably the best known locally gathered herb, followed closely by dandelion greens. See also *sulphur and molasses*.

The practice of taking tonics in the spring, perhaps for two weeks or so, was fairly widely established by the nineteenth century. The reasons for the emergence and persistence of spring tonics are complex. One thread seems to have been the long-standing notion that the body was suffering from a plethora, an over-abundance, of vitiated or bad blood. This was commonly treated by blood-letting, until the nineteenth century when various other forms of "blood purification" (q.v.) emerged. In fact the value of losing blood is found in the recently recorded Newfoundland oral tradition. One example involved a cut on the foot to let out bad blood; it was also said that "a good nosebleed now and then gets rid of dirt in the blood and is a great help to a person." Although no clear evidence has been found, it is possible that nosebleeds were also thought to remove "too much blood," a notion that explained the link between blood and headaches, backaches, strokes, dizziness, and swelling of the feet. "Too much blood" has, at times, been treated with taking vinegar to "dry up" the blood.

Whether the often inclement springtime of Newfoundland or other factors encouraged greater use of tonics than elsewhere is unknown, but possible. It was reported in 1921 that the "first seasonal signs of the effect of restricted diet appeared at the end of March and beginning of April ... A sudden increase in nervous instability was evident at this season." There was also a sense that certain spring customs had health associations. For some people, the culinary rite of eating a plate of dandelions was as much a celebration of spring as a health rite; at least one influential social reformer, Wilfred Grenfell, promoted dandelions for nutrition.

Spring tonics – mostly regarded as "blood purifiers" (q.v.) or laxatives – were employed as tonics at other times of the year (perhaps "after flu or something, no get up and go, didn't care whether you ate or no.") Ingredients in one compounded tonic/blood purifier or "cleanser" recorded in the oral tradition contained medicinal plants that were all well known in Newfoundland: "ground juniper, tansy, blackberry, juniper herb and black spruce." Other widely known tonics were dogberry (q.v.) – sometimes specified as the inner bark – "cherry tree bark" (see *wild cherry*), sarsaparilla (q.v.), sulphur and molasses (q.v.), and cod liver oil (q.v.). Seaweed has also been mentioned as a spring tonic "to clean the blood and increase the milk supply." The latter presumably refers to the "galactagogue" action or the increase of milk supply of a nursing mother. Seaweed is not generally recognized as having such an action.

As in other areas of self-care, commercial preparations, by invoking new medical concepts, often extended the tonic market, as did a number of physicians who recommended them. The records of Newfoundland physician George Cross for 1930 indicate that he prescribed many so-called tonics, although these are not named. Many physicians still saw a role for these preparations in the 1950s.

At the time of McMurdo drugstore's 1925 promotion of spring tonics, both the listed hypophosphite preparation and the Quinine Iron Tonic had been popular for some time. Lay and, to some extent, professional interest in hypophosphites was linked to the view that phosphorus was a nerve and brain food as well as having a generally favourable influence on nutrition; it was also said to be of special value against tuberculosis. As such, hypophosphites were included in many tonics.

Preparations such as Quinine Iron Tonic added another concept to blood purification – that of a strengthener. This preparation, like many tonics, was very bitter. In this case, that was due to the presence of quinine, a constituent of the bark of the cinchona tree, which had long been employed as a general tonic, albeit better known for the treatment of malarial fevers. But the presence of iron was seen by many as especially valuable. Preparations with iron – with the implicit, if not explicit, analogy to the strength of the metal – deserve special mention because of their popularity in Newfoundland, at least those that were intensively advertised. The use of iron, well established in the nineteenth century, had a veritable reputation as a cure-all for "weakness, inactivity, depression, loss of appetite, dyspepsia, indigestion, neuralgia, hysteria, and all diseases so distressing to ladies," and so on. In the twentieth century, it came to be linked with the treatment of iron-deficiency anaemia, although Newfoundlanders sometimes spoke of a "shortage of blood" or of being as "white as a sheet."

In Newfoundland during the early 1900s, Dr. Bovel's Iron Tonic Pills, said to make "rich red blood," were promoted for many conditions, including the needs of weak women. There was also Nuxated Iron (red blood food; organic iron as in vegetables). But more long lasting in Newfoundland, and still widely remembered, was Parrish's Chemical Food. It contained, according to McMurdo & Co's brand available around 1910, "Syrup of the Phosphates of Lime, Iron, Potash and Soda." Aside from the iron, the phosphate content was viewed as beneficial. It is difficult to assess the overall importance of iron preparations, but certainly iron-deficiency anaemia was probably a not uncommon condition.

As a footnote, Dr. Williams Pink Pills have served as another long-lasting and popular commercial tonic in Newfoundland. At various times, the advertisements have proclaimed that "Spring blood is bad blood" and that the pills take "the lead feeling out of your legs." The Pink Pills were often thought to contain iron. That an analysis early in the century found only the laxative aloes to be present is yet another instance of the current difficulty in assessing the value (if any) of many over-the-counter medicines.

Iron, like all older tonics, has been pushed to one side in recent decades by vitamins (q.v.), although the persistent and growing emphasis on mineral supplementation ensures a continuing market for iron tonics even when there is no obvious clinical justification. Current interest in herbal medicine is also refocusing attention on spring tonics and tonics in general. Swedish Bitters, for instance, one of a number of so-called tonics now on the market, was described in April 1991 as "Your perfect partner for spring cleansing."

NOTES
See: Day, R., for information on Dr. George Cross; Bergen (1899) 163, for note-worthy contemporary comment; Appleton (1921), for springtime nervous instability; Waldo (1920) 20, for one instance of Grenfell's promotion of dandelion; Creighton (1968) 231, on dandelion greens in Nova Scotia (one comment: "as good as iron pills); Wicks (n.d.), for Newfoundland advertisements promoting beer, and so on, as tonic; Harris (1989), for general background on iron; *Alive*, 21 April 1991, for Swedish bitters advertisement.

Representative MUNFLA references: 68-016D (shortage of blood), 69-12/3 (value of nosebleed), 73-189 (seaweed), 76-249 (juniper, sarsaparilla, cherry bark, spruce beer tonics), 78-195 (wormwood and salt), 78-200 (cut feet to let out bad blood), 82-121 (cod liver oil, rum as tonics), 82-158 (dogwood tree, cherry tree).

Personal communication: R. Day (1991), for information on Dr. George Cross.

## TOOTHACHE AND TEETHING

Graphic recollections, even if embroidered, testify to the once common-place extraction of teeth by physicians rather than dentists in Newfound-land outports. "In those days wild screams would come from the surgery as some poor unfortunate went through the ordeal of tooth extraction, and how occasionally the quiet voice of the doctor would float through the hallway. 'If you will kindly let go of my beard madam, I will proceed with the extraction!'" As one physician wrote on 10 March 1922: "I am gathering quite a reputation as a dentist, or tooth extractor. I give nothing and take everything, then soak them 50 cents afterwards. Have removed more than a dozen to now and like it less all the time."

The poor state of Newfoundlanders' teeth until recent times has often been mentioned: "You'd see people every day with old scraggy teeth and they'd be dark and black and then poison in the gums." Suggested reasons were that "the constant diet of bread and tea, tea and bread is hard on the teeth" (1920), and "the dentists used to come in the summer, but being no dentist around here your teeth got bad and rotten." The extent of the use of commercial cleaners – powders and pastes – is not clear, although they were certainly being widely advertised at the time of this comment.

There is a sense that until recent decades many Newfoundlanders felt that extracting a bad tooth was the best way to get rid of the problem once and for all; this reflected expediency and self-reliance, given that "gum-ming" food was satisfactory for many. Even so, innumerable ways of

relieving or attempting to relieve toothache were tried. People expreri-
mented while waiting for their next trip to St. John's and the dentist. Still
well known is the application of clove oil to the aching tooth. (Applying a
clove, if in fact carried out, was a poor substitute). Other apparently popular
suggestions involved the use of Gillett's Lye or Jeyes' Fluid. Alternative
applications were iodine, zap (tobacco juice from pipe), "hot, coarse pieces
of salt," warm hard bread, tow impregnated with pepper, gunpowder, and
tobacco. Of these, the application of warmth was more in line with
professional care. One feature of the recommendations was the general
availability of the items: "And then if you had a cavity. Jeyes' Fluid. Actually
what we used to do with it when I was young keeping house, there were
no bathrooms in the house so there would be a pail in the grandfather's
room and there'd be a pail somewhere else and there'd always be a chamber
pot under the children's bed. They had to be washed in the morning and
brought away to a big hole dugout. That went in everywhere."

A number of applications were recommended for the side of the face
over the aching tooth: hot tansy or pepper poultice, heated hard bread, a
warm plate, or a warm lamp, all of which probably gave ease on occasions.
Again, these are instances of the reputed therapeutic benefit of warmth.

Newfoundlanders also visited charmers. A common pattern of events was
for the charmer to write some "mysterious message" on a piece of paper,
roll it tightly, and instruct the person to wear it around the neck until the
toothache stopped. A "please" or "thank you" was not allowed, nor was
looking at the charm, "or it wouldn't work." Some charmers touched the
tooth, sometimes while saying a few words.

Innumerable charms and amulets were also tried without the intervention
of a charmer. They included a string, sometimes described as a toothache
string. Visiting the graveyard could also be useful: there one picked a grass
straw or bunch grass, alone at night, and pushed it into the tooth. Perhaps
this allowed one to forget the toothache for a while. A more common
practice, which some considered a way of invoking the Trinity, was to take
a pebble from a grave newly dug for a good person.

A frustrating, sometimes worrying, period for parents was (and is) the time
of children's teething. In the past, parents worried that teething might
seriously undermine the health of the infant. Even so, few recommendations can be found in the oral record, although "biting" on a teething stick
or other items was a well-known suggestion. There was, however, no
shortage of over-the-counter recommendations for teething, such as Steedman's Powders. Perhaps, too, at least in the early years of the century,
Newfoundlanders, as elsewhere, tried the opium preparation, laudanum. If
nothing else, these practices underscore how radically the increasing availability of professional dentists (and other painkillers) and the emphasis on

dental health after the 1950s have changed the management of many dental problems.

Despite the long history of poor teeth in Newfoundland, the fluoridation of the St. John's water supply, first raised in the 1950s, has still not taken place. If this approach is supposed to encourage the sense of individual responsibility that marks self-care, it ignores the hard-earned lessons of failure to use dentifrices and matters of benefit to a community overall.

NOTES
See: Fitz-Gerald (1935) 170, for opening quotation; Dr. T.M. Yates correspondence, 1922 letter; Waldo (1920) 95, for quotation on diet; Brown collection (Hand 1961, vol. 6) 301–7, for many items, and indication that tobacco and salt were well known; *Evening Telegram* 21 January 1955, concerning fluoridation; CMG (1992) 008, on Jeyes Fluid and no dentist; CMG (1992) 001, on scraggy teeth.

Representative MUNFLA references: 65-4/58 (graveyard straw), 68-13/19 (written charm around neck), 68-13/20 (bunch grass), 76-249 (tansy poultice, warm hard bread, side of face, charmers, touching tooth), 77-87 (vinegar), 78-195 (oil of cloves), 78-250 (zap from pipes, vinegar), 82-218 (gunpowder, pepper, or tobacco worked into piece of food), 82-238 (charmed by seventh son), 84-361B (graveyard pebbles).

TUBERCULOSIS

An advertisement in the *Evening Telegram* (14 November 1900) stated:

One in seven dies ... of consumption
And consumption begins with a cold
that could be cured by Dr. Chase's
Syrup of Linseed and Turpentine

Such advertisements heralded a half-century or more of fear-mongering in Newfoundland about consumption – increasingly called "tuberculosis" as the disease came within the framework of scientific medicine. Fear was easy to arouse, because of the high incidence of the disease on the island. In fact, tuberculosis can be said to have existed in epidemic proportions. It is therefore surprising that, while deaths are remembered, relatively few suggestions for treatment exist in the recently recorded Newfoundland oral tradition.

Aside from the growing belief in the value of treatment (including surgery) in the "san" – although not entirely eclipsing doubts of the value of professional care – the lack of information on self-treatment could be traced to the tendency to silence. In 1936, it was said that "there is a belief in specific cures for consumption [and] many reports of cures wrought on persons 'given up by the doctor.' The workers of such miracles seem loath to give up their secret." Tuberculosis was certainly a disease that might inhibit discussion between neighbours or even within families because of the fear and stigma associated with the disease. Some of the dilemma concerning self-treatment of tuberculosis is glimpsed in Aubrey Tizzard's recollections about the death of his sister in 1939: "In the five years she was confined to the house she tried different kinds of medication, patent medicine and cod liver oil. The last medicine she received arrived a few days before she died. There were several bottles from a distributor in Change Island. Some were to be taken orally and others to be rubbed on the flesh. She took a little and my mother rubbed her with the liniment a few times but it proved of no avail. Perhaps it came too late, I do not know."

It must, of course, be said that there was no certain medical cure until chemotherapy (late 1940s). The few treatment suggestions in the oral record for pulmonary tuberculosis were, in fact, typical chest remedies and tonics or blood purifiers: "turpentine buds" (myrrh [q.v.]) or "balsam buds" (perhaps steeped in rum for three or four weeks and taken in tablespoon doses); wild cherry bark (q.v.), fresh air, blackstrap molasses and milk, rum and molasses, and juniper. Other familiar treatments for the chest were no doubt used, such as juniper (q.v.), an ingredient in a recipe for "Syrup for Consumptives," described as "very successful" in Chase's *Book of Recipes*.

Cod liver oil (q.v.) was also considered helpful, if not a cure, by physicians and lay people alike. Its popular reputation for health-giving properties, supported by long familiarity, was reinforced in the early twentieth century by various advertisements, such as for Scott's Emulsion of Cod Liver Oil, which carried the heading "Consumption Panic" (1910). By then cod liver oil was partly seen as a strengthener and had become part of public-health teachings concerning diet. The notion that TB was linked to starvation (or poor diet) was a significant impetus to public-health educators on the island, and elsewhere, to improve nutrition in various ways.

A number of over-the-counter medicines focused attention on the disease, at least until such therapeutic claims were curtailed. In the late 1800s and early 1900s, reference to the disease appeared in Newfoundland advertisements and, in 1907, Sprucine was said to be invaluable when taken with cod liver oil "in the first stages of consumption." Alternatives were Ayer's Cherry Cordial, Dr. Pierce's Golden Medical Discovery, Nerviline, and Dr. Strandgard's T.B. Medicine. The island, however, seems to have missed some of the blatant tuberculosis quackery found in, say, the United States, although readers of the *Evening Telegram* in 1898 could write off for a prescription for many ailments, including consumption, to a Rochester, New York, address.

Even after specific claims for tuberculosis disappeared from over-the-counter medicine promotion, subtle implications remained in advertising for colds. Such statements as "Every cold is serious," for instance (in an advertisement for Dr. Chase's Syrup of Linseed and Turpentine), carried worrisome overtones given the widespread nature of the disease. Once (11 January 1930) the advertisement was juxtaposed to a news item, "Sugar as Possible Cure [for] Tuberculosis," which described a new sugar "produced by tuberculosis germs."

No discussion on home-management would be complete without mention of a regimen suggested by some physicians, namely the application of ice to the chest to reduce haemorrhage. "When she'd get these haemorrhages she'd have to lie down and there was nothing the doctor could do for her. The only suggestion he had, and this went on for years, that they'd put ice on her chest. She had a rubber sheet underneath her. When she would get these attacks, we had a red blanket and we'd put that over her so we wouldn't see the blood, when she'd be throwing up."

Treatments with specific magical or religious associations have not been found in the Newfoundland record, unless it be drinking from Coffen's Cove. Nevertheless, the protracted nature of the condition – often suspected if not diagnosed – led to treatments for the various symptoms, such as weight loss and spitting blood.

NOTES
See: Parsons (1936), for quote on secrecy in 1936; Tizzard (1984) 81; Green (1990) 1156, for discussion of the flaxseed well known to Newfoundlanders through Chase's Syrup of Linseed and Turpentine; Chase (1862) 102, for juniper (tamarack); MCG (1992) 008, concerning ice.

Representative MUNFLA references: 63-1/17 (myrrh bladders for tuberculosis), 68-19/4 (myrrh and sugar for tuberculosis), 68-26/23 (Coffen's Cove brook), 78:200 (cod liver oil, rum and molasses, blackberry bushes, cherry-tree bark).

Personal communication: I. Rusted (1991), concerning ice.


TURPENTINE

As noted under cuts (q.v.), commercial turpentine – a preparation from pine trees (not the myrrh [q.v.] which is often called turpentine in Newfoundland) – has been used extensively in Newfoundland. This popularity echoes the recommendations in countless regular and domestic medicine texts, until at least the 1940s.

Interest in turpentine was evident at the end of the seventeenth century. In *Currus Triumphalis* (1679), James Yonge, who is part of Newfoundland history because of his voyage to, and account of, Newfoundland, promoted the product for treating and dressing wounds. Yonge noted its past "astringing" reputation and employment for the treatment of chest complaints.

At a later time, turpentine was frequently noted in Newfoundland, and elsewhere, for coughs and colds (perhaps in conjunction with wild cherry, q.v.), for urinary problems, and for aches and pains. Turpentine was included in a number of apparently effective over-the-counter diuretic preparations as well, such as Haarlem Oil (see under *kidney complaints*). One phrase used by an informant about the application to cuts – "turpentine kills the soreness and kills the germ inside it" – seems to summarize the widespread confidence.

NOTES
See Yonge (1679); MCG (1992) 002, for quotation.

Personal communication: J. O'Mara (1990), for confirmation of considerable over-the-counter sales of commercial turpentine for uses noted above.

## TWINFLOWER

Little information has been found concerning Newfoundlander's usage of the small but attractive plant, *Linnaea borealis*. In fact, few references attest to its usage anywhere, although occasional mention can be found of the plant's bitter, sudorific, and diuretic properties. In 1899, it was reportedly used in Newfoundland as a remedy for coughs. Only one subsequent reference has been found for the province – in fact from someone who grew up in Labrador: "Well for fever, Daddy always went and picked a twinflower; it was a little flower growing along the ground and steeped it out if we got sick, if we were running a temperature. And it always did us good." Although this is in line with other reports, it is noteworthy that the informant indicated that aspirin might also be taken at the same time.

NOTES
See: Bergen (1899) 113; Erichsen-Brown (1979) 338, nineteenth- and twentieth-century; MCG (1992) 008.

## URINE (SEE ANIMAL PRODUCTS)

## VASELINE, VICKS VAPORUB

Although relatively few over-the-counter medicines are considered specifically in the entries, the two noted here were among the mainstays in many a Newfoundland home. Vaseline is best known as a general skin emollient. In Newfoundland, aside from its role as an application for burns, it was used to "soften" haemorrhoids and to "grease the tubes" for whooping cough. Perhaps the latter was one of the medicated vaselines popular until at least the 1920s as a rub for the chest, as well as for colds and skin conditions. Borated, carbolated, and mentholated products were sold. Newfoundlanders added their own medications (for example, juniper) as well.

The strongly aromatic "Vicks" has been used as widely in Newfoundland for colds and coughs (q.v.) and croup (q.v.) as elsewhere, following the introduction of Vaporub during 1890. It has been recently reported that despite falling sales, more than a million dollars worth of Vaporub is still sold worldwide. Stories in Newfoundland illustrate ingenuity in its applications (for example, see *croup*). Noteworthy, too, is the grandmother who "would apply Vick's Vaporub to the tip of a lighted cigarette and proceed to smoke it." The informant, however, felt that it was an excuse to smoke at a time when few women smoked. Some Vicks Vaporub promotions (for instance, *Daily News*, 3 January 1930) stressed that dosing should be avoided, just one indication that concerns over side-effects of many medicines are not new.

NOTES
See: "Vicks Vaporub Observes 100 Years," *Daily Reflector*, 24 December 1990.
    Representative MUNFLA references: vaseline: 82-122 (haemorrhoids, whooping cough), 84-149 (burns), 84-321B (juniper); 84-355A/B (smoking Vicks).

## VINEGAR, VINEGAR PLANT

Vinegar had already had a long history as a deodorizer and an "antiseptic" for purifying the air before the germ theory of disease was generally established around the 1880s. The acid product was also popular as an ingredient in smelling salts, and its professional medical usage was varied. As well, the product's aromatic properties are reflected in the suggestions found in the recently recorded Newfoundland oral tradition for treating headache (for example, soaking a cloth in vinegar and wrapping it around the head). As elsewhere, the acetic acid content has been viewed as significant – a rationalization, even if the precise nature of the acid is not always understood: "There's an acid in it see, there's phosphoric acid and it kills germs and then it heals. If you have a cut now and you get some inflammation in it, give it a wash and put some vinegar on and it kills it."

Employment of vinegar for toothache is also noted, as is its usage for improving blood and removing "membranes" from the back of throats (in cases of diphtheria [q.v.]), which can lead to suffocation.

The vinegar plant – perhaps kept in a crock or teapot – yielded home-fermented vinegar (an acetobacter culture). This was started with toasted bread, molasses, yeast, and water. Its use for treating headache has been recorded.

NOTES
See: MCG (1992) 002, for acid and germs.
    Representative MUNFLA references: 77-87 (toothache), 78-195 (headache).

## VITAMINS

Various entries show the influence of vitamins on self-care; for instance, the B vitamins in nerve preparations and vitamins A and D in cod liver oil. There is a clear sense that although in the 1920s and 1930s vitamins became medicinals, more recently, they have generally been promoted as nutrition supplements. As noted under *tonics*, vitamins have pushed aside many "old time" tonics. For example, Doyle, the great promoter of over-the-counter products, had Seatone in his line – a preparation of vitamins, minerals, and dulse. ("Health and growth for all the family.") And no longer do many Newfoundlanders take cod liver oil regularly (even in relatively tasteless capsules), whether as a preventative or treatment. More likely they are consumers in the large market for the countless vitamin preparations promoted for a host of existing or potential complaints.

It is hard to overestimate the impact of vitamins in twentieth-century medicine: they have changed not only many therapies, including self-treatments, but also nutritional practices. Much uncertainty and conflicting information have arisen, however, along with issues that have become increasingly conspicuous in self-care. On 10 May 1956, a cartoon in the *Evening Telegram* featured a woman talking to a cashier at Ayre's Supermarket: "I think I have carbohydrates and vitamins straight. Now tell me about calories and minerals." Added to such a question are today's queries about whether vitamin (and mineral) supplements can improve children's IQ values. Questions also exist about their value for enhancing memory, something for which a variety of products are being promoted. Lecithin and ginkgo, for instance, are gaining adherents, if less so in Newfoundland than elsewhere.

NOTES
See: Davis (1982), for background; Schoenthaler et al. (1991).

## WARTS

Recommendations for treating warts have been, in Newfoundland as in other cultures, extraordinarily commonplace. Today, although little confidence is placed in past practices, some Newfoundlanders still claim, "They worked if you believed in them." Some people, of course, remain uncertain. Among elderly informants, recollections of, and testimonials to, the cure of warts abound:

When I went to work in St. John's I had a lot of warts on my hands. At that time the Gerald S. Doyle news bulletin was on and during my dinner hour we'd be up in the main office and this fellow came in and he asked me if I would take a note to put on the news in the night time. He turned out to be an American. He was in the forces and he had lost his passport and he wanted to put it on the radio. While I was writing it out, he said you got an awful lot of warts, can you count them. Another fellow was there that worked with me, he said go ahead, count them, and we started counting and I had ninety-two, all little ones, big ones here, there's marks there yet. He said can you get a bit of bread and I said yes, I can get a bit of bread, so I ran across the street to the Stirling Restaurant and came back with the piece of bread. He took a tissue and he put a piece of bread between it and he crossed everyone of them, so he wrapped it up and put it in his shirt pocket. He said if I touch that bread I'll get everyone you got. He said they'll go, the big ones might take a little longer than the others. (1992)

It has been said that the apparent, occasional success of one method was simply that it had been employed at the time of natural recovery from warts and after the failure of other approaches. One study suggested that two-thirds of patients lose existing warts naturally over two years. Such information sidesteps the question of faith (or confidence) in a treatment procedure, which some suggest might enhance the body's normal immunologic response of combating the wart virus. This applies to lay regimens as well as to current professional medical approaches, ranging from salicylic acid applications (many available over-the-counter) to electrocauterization. Increasingly, over-the-counter items and "doctors'" treatments have, in recent decades, pushed aside many long-standing practices, although some continued to be advertised to Newfoundlanders (for example, Dr. E. Deighton's Wart Remover, made from herbs in 1952).

Faith in a treatment was perhaps of special significance to the reputation of charmers, who "put away" warts. As in the opening quote, charmers' treatments, once conspicuous in Newfoundland, included what is commonly known as "transference." Another example is the application of fat pork and grease to the wart; the mixture is then put out for a cat or a dog to eat. Although it has been said that charmers sometimes employed a form of hypnosis in treating warts, no clear evidence exists that this was so in Newfoundland.

The transference of warts was often tried in the home, without the intervention of a charmer. Substances employed included fat or salt pork, worms, butter, green grass, potatos, bread, or a specific number of beans (one for each wart). Methods included being touched by a corpse in a way described for birth marks (q.v.), or knotting a string (one knot for each wart) and burying the string.

Additional approaches invoked calls to religious sensitivities. Common suggestions were to make the sign of a cross over the wart or to draw crosses with chalk (one for each wart) in an oven. It was said that by the time the crosses had burned off, the warts would disappear. Some practices merely required the reciting of sayings, biblical passages, Christian liturgy, or certain words. These, when used by charmers, were often unintelligible to the sufferer. However, one seventh son of the seventh son was reported to say: "Go home, say your prayers and do not look at your warts for two weeks. Your warts will disappear."

Amid the magical and religious approaches were a few suggestions for applying substances to warts: "juice from knobs on kelp," potato peelings, and dandelion milk or latex. While some people viewed magic as the rationale (for example, the disappearance of a wart as the potato rotted), some believed that the effectiveness lay in excluding the air. Aside from testimonials, however, clear evidence of a cure is generally wanting.

NOTES
See: Brown Collection (Hand 1961, vol. 6) 309–50, for extensive list of treatments, many described in Newfoundland; Massing and Epstein (1963), for natural remission; Johnson and Barber (1978); MCG (1992) 115, for narrative about bread; Burns (1992), for general review of warts, including the suggestion that the notion of transference recognized contagion.

Representative MUNFLA references: 68-21/30 (juice from kelp), 68-22/11 (dandelion "juice," said not to work), 69-2/24 (transference via fat pork), 69-2/27 (transference by butter), 69-7/11 (transference via worms), 69-19/1 (transference via alder leaves), 69-22/5 (chalk crosses), 82/316 (charmer for warts), 84-353B (seventh son, words).

## WATER ON THE KNEE

Water on the knee (synovitis, inflammation of the synovial membrane in joints), not an uncommon complaint, was generally managed by a physician "tapping" the water and applying a firm bandage; this often had to be repeated. Many found this treatment inconvenient during a busy fishing season, even when readily available. Alternatives were sought. One Newfoundlander has described graphically how his knee, in turn, was painted with iodine, had a cabbage leaf applied, and then benefited from the services of a charmer. Poultices were also tried.

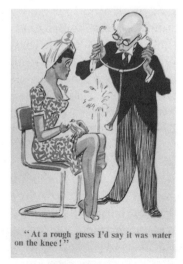

"At a rough guess I'd say it was water on the knee!"

Postcard, 1930s

NOTES
See: Troake (1989) 20, for iodine and cabbage leaf.
    Representative MUNFLA reference 78-200 (cabbage, iodine).

## WATER LILIES (SEE BEAVER-ROOT)

## WATER PUPS (GURRY SORES)

"Water pups," long a recognized occupational hazard of Newfoundland fishermen, generally refer to sores around the wrists. They arise when the cuff of a sleeve, especially when wet, rubs on the skin. "A string of boils [were] between his elbows and wrists where the wet jersey and oil skins cut into the flesh. The salt water stung them unpleasantly, but when they were ripe Domn treated them with Disko's razor, and assured Harvey that he be a 'blooded Banker;' the affliction of the gurry sores being the mark of the cast that claimed him." (*Captains Courageous* [1897]).

Protection of the wrist took many forms, but one of the commonest was to wear wrist-chains (bracelets) of copper or brass (three strands or a wide band were often tried). Flannel and raw wool were other items that provided physical protection.

The application of a pad covered with a "stick salve" called "ox-blood" (probably dragon's blood [q.v.], which was certainly used) was perhaps as much treatment as protection, as were other thick salves or poultices (for example, molasses and flour). Washing the wrists in a "potion" of alder leaves is also noted; if this was done frequently, the tannin content might well "toughen" the skin.

NOTES
See: *Dictionary of Newfoundland English* (1990), under water pup.
    Representative MUNFLA references: 72-41 (alder leaves and wool), 76-249 (copper or brass chain), 78-200 (worsted yarn wound around wrist thirteen times or for as many turns as water pups, silver, copper, and brass chains), 82-122 (apply red flannel or salt water to welps), 84-323B (molasses and flour).
    Personal communication: Troake (1990); Anita Best (1991), for use of chains as both prevention and cure.

## WHITLOW

A whitlow, also called "run-around" in Newfoundland as elsewhere, was probably treated with a Sunlight soap poultice more than any other. Some said it was something in the soap, a reflection of the widespread confidence in this product.

NOTES
See: MCG (1992) 108.


## WHOOPING COUGH

Among the medicines employed for colds and coughs, Friar's balsam (as an inhalation) was one specifically mentioned in the oral record for whooping cough (pertussis), at least when combined with Jeyes' Fluid. Such an inhalation regimen can perhaps be viewed as an "updated" version, with disinfectant, of such earlier whooping-cough treatments as "a change of air" or the breathing in of natural or man-made odours.

Over-the-counter preparations specifically promoted at times for Newfoundland sufferers included preparations of wild cherry such as Dr. Wistar's Balsam of Wild Cherry, Vapocresoline, and Vicks Vaporub (q.v.). In 1925, one Newfoundland advertisement for the latter stated it was not to be taken as a cure for whooping cough, but to help "reduce the paroxysms of coughing." Not everyone appreciated the limitation.

Non-medicine recommendations in the recently recorded Newfoundland oral tradition include transference of the disease. The employment of a trout was apparently well known: a live trout was held up to the mouth and the patient coughed over it; the fish was then returned to the water. A variant was merely to hold the fish to the sufferer's throat, before returning it to the water. One is tempted to think that such complicated methods were rarely used, even bearing in mind that whooping cough elicited much parental worry.

A simpler transference approach was to take an egg and bury it in the ground. It was said that the whooping cough disappeared as the egg rotted. Also reported more than once was the value of eating bread baked by a woman who had not changed her surname at marriage.

Although whooping-cough vaccines became available in the 1920s, their variable effectiveness, plus other factors, meant that deaths from whooping cough were not controlled for some time – hardly testimony to the effectiveness of home treatment. Between 1940 and 1944, 260 such deaths were recorded in Newfoundland. Although a dramatic decline occurred over the next twenty years, outbreaks have remained a public-health and self-care issue.

NOTES
See: Brown Collection (Hand 1961, vol. 6) 351–53, for many beliefs, especially use of general cold medicines and swallowing a fish alive (variant of the use of fish noted above); Hand (1968), for change of air and inhaling odours; Severs (1979), for immunization.

Representative MUNFLA references: 66-10/30 (rotting egg, bread from woman who did not change name, 67-3/53 (inhale mixture Jeyes' Fluid and Friar's balsam), 68-19/27 (bread baked), 69-20/2 (cough at trout).

## WILD CHERRY

Many references exist in the Newfoundland oral record to the medicinal use of "wild cherry," as is the case throughout North America. On the island, the vernacular name (as well as "cherry bark" when used in a medical context) refers to both *Prunus virginiana* (also known as sloe-tree, choke cherry, chuckley plum) and, more usually, to *Prunus pensylvanica* (pin cherry).

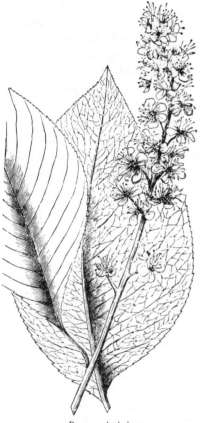

*Prunus virginiana*

Newfoundland usage of wild cherry for coughs and colds, even if commonly combined with turpentine ([q.v.], another well-known remedy for coughs), mirrors considerable popularity in the past, both within and outside professional medicine. Many tried wild cherry bark: "My cousin, he was supposed to have TB, they were testing him, I suppose his lungs must be weak or something ... but he got right thin and miserable looking ... He drank more cherry bark than anyone and he's alive up in his 80s."

This popularity of *P. virginiana* for chest conditions has been rationalized by its known constituents, the principal one being glycosides which yield hydrocyanic acid. It is unlikely, however, that any of this acid remained after the manufacture of the medicines. The following home preparation probably had no residual hydrocyanic acid, though the astringency may have been the reason for its treatment of lack of appetite. "Granny would get a cherry stick ... and she'd peel it and boil it and put some sugar in it and give me that to drink and you get your appetite back."

The recommendations for using wild cherry as a tonic (and a blood purifier), as in the Newfoundland record, were once established in the professional medical literature. In contrast, the bark was not generally recommended for diarrhoea, as in some Newfoundland records. A tea, however, especially if boiled in sufficient quantity, could have an anti-diarrhoeal effect because of the tannin content.

Undoubtedly, some of the lay popularity of wild cherry, and confidence in its effectiveness, came from the promotion of numerous commercial wild cherry preparations. Before 1900, Dr. Wistar's Balsam of Wild Cherry, widely known throughout North America, was promoted in the St. John's newspapers (for example, by McMurdo drugstore). Supporting testimonials such as the following (Daily News, 12 June 1894) probably had an impact as well:

From G.W. Thomas of Battleboro', Vt.,
For ten or twelve years past I have been troubled much of the time with Catarrh, which has kept up a continual irritation of the throat and lungs, attended with a severe cough. During this time I have tried many of the popular remedies of the day without the least benefit. The past winter I commenced the use of Dr. Wistar's Balsam of Wild Cherry, the beneficial effects of which have been very great, as after having used three bottles I find myself entirely cured of my disease.

Soon Wistar's competed with other wild-cherry preparations such as the "local" Macs Compound Cherry Bark Cough Syrup. The declining usage – noticeable by the 1950s – was linked not only to competition from other products, but also to the decreasing popularity of liquid medicines.

NOTES
See: Introduction to bibliography for general history and background information; MCG (1992) 002, for cherry stick and appetite, 008 for TB.

Representative MUNFLA references: 77-87 (with spirits of turpentine for coughs), 78-200 (cherry-tree bark for tuberculosis, tea of leaves and root for headache, cherry bark to clean blood).

WILD-PARSNIP

In Newfoundland, "wild-parsnip" generally refers to *Heracleum lanatum*, also commonly known as "cow-parsnip," which is a coarse, umbelliferous weed; some people liken the strikingly large leaves to rhubarb leaves. Other common names include eltrot, helltrot, health root, and dock. Although dock is used for large leaved plants, it generally refers to *Rumex* spp.

Given the many popular names, it is not altogether surprising that wild-parsnip was generally well known in traditional medicine, wherever it was grown. Principal uses have been as an application (in the form of a poultice or fomentation of the leaves or roots) for skin ailments, as a poultice tied on to the forehead with a band for headaches, or as a decoction of the roots for rheumatism or stomach ailments.

The Newfoundland record covers these uses (as well as seasickness), although there is little evidence that the plant was widely used. Despite fairly extensive popular knowledge about the plant, it attracted little interest within professional medicine, possibly an indication of its non-specific pharmacological properties. (Reported Micmac usage for smallpox and cholera may not have been well established). Its reputation as an internal remedy is perhaps linked to the aromatic character of the plant and its presumed carminative properties. See under *burdock* for possible confusion with the plant.

NOTES
See: Introduction to bibliography, for history and background infromation; Bergen (1899) 112, for various uses; Chandler et al (1979), for Micmacs.
    Representative MUNFLA reference: 68-10/9 (el-trot for headache).


## WINTERGREEN

Wintergreen has been widely discussed in past professional and popular medical literature. *Gaultheria procumbens* (uncommon in Newfoundland) is generally referred to, although the name has been used for other plants (for example, *creeping snowberry* [q.v.]). Newfoundland interest, as elsewhere, has focused on the commercially available oil of wintergreen, primarily as a rub for rheumatism. Employment of a tea of the leaves as a carminative is rationalized by the essential oil present.

NOTES
See: Introduction to bibliography for general history and information.


## WITCHHAZEL

Many Newfoundlanders purchased witchhazel ointment or other preparations from local stores – mostly for bruises or minor skin ailments. However, that witchhazel (*Hamamelis virginiana*) is not to be confused with what many Newfoundlanders have for a long time called witchhazel. The latter is yellow or grey birch, *Betula lutea*. Like other birches (see *birches*), little interest has been expressed in possible medical uses. Recent Micmac informants, however, recollect that the inner bark was steeped to make a tea that was drunk to treat diarrhoea or a sore throat.

NOTES
See: Introduction to bibliography for general history and information; MCG (1993) 2, for Micmac information; *Dictionary of Newfoundland English* (1990), under witch-hazel.

## WORMS

Suggestions for treating "worms" (mostly in children), found in the recently recorded Newfoundland oral tradition, include herbal preparations of snakeroot (q.v.), bogbean (q.v.), and dogwood (q.v.). None of these is generally recognized as a vermifuge or anthelmintic (that is, preparations to remove worms); nor have the recorded gunpowder and molasses, cabbage and molasses, or various laxatives (for example, senna and castor oil) been generally recognized as treatments. That does not mean that they were not promoted with great enthusiasm on occasions: "Everybody knew about burnt cabbage leaves for worms."

Additionally, there were the tall stories, common in Newfoundland and elsewhere and dating from the 1960s if not before, about treating tapeworms: "I have heard of several instances of people advising tapeworm carriers to fast for several hours. Then the victim has only to open his mouth and hold his head over a saucer of evaporated milk which has just been boiled. The tapeworm would come up after the milk." Other Newfoundland accounts report using boiled milk to attract worms out of the mouth. The sufferer could even make the worms "drunk," by taking shots of rum or whisky.

Another suggestion was to take a mixture of butter, bread, molasses, and human hair. Small pieces of hair are put onto a half slice of buttered bread and molasses is spread on top. The whole is eaten before going to bed. Although this form of treatment – at least the use of hair – was seemingly well known, the notion of trapping the worm is hardly valid, nor was the similar concept of swallowing a lump of dough in which the worms were supposedly collected and passed with faeces.

Commercial vermifuges – prescribed or purchased over-the-counter and undoubtedly generally effective – were widely used; unlike recommendations in the oral tradition, specific treatments were (and are) directed to specific worms. Keating's Worm Tablets – "a purely vegetable sweet meat" for the common (or pin) worms – was promoted in St. John's before 1900. Such worms, initially suspected because of intense irritation around the anus, were commonplace. Indeed, there was much agreement with a statement made in a 1927 Gerald Doyle advertisement: "Most children are more or less infested with worms and these parasites sap the strength of the little ones." In this case, the answer was Dr. Hobson's Pink Worm Wafers (they "taste like candy.") But making choices was not easy, and some tried Dr. McKenzie's Dead Shot Worm Candy in the 1950s, or other preparations from the local store.

Worms are still a common problem today. Depending on the type of worm infestation, drug treatment can range from being very effective to moderately so. General hygienic precautions, not reported in the oral tradition, remain important considerations in prevention and control.

NOTES

See: Coish (1985), for tapeworm stories; MCG (992) 002, on cabbage and molasses.

Representative MUNFLA references: 66-10/25 (gun powder and molasses), 67-3/55 (senna), 68-23/12 (dogwood), 73-189 (dough), 82-121 (bogbeans, snakeroot), 82-122 (castor oil), 82-218 (sugar and tapeworms), 84-296B (hair).

## WORMWOOD

Wormwood, generally *Artemesia absinthium*, although other species (*A. abrotanum, A. borealis, A. vulgaris,* and others) have been called by the same name, is perhaps best known as an ingredient in the alcoholic beverage absinthe. Long known and used as a medicinal plant, wormwood, after a long-standing reputation as a veritable panacea, was generally viewed as a tonic by the end of the nineteenth century.

The Newfoundland record (probably for *A. absinthium,* but other wormwoods have been cultivated on the island) notes its use primarily as a tonic – usually a spring tonic – and appetite restorer (q.v.), due to the bitterness; it is also noted for the treatment of beriberi (q.v.), but perhaps this was more for stimulating general malaise.

Other recommendations which persisted in many oral traditions – as a vermifuge for worms, for amenorrhoea, and as an external application for bruises, sprains, and inflammation – are not found in the Newfoundland record. Usage over time can produce toxic effects.

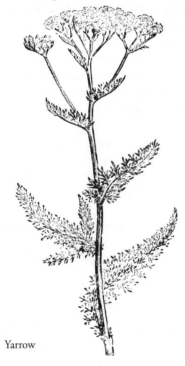

NOTES

See: Introduction to bibliography for general history and background information.

Representative MUNFLA references: 76-249 (restore appetite), 78-195 (wormwood and salt as tonic, for poor appetite).

## YARROW

Yarrow (*Achillea millefolium,* also popularly known as "deadman's daisy," "deadman's posy," or "fern tansy") – once fairly popular as a medicinal plant – has long been recommended for diarrhoea and unsettled stomachs. Its reputation,

Yarrow

however, has been uneven, as reflected perhaps in the paucity of information in the Newfoundland record, even though it grows commonly on the island. At least its astringency, rather than its odour, might rationalize one Newfoundland usage – putting it in a bath for the treatment of haemorrhoids.

Tonic properties were reported for yarrow throughout the nineteenth century and to a lesser extent since. A reputation for treating wounds and haemorrhoids, however, had generally faded by around 1900. Since the plant, apart from the flowers, looks like tansy (q.v.), it is quite possible that some of the many Newfoundland references to tansy actually referred to yarrow.

NOTES
See: Introduction to bibliography for general history and background information.

### ZAM-BUK OINTMENT

Usage of Zam-Buk ointment – a well-known green ointment based on oil of elder – has already been noted (for example, under *antiseptic ointments.*) It is mentioned again as a final entry in our alphabetical listing. Like many numerous items already considered, the large number of past claims are no longer credible, even if they were when first made. Extravagant claims often reflect rampant commercialism and/or fraud – appropriately called "quackery." Nevertheless, as many entries have made clear, some of these unacceptable claims merely reflect theories and concepts of the time. And those concepts, past and current, may or may not rationalize empirical observations. Any evaluation of the value of, and roles for, remedies is complex and may need to be considered in terms of their place in a family or community as well as their usage by the individual person.

# Notes

PART I

1  Little (1908a), emphasis added.

2  Olds (1967).

3  Benoit (1990) 180, quotation from widow born 1909.

4  Anon. (1945). Reinforces Adamson et al (1945) who noted that "public health in Newfoundland is far from satisfactory;" also Metkoff, J. (1945). For a significant issue reinforcing notions that poor state of health was the concept of "subclinical dietary deficiency disease," see Dove (1943).

5  Miller (1950).

6  Alexander (1983), especially 32–43.

7  Sharpe (1988).

8  Various published and manuscript sources (for instance, MCG files) support this view. Myra Bennett, for instance, wrote of her experiences in the 1920s and 30s: "Of course there was poverty! And where was there not poverty during a world depression? But here every family owns its own home, and since they built it themselves they do not have to pay rent. When starvation was rife in other countries, the inhabitants here lived well with their homegrown vegetables, their own cows to provide milk, cream and butter. Every family had a good supply of meat, either home raised or hunted. Moose, caribou, rabbits all helped the food supply." Green (1973), 80.

9  MCG (1992), 108.

10  For information on Dr. De Jongh's "Cod Liver Oil," sung by Walter Laburnun (c. 1890), which precedes the cod-liver-oil song well known in Newfoundland, I am grateful to the W.H. Helfand Collection.

11  Royal Commission (1930), 18. Earlier comments suggest that commercial trends had been underway for some time. For instance, physician Eliot Curwen, working for the Grenfell mission, records in his 1893 journal comments from colleague Albert Bobardt: Those living at and arriving in Battle Harbour "are

rather uneducated, and there is amongst them an abundant element of faith and reliance in quack remedies, for which they pay extravagant prices." (Thanks to R. Rompkey for access to his transcript of the journal.)

12   For some reminiscences, see Saunders (1986), 136. Merchants generally carried supplies of well-known over-the-counter remedies and often provided them on credit. The scope is reflected in the following, advertised by G. Knowling (*Evening Telegram,* 6 March 1922):

| | |
|---|---|
| Kay's Essence Linseed – For Coughs and Colds | 27 cts. bottle |
| Owbridge's Lung Tonic – Known the World Over for Coughs, Colds, Asthma and Bronchitis | 40 cts. bottle |
| Antiseptic Throat Pastilles For Hoarseness, Sore Throat, etc. | 30 cts. box |
| Radway's Ready Relief – For Internal and External Use | 37 cts. bottle |
| Steedman's Soothing Powders – For Babies Teething | 28 cts. pkg. |
| Phosforene – The great English tonic | 30 cts & 80 cts. bottle |
| Ayer's Cherry Pectoral – For Coughs and Colds | 50 cts. bottle |
| Linseed, Liquorice and Chlorodyne – Lozenges; Eibsen's Genuine | 06 cts. oz. |
| Bromo Quinine Tablets – Grove's; The Remedy for LaGrippe | 32 cts. |
| Colman's Mustard Oil – For Rheumatism | 16 cts & 34 cts. bottle |
| Eucalyptus Oil – Genuine Platypus brand | 50 cts. bottle |
| Keating's Cough Lozenges | 47 cts. tin |
| Medicamentum – The genuine Dutch drops for the kidneys, etc. | 15 cts. bottle |
| Mentholatum | 30 cts. |
| Powel's Balsam of Aniseed – For Coughs and Colds | 50 cts. bottle |
| Pyny Balsam – For Coughs and Colds | 40 cts. bottle |
| Red Spruce Gum | 34 cts. bottle |
| Scott's Emulsion of Cod Liver Oil | 65 cts. bottle |
| Syrup of Tar and Cod Liver Oil | 40 cts. bottle |
| Chase's Syrup of Linseed and Turpentine | 30 cts & 60 cts. bottle |
| White Pine and Tar Compound | 28 cts. bottle |
| Stafford's Phoratone | 35 cts. bottle |
| Stafford's Liniment | 35 cts. bottle |
| Minard's Liniment | 20 cts. bottle |

13   For a 1960 study, see Girt (1970), 181.

14   Aspects of the story of what are commonly called patent medicines have been told a number of times, most fully for the United States: Young (1967, 1974). The Canadian story has not been written, but for some sense (including mention of Buckley's Medicine) see Rasky, F. (1988). For influence elsewhere in the twentieth century, as in Newfoundland (discussed below), see a southern Appalachian story: Crellin and Philpott (1990, vol. 1) 75–9 and other pages.

15  Dearin advertisement, from Smallwood and Pitt (1981), 604. Assessment of Ayer's products, J. O'Mara, unpublished ms.

16  Quotations from reminiscences of the medical practice of John Heath, unpublished ms., courtesy Dr. R. Day.

17  For Pratt, Pitt (1984, vol. 1) 74–5, 78–9. Bottle for Arctic Indigestion Cure in Apothecary Hall, Newfoundland Pharmaceutical Association.

18  For some notes on McMurdo and Stafford, see J. O'Mara, unpublished ms.

19  Illustration from Adams (1988).

20  Tucker (1988), 82. For background: see Hiscock (1987).

21  Saunders (1986), 138. For other information on Doyle, see Deir (1983).

22  Pitman ms., courtesy I. Rusted.

23  Piercey (1992), 5; see also Mifflen (1983), 84–9 ("Our Friend the Almanac").

24  Advertisement, *Canadian Pharmaceutical Journal*, October 1926.

25  MUNFLA-NAC tapes 83/B/C.

26  For background to books such as by Chase and Pierce, see Gevitz (1990). Perhaps of relevance to Newfoundland are domestic- and sea-medicine chest guides, see Gordon (1993).

27  Redfearn/Smith ms., Newfoundland Provincial Archives, #P6/A/23 Smith Collection, Box 7.

28  For general discussion on autointoxication, see Hudson (1989).

29  Information on cervix as site of infection, see I. Rusted, personal communication, 1991. Quotation from Ephraim (1937), 179.

30  For general context concerning cleanliness in the United States (some of which seeped to Newfoundland), see Vinikas (1992).

31  Parsons (1936), for turning of the blood; MCG (1992) 002, for explanation of the latter. Also Hufford (1982).

32  Information kindly provided by Gary Saunders from his forthcoming book on Dr. John Olds.

33  MCG (1992), 116.

34  Quoted from Debus (1991), 17.

35  For some background: Soucy (1953); and for recent discussion on various current problems in Canada: Lexchin (1990).

36  Relevant writings can be found in Hunter and Wotherspoon (1986).

37  For instance, in Grenfell (c. 1920), p. 116, and Rieti (1991b), 163–4, note the reputations of two practitioners who encouraged stories about their fairy connections. See also Rieti (1991a), 287, for another story which, although open to various interpretations, may reflect similar attitudes.

38  Kerr (1959), 71.

39  Grenfell (1932), 96.

40  For some indication of attitudes toward government physicians, see Harris (1990). Various comments in the records housed in MUNFLA suggest some elderly informants "didn't like doctors very much" (MUNFLA 72-64, 73-142 as examples; for quote about Jim: 73-142). Some Newfoundlanders perhaps visited doctors only at the insistence of their children.

41  Quoted from Young (1967), 26.

42  MUNFLA references 88-281 (cold cabbage), 75-21; for background toward attitudes about germs, see Tomes (1990); for a sense of the resistance to antiseptics in Newfoundland, see Musson (1910).

43  For "ounce of prevention" example, see MUNFLA reference 84-311B.

44  This is clear from a survey carried out in 1992. See MCG (1992) files.

45  MUNFLA references 63-1/298 and 350 (carrots and towels).

46  Quoted from manuscript on John Olds by G. Saunders. A belief in hard work and rough food, albeit shaped by nostalgia, is clear from MCG files.

47  Rutherford manuscript, deposited in Newfoundland files, History of Medicine, Faculty of Medicine, Memorial University of Newfoundland.

48  Cavender (1990); Hadlow and Pitts (1991). Many accounts highlight particular issues among ethnic groups; for example, Roedor (1988), 188.

49  *Dictionary Newfoundland English* 1990, xiii.

50  For one example of the malapropism, see Sugerman and Butters (1985).

51  Mifflen (1983), 95, for stomach quote; for some discussion of ethnomedical issues, see Nations et al. (1985).

52  Blumhagen (1980).

53  Examples from *Dictionary Newfoundland English* and MUNFLA reference, 84-330B.

54  Freeman (1987); Demak and Becker (1987) for more general background, but with a central focus on communication.

55  Goldstein (1991), for discussion on experience in another context.

56  Rieti (1991b); various papers in Narváez (1991); Bennett (1989) 128–9, "Indians as Witches."

57  MUNFLA reference 86-254. Many discussions exist concerning lay theories of illness; Helman (1990) is noted here, but is also useful for general background to this volume.

58  MUNFLA reference 72/64.

59  Although we cannot elaborate on the notion of the life-force, it is noteworthy that the use of this concept in many forms of alternative medicine attracts Newfoundlanders even today.

60  Osler (1985), 16.

61  It is outside the scope of the present account to detail the historical roots of the practices considered. For some European roots, see Opie and Tatem (1989); also consult sources noted in introduction to bibliography. Some sense of the eclectic conceptual background in the nineteenth century can be acquired from Cooter (1988).

62  Cramp (1936), 69.

63  MUNFLA reference 68-7.

64  Persistence of magical treatments in North America is highlighted by Hand (1980). Debate about the displacement of traditional beliefs by more rational ideas and values provide a significant context to this volume. Superstitions are increasingly viewed as performing social and psychological functions.

65  Rieti (1991b), 213, for priests and place in fairy narratives.

66  MUNFLA reference 72-90 ms.

67  For recent discussions on lifestyles and change indicating conflicting interpretations, see Davis (1983); Pocius (1991).

68  Piercey (1992) ms.

69  For an example of a male who "stitched up a huge cut made by axes or saws," see Squire (1974), 63. Butler (1980), 13, mentions other practitioners without training, but skilled.

70  The quote from William Faulkner is used by James Breedon in a book of much relevance to the issue of distinctiveness: Savitt and Young (1988). Relevant information is also found in Numbers and Savitt (1989).

71  Mitchell and Matthews, cited in Kirkland et al (1992), 8. The figure is in line with others published. In 1991, it was reported (Kasparek [1991] quoting unpublished Berger, E., *Canada Health Monitor Overview Report*, Price Waterhouse 1990) that "one in five Canadians used some form of alternative therapy." Besides herbalism, this includes chiropractic, acupuncture, and homeopathy. A recent U.S. study, Eisenberg et al. (1993), concluded: "One in three respondents (thirty-four per cent) reported using at least one unconventional therapy in the past year, and a third of these saw providers for unconventional therapy." See also Brown and Marcy (1991).

72  Rieti (1990), 564, cites an informant who changed explanations.

73  *Newfoundland Health Review* (1986, St. John's: Department of Health) highlights many issues.

74  For relevant discussion, see Aakster (1986). See Snow and Johnson (1977) for comments on patients deliberately withholding information from doctors, and health hazards; Burnham (1984) for background on outmoding of beliefs.

75  Segall, A., and Goldstein (1989).

76  For recent references indicating increasing usage, see, for example, Eisenberg et al. (1993).

77  See, for instance, Cayleff (1990) for references to women and self-care in general; and Fuller (1989) for spiritual well-being in North America.

78  Although calls for academic research on self-care have been increasing in recent years, only occasionally does such research look at "traditional" or "alternative" practices. For example, see Brown and Marcy (1991).

79  Such specific aspects of self-care have been explored to some extent. See Bakx (1991); Hufford (1988).

## PART II

1  Micmac health beliefs and their present-day roles are the subject of a separate study by the Medical Communication Group, Memorial University of Newfoundland.

2  MCG (1992) 001.

3  Green (1974), 94.

4 MUNFLA reference 67-4. Many other accounts list religious cures (for example, 73-189).

5 See Rieti (1990, 1991a, 1991b) for background to fairies; Rieti (1989) on black magic. A spell in the recent record of the Newfoundland tradition states that "if a person believes he is witched, he will fill a bottle with his urine, insert the stopper filled with pins (cork stopper), hang it up on the back of the stove in the heat until all the urine has evaporated." When this was done the witch would be unable to pass water and therefore remove the spell. See Patterson (1895) for another example of a spell, albeit not medical.

# Bibliography

## INTRODUCTORY COMMENTS

It is impossible to give a detailed background for all the various medications considered. However, further information to help evaluate many herbs and other home medicines considered in Part II is relatively easily available from a number of texts listed in the bibliography. These include Crellin and Philpott (1990), Evans (1989), Moerman (1986, for native Indian uses), *Reader's Digest* (1986), Duke (1985), Tyler (1982, 1987), Leung (1980), and Erichsen-Brown (1979). Older writings published when the medicines were in common usage are of special value; for example, Foster (1890–94, 1897), and Millspaugh (1892).

Information on self-care practices elsewhere around the world, generally similar to those found in Newfoundland, can be located in various compilations. These include the well-known Brown Collection (Hand 1961), which is frequently footnoted in the text to illustrate similarities. Other regional compilations which can be used in the same way include Bergen (1899), Browne (1958), Creighton (1968), Hand (1980), Hand et al. (1981), and Green (1990).

The major manuscript collections used were the T.M. Yates correspondence (Folklore and Language Archive, Memorial University of Newfoundland), the John Little letters (courtesy Mr. Charles Smith), the John Heath ms. (courtesy Dr. R. Day), the Pitman ms. (courtesy Dr. I. Rusted), and the Redfearn/Smith ms. (Newfoundland Provincial Archives). Copies of some manuscript materials are also housed with the files of the Medical Communication Group, History of Medicine, Faculty of Medicine, Memorial University of Newfoundland.

Aakster, C.W. 1986. "Concepts in Alternative Medicine." *Social Science and Medicine* 22: 265–73.

Adams, F. 1988. *St. John's – The Last 100 Years*. St. John's: Creative Publishers.

Adamson J.D., J.D. Jolliffe, H.D. Kruse, O.H. Lowry, P.E. Moore, B.S. Platt, W.H. Sobrell, J.W. Tice, F.F. Tisdell, R.M. Wilder, and P.C. Zamecnik. 1945. "Medical Survey of Nutrition in Newfoundland." *Canadian Medicine Association Journal* 52: 227–50.

Alexander, D.F. 1983. "The Political Economy of Fishing in Newfoundland," in *Atlantic Canada and Confederation. Essays in Canadian Political Economy*, compiled by E.W. Sager, L.R. Fischer, and S.O. Pierson, 32–43. Toronto: University of Toronto Press.

Andrieux, J.P. 1983. *Prohibition and St. Pierre*. Lincoln: Rannie.

Apple, R.D. 1987. *Mothers and Medicine. A Social History of Infant Feeding*. Madison: University of Wisconsin Press.

– ed. 1990. *Women, Health, and Medicine in America. A Historical Handbook*. New York: Garland.

Appleton, V.B. 1921. "Observations on Deficiency Diseases in Labrador." *American Journal Public Health* 11: 617–21.

Arrindell, W.A., M.J. Pickersgill, H. Merckelbach, A.M. Ardon, and F.C. Cornet. 1991. "Phobic Dimensions: III. Factor Analytic Approaches to the Study of Common Phobic Fears; An Updated Review of Findings Obtained With Adult Subjects." *Advanced Behaviour Research and Therapy* 13: 73–130.

*Audubon Society Field Guide to North American Wildflowers*. 1983. New York: Knopf.

Aykroyd, W.R. 1928. "Vitamin A Deficiency in Newfoundland." *Irish Journal Medical Science* 28: 161–5.

– 1930. "Beriberi and Other Food-deficiency Diseases in Newfoundland and Labrador." *Journal Hygiene* 30: 357–86.

Bader, D.L., ed. 1990. *Pressure Sores – Clinical Practice and Scientific Approach*. London: Macmillan Press.

Bakx, K. 1991. "The 'Eclipse' of Folk Medicine in Western Society." *Sociology, Health, Illness* 13: 20–38.

Baldwin, C.A., L.A. Anderson, and J.D. Phillipson. 1987. "Storm in a Herbal Teacup." *Pharmaceutical Journal* 239 (Oct. 10): R10.

Bell, S.E. 1987. "Changing Ideas: The Medicalization of Menopause." *Social Science and Medicine* 24: 535–42.

Bennett, M. 1989. *The Last Stronghold. Scottish Gaelic Traditions in Newfoundland*. St. John's: Breakwater.

Benoit, C. 1983. "Midwives & Healers. The Newfoundland Experience." *Health Sharing* 5: 22–6.

– 1989. "The Professional Socialisation of Midwives: Balancing Art and Science." *Sociology, Health, Illness* 11: 160–80.

– 1990. "Mothering in a Newfoundland Community: 1900–1940," in *Delivering Motherhood. Maternal Ideologies and Practices in the 19th and 20th Centuries*, edited by K. Arnup, A. Lévesque, and R.R. Pierson, 173–89. London: Routledge.

Bergen, F.D. 1896. *Current Superstitions Collected from the Oral Tradition of English-Speaking Folk*. Boston: The American Folk-Lore Society.

– 1899. *Animal and Plant Lore. Collected from the Oral Tradition of English-Speaking Folk*. Boston: The American Folk-Lore Society.

Black, G., ed. 1927. *The Doctor at Home and Nurse's Guide*. London: Ward, Lock & Co.

Blumhagen, D. 1980. "Hyper-tension: A Folk Illness with a Medical Name." *Culture, Medicine, Psychiatry* 4: 197–217.

Bourke, J.G. 1891. *Scatologic Rites of All Nations; A Dissertation Upon the Employment of Excermentitious Remedial Agents in Religion, Therapeutics, Divination, Witch-craft, Love-Philters*. Washington: Laudermilk.

Bricklin, M. 1990. *The Practical Encyclopedia of Natural Healing*. London: Penguin.

British Medical Association. 1909. *Secret Remedies. What They Cost and What They Contain*. London: British Medical Association.

Brooks, P.M. 1985. "Patient Education in Chronic Arthritis." *Medical Journal of Australia* 143: 186–7.

Brown, J.H., P.W. Spitz, and J.F. Fries. 1980. "Unorthodox Treatments in Rheumatoid Arthritis." *Arthritis Rheumatism* 23: 657–8.

Brown, J.S., and S.A. Marcy. 1991. "The Use of Botanicals by Members of a Prepaid Health Plan." *Research in Nursing and Health* 14: 339–50.

Browne, R.B. 1958. *Popular Beliefs and Practices from Alabama*. Berkeley: University of California Press.

Buckley, A.K., with C. Cartwright. 1983. "A Good Wake: A Newfoundland Study." *Culture and Tradition* 7: 6–16.

Burgess, I. 1990. "Carbaryl Lotions for Head Lice – New Laboratory Tests Show Variations in Efficacy." *Pharmaceutical Journal* 245: 159–61.

Burnham, J.C. 1982. "American Medicine's Golden Age: What Happened to it?" *Science* 215: 1474–9.

– 1984. "Change in the Popularization of Health in the United States." *Bulletin History Medicine* 58: 183–97.

Burns, D.A. 1992. "'Warts and all' – the History and Folklore of Warts: A Review." *Journal Royal Society Medicine* 85: 37–40.

Butler, G.F. 1900. *A Text Book of Materia Medica, Therapeutics and Pharmacology*. Philadelphia: Saunders.

Butler, V. 1977. *Sposin I Dies In D'Dory*. St. John's: Jesperson.

– 1980. *The Little Nord Easter: Reminiscences of a Placentia Bayman*, edited by W.W. Wareham. St. John's: Breakwater.

Campbell, C.M. 1924. *The Lazy Colon*. New York: Blue Ribbon Books.

Campbell, R.L., J.L. Seymour, L.C. Stone, and M.C. Milligan. 1988. "Effects of Diaper Types on Diaper Dermatitis Associated with Diarrhoea and Antibiotic Use in Children in Day-Care Centers." *Paediatric Dermatology* 5: 83–7.

Camporesi, P. 1988. *The Incorruptible Flesh. Bodily Mutation and Mortification in Religion and Folklore*. Cambridge: Cambridge University Press.

*Canadian Drug Identification Code*. 1993. Ottawa: Health and Welfare Canada.

Carpenter, K.J. 1986. *The History of Scurvy and Vitamin C.* Cambridge: Cambridge University Press.

Carter, K.C. 1982. "Nineteenth-Century Treatments for Rabies as Reported in the Lancet." *Medical History* 26: 67–78.

Cassidy, M., A. Jacobs, and B. Bresnihan. 1983. "The Use of Unproven Remedies for Rheumatoid Arthritis in Ireland." *Irish Medical Journal* 76: 464–5.

Cassileth, B.R., E.J. Lusk, D. Guerry, A.D. Blake, W.P. Walsh, L. Kascius, and D.J. Schulz. 1991. "Survival and Quality of Life Among Patients Receiving Unproven as Compared with Conventional Cancer Therapy." *New England Journal Medicine* 324: 1180–5.

Cassileth, B.R., E.J. Lusk, T.B. Strouse, and B.J. Bodenheimer. 1984. "Contemporary Unorthodox Treatment in Cancer Medicine: A Study of Patients, Treatments and Practitioners." *Annals Internal Medicine* 101: 105–12.

Cavender, A., ed. 1990. *A Folk Medical Lexicon of South Central Appalachia.* Johnson City, Tenn: History of Medicine Society of Appalachia, Miscellaneous papers no. 1.

Cayleff, S.E. 1990. "Self-Help and the Patent Medicine Business." In *Women, Health and Medicine in America. A Historical Handbook*, edited by R.D. Apple, 311–36. New York: Garland.

Chandler, R.F., L. Freeman, and S.N. Hooper. 1979. "Herbal Remedies of the Maritime Indians." *Journal Ethnopharmacology* 1: 49–68.

*Chase Almanac.* 1993. n.p.

Chase, A.W. 1862. *Dr. Chase's Recipes or Information for Everybody: An Invaluable Collection of About Eight Hundred Practical Recipes.* Ann Arbor: author.

– 1887. *Dr. Chase's Third, Last and Complete Receipt Book and Household Physician.* Detroit: F.B. Dickerson.

Clute, W.N. 1942. *The Common Names of Plants and Their Meanings.* Indianapolis, Clute & Co.

Coish, C. 1985. "Molasses, Myrrh, and Maggots – Newfoundland Folk Medicine." *Atlantic Advocate* 81: 182–4.

Cooter, R. 1988. "Alternative Medicine, Alternative Cosmology." In *Studies in the History of Alternative Medicine*, edited by R. Cooter, 63–78. New York: St. Martin's Press.

Cormack, W.E. 1856 [1873]. *Narrative of a Journey Across the Island of Newfoundland.* St. John's: Morning Chronicle.

– 1928. *Narrative of a Journey Across the Island of Newfoundland in 1922*, edited by F.A. Bruton. London: Longman's, Green.

Couzens, G. 1993. *House Calls.* New York: Simon and Schuster.

Cramp, A.J. 1936. *Nostrums and Quackery and Pseudo-Medicine.* Vol. 3. Chicago: American Medical Association.

Creighton, H. 1968. *Bluenose Magic. Popular Beliefs and Superstitions in Nova Scotia.* Toronto: Ryerson Press.

Crellin, J.K., and J. O'Mara. 1990. *A Store Mixt, Various Universal. Community Pharmacy Past and Present.* St. John's: Faculty of Medicine, Memorial University of Newfoundland.

Crellin, J.K., and J. Philpott. 1990. *Herbal Medicine Past and Present.* 2 vols. Durham: Duke University Press.

Dana, W.S. 1989 [1893]. *How to Know the Wild Flowers.* Boston: Houghton Mifflin.

Davis, A.B. 1982. "The Rise of the Vitamin-Medicinal as Illustrated by Vitamin D." *Pharmacy in History* 24: 59–72.

Davis, D.L. 1983a. "The Family and Social Change in the Newfoundland Outport." *Culture* 3: 19–32.

– 1983. *Blood and Nerves. An Ethnographic Focus on Menopause.* St. John's: ISER.

– 1984. "Medical Misinformation: Communication Between Outport Newfoundland Women and their Physicians." *Social Science and Medicine* 18: 273–8.

– 1988. "Folk Images of Health and Menstrual Patterns among Newfoundland Outport Women." *Health Care International* 9: 211–23.

– 1989. "George Beard and Lydia Pinkham: Gender, Class and Nerves in Late 19th Century America." In *Gender, Health and Illness. The Case of Nerves,* edited by D.L. Davis and S.M. Low, 1–22. New York: Hemisphere.

Davis, D.L., and S.M. Low. 1989. *Gender, Health and Illness. The Case of Nerves.* New York: Hemisphere.

Debus, A.G. 1991. *Drugstore Cabaret. Reflections of Pharmacy in Popular Music.* Madison: American Institute History of Pharmacy.

Deir, G. 1983. "We'll Rant and We'll Roar, The Gerald Doyle Songbooks." *The Livyere* 1(3–4): 38–40.

Demak, M.M., and M.H. Becker. 1987. "The Changing 'Patient-Provider Relationship: Clarifying the Future of Health Care." *Patient Education and Counselling* 9: 5–24.

Denis, J.E. 1888. *Contribution à l'étude de la géographie médicale campagne de Terra-Neuve en 1886.* MD thesis, University of Bordeaux, France.

Devine, P. K. 1937a. *Devine's Folk Lore of Newfoundland.* St. John's: Robinson.

– 1937b. "Newfoundland Folk-lore." In *The Book of Newfoundland,* Vol. 1, edited by J.R. Smallwood, 230–3. St. John's: Newfoundland Book Publishers.

*Dictionary of Newfoundland English.* 1990. Edited by G.M. Story, W.J. Kirwin, and J.D.A. Widdowson. Toronto: University of Toronto Press.

Dinham, P.S. 1977. *You Never Know What They Might Do. Mental Illness in Outport Newfoundland.* St. John's: ISER.

*Dodd's Almanac.* c. 1910. n.p.

Doherty, F. 1990. "The Anodyne Necklace: A Quack Remedy and Its Promotion." *Medical History* 34: 268–93.

– 1992. *A Study of Eighteenth-Century Advertising Methods: The Anodyne Necklace.* Lewiston: Edward Mellen.

Dove, R.F. 1943. "The Diagnosis and Treatment of the Subclinical Dietary Deficiency Diseases." *Northern Medical Record* 1: 7–9.

Doyle G.S., ed. 1927. *Old-Time Songs and Poetry of Newfoundland.* St. John's: author.

– 1940. *Old-Time Songs and Poetry of Newfoundland.* St. John's: author.

– 1955. *Old-Time Songs and Poetry of Newfoundland.* St. John's: author.

– 1966. *Old-Time Songs and Poetry of Newfoundland.* St. John's: author.

Duke, J.A. 1985. *CRC Handbook of Medicinal Herbs.* Boca Raton: CRC Press.

Eisenberg, D.M., R.C. Kessler, C. Foster, F.E. Norlock, D.R. Calkins, and T.L. Delbanco. 1993. "Unconventional Medicine in the United States: Prevalence, Costs, and Patterns of Use." *New England Journal Medicine* 328: 246–52.

Entract, J. P. 1970. "'Chlorodyne' Browne." *London Hospital Gazette* 73: 7–11.

Ephraim, J.W. 1937. *Take Care of Yourself.* New York: Simon and Schuster.

Erichsen-Brown, C. 1979. *Use of Plants for the Past 500 Years.* Aurora: Breezy Creek Press.

Estes, J.W. 1988. "The Pharmacology of Nineteenth-Century Patent Medicines." *Pharmacy in History* 30: 3–18.

Evans, W.L. 1989. *Trease and Evans' Pharmacognosy.* London: Baillière Tindall.

Fitz-Gerald, C. 1935. *The "Albatross." Being the Biography of Conrad Fitz-Gerald 1847–1933.* Bristol: Arrowsmith.

Fizzard G. 1987. *Unto the Sea: A History of Grand Bank.* Grand Bank: Grand Bank Heritage Society.

– 1988. *Master of His Craft. Captain Frank Thornhill.* Grand Bank: Grand Bank Heritage Society.

Foster, F.P., ed. 1892–94. *An Illustrated Encyclopedic Medical Dictionary.* 4 vols. New York: Appleton.

– ed. 1897. *Reference-Book of Practical Therapeutics.* 2 vols. New York: Appleton.

Francis, A. 1968. *A Guinea a Box: A Biography [of Thomas Beecham].* London: Hale.

Freeman, S.H. 1987. "Health Promotion Talk in Family Practice Encounters." *Social Science and Medicine* 25: 961–6.

Fuller, R.C. 1989. *Alternative Medicine and American Religious Life.* Oxford: Oxford University Press.

Gabe, J., U. Gustafsson, and M. Bury. 1991. "Medicating Illness: Newspaper Coverage of Tranquilliser Dependence." *Sociology, Health & Illness* 13: 332–53.

Gerard, J. 1633. *The Herball or Generall Historie of Plantes.* London: Reprint Dover Publications, 1975.

Gerhardt, U. 1989. *Ideas about Illness. An Intellectual and Political History of Medical Sociology.* New York: New York University Press.

Gevitz, N. 1990. "Domestic Medical Guides and The Drug Trade in Nineteenth-Century America." *Pharmacy in History* 32: 51–6.

Gillan, J.G. 1991. *Through Northern Eyes.* Calgary: University of Calgary Press.

Giovannini, M. 1988. *Outport Nurse.* St. John's: Faculty of Medicine, Memorial University of Newfoundland, Occasional papers in the History of Medicine.

Girt, J.L. 1970. A Consideration of Some Relationships of Environment to Disease in Leeds and Newfoundland. Ph.D. thesis, Leeds University, England.

Goldstein, D.E. 1991. "Perspectives on Newfoundland Belief Traditions: Narrative Clues to Concepts of Evidence." In *Community and Process,* edited by G. Thomas and J.D.A. Widdowson, 27–40. St. John's: Breakwater.

Goodenough, J. 1909. *The Favorite Medical Receipt Book and Home Doctor.* Toronto: Dominion Book Co.

Gordon, E.C. 1993. "Sailors' Physicians: Medical Guides for Merchant Ships and Whalers, 1774–1864." *Journal History of Medicine and Allied Sciences* 48: 139–56.

Graedon, J., and T. Graedon. 1991. *Graedons' Best Medicine.* New York: Bantam.

Gray, D. 1983. "'Arthritis': Variation in Beliefs About Joint Disease." *Medical Anthropology* 7: 29–45.

Green, H.G. 1974. *Don't Have Your Baby in the Dory. A Biography of Myra Bennett.* Montreal: Harvest House.

Green, P. 1990. *Paul Green's Wordbook. An Alphabet of Reminiscence.* 2 vols., edited by R.H. Wynn. Boone: Appalachian Consortium Press in association with the Paul Green Foundation.

Greenish, H.G. 1909. *A Text Book of Materia Medica.* London: Churchill.

Grenfell, W. c. 1920. *The Story of a Labrador Doctor.* London: Hodder and Stoughton.

– 1932. *Forty Years for Labrador.* Boston: Houghton Mifflin.

Grindstaff, C.F. 1980. *The Pharmacist and Family Planning: New Roles and Responsibilities.* North Quincy: Christopher Publishing House.

Gunn, J.C. 1869. *Gunn's New Family Physician.* New York: Moore, Wilstach & Moore.

Hadlow, J., and M. Pitts. 1991. "The Understanding of Common Health Terms by Doctors, Nurses and Patients." *Social Science and Medicine* 32: 193–6.

Hall, L.A. 1991. *Hidden Anxieties. Male Sexuality, 1900–1950.* Cambridge: Polity Press.

Hand, W.D., ed. 1961. *The Frank C. Brown Collection of North Carolina Folklore.* Vols. 6 and 7. Durham: Duke University Press.

– 1968. "Folk Medical Inhalants in Respiratory Disorders." *Medical History* 12: 153–63.

– ed. 1976. *American Folk Medicine. A Symposium.* Berkeley: University of California Press.

– 1980. *Magical Medicine.* Berkeley: Berkeley University of California Press.

Hand, W.D., A. Cassetta, and S.B. Thiederman. 1981. *Popular Beliefs and Superstitions. A Compendium of American Folklore from the Ohio Collection of Newbell Niles Puckett.* 3 vols. Boston: Hall.

Harris, B.P. 1990. *Good as the Sea. Rural Newfoundland: Medical and Other Experiences, 1955–58.* St. John's: Faculty of Medicine, Memorial University of Newfoundland, Occasional papers in the History of Medicine.

Harris, M.R. 1989. "Iron Therapy and Tonics." In *Fitness in American Culture. Images of Health, Sport and the Body, 1930–1940,* edited by K. Grover, 67–85. Amherst: University of Massachusetts Press.

Harris, M.R. 1983. "When Pharmacists Applied Their Own 'OTC' Labels." *Pharmacy in History* 25: 40–1.

Hartnett, J.C. 1974. "The Cobweb or Spider's Web. The Dreamy Stuff of 19th Century Pharmacy and Therapeutics." *Pharmacy in History* 16: 11–17.

Havard, C.W.H. 1990. *Black's Medical Dictionary.* London: A.C. Black.

Health News. c. 1910. *Exposures of Quackery.* London: Savoy Press.

Helfand, W.H. Collection. 1991. *The Picture of Health. Images of Medicine and Pharmacy.* Philadelphia: Philadelphia Museum of Art.

Helman, C.G. 1990. *Culture, Health and Illness. An Introduction for Health Professionals.* London: Wright.

– 1981. "'Tonic,' 'Fuel' and 'Food': Social and Symbolic Aspects of the Long-Term Use of Psychotropic Drugs." *Social Science and Medicine* 15B: 521–33.

Herzlich, C. 1973. *Health and Illness. A Social Psychological Analysis.* London: Academic Press.

Hiebert, C.A. 1989. "Seldom Come By. The Worthwhileness of a Career in Surgery." *Archives Surgery* 124: 530–4.

Higman, C., and M.I.V. Jayson. 1982. "Nonprescribed Treatments in Rheumatic Patients." *Annals Rheumatic Diseases* 41: 203.

Hiscock, P. 1987. *Folklore and Popular Culture in Early Newfoundland Radio Broadcasting.* MA thesis, Memorial University of Newfoundland, St. John's, Newfoundland.

Hudson, R.P. 1989. "Theory and Therapy: Ptosis, Stasis and Autointoxication." *Bulletin History Medicine* 63: 392–413.

Hufford, D. 1982. *The Terror That Comes in the Night.* Philadelphia: University of Pennsylvania Press.

– 1988. "Contemporary Folk Medicine." In *Other Healers*, edited by N. Gevitz, 228–64. Baltimore: John's Hopkins Press.

Hunter, I., and S. Wotherspoon. 1986. *A Bibliography of Health Care in Newfoundland.* St. John's: Faculty of Medicine.

Ihde, A.J. 1975. "The Roles of Cod Liver Oil and Light (Studies on the History of Rickets II)." *Pharmacy in History* 17: 13–20.

Jabeer, R., S. Steinhardt, J. Trilling. 1991. "Explanatory Models of Illness – A Pilot Study." *Family Systems* 9: 39–51.

Jackson, W.A. 1974. "Bear's Grease and Its Containers." *History Medicine* (E.R. Squibb) 5(4): 16–21.

Johnson, R.F., and T.X. Barber. 1978. "Hypnosis Suggestions, and Warts: An Experimental Investigation Implicating the Importance of 'Believed-in Efficacy.'" *American Journal Clinical Hypnosis* 20: 165–74.

Kasparek, M.C. 1991. [Bureau of Nonprescription Drugs, Department of National Health and Welfare], "Harmonisation of International Testing Requirements and Standards," presented to Drug Information Association, Paris, October 28. Unpublished.

Kerr, J.C. 1959. *Wilfred Grenfell. His Life and Work.* New York: Dodd, Mead & Co.

Kestin, M., L. Miller, G. Littlejohn, and M. Wahlqvist. 1985. "The Use of Unproven Remedies for Rheumatoid Arthritis in Australia." *Medical Journal Australia* 143: 516–8.

Kipling, R. 1939 [1897]. *Captains Courageous.* Toronto: Macmillan.

Kirkland, J., H.F. Matthews, C.W. Sullivan III, and K. Baldwin, eds. 1992. *Herbal and Magical Medicine. Traditional Healing Today.* Durham: Duke University Press.

Leung, A.Y. 1980. *Encyclopedia of Common Natural Ingredients Used in Food, Drugs, and Cosmetics*. New York: Wiley.

Levenstein, H.A. 1988. *Revolution at the Table. The Transformation of the American Diet*. New York: Oxford University Press.

Lexchin, J. 1990. "Drug Makers and Drug Regulators: Too Close for Comfort. A Study of the Canadian Situation." *Social Science Medicine* 31: 1257–63.

Lind, J. 1772. *A Treatise on the Scurvy*. London: Crowder.

Little, J.M. 1908a. "A Winter's Work in a Subarctic Climate." *Boston Medical Surgical Journal* 158: 996–7.

– 1908b. "Medical Conditions on the Labrador Coast and North Newfoundland." *Journal American Medical Association* 50: 1037–9.

– 1912. "Beriberi Caused by Fine White Flour." *Journal American Medical Association* 58: 2029–30.

Lysaght, A.M. 1971. *Joseph Banks in Newfoundland & Labrador, 1766. His Diary, Manuscripts and Collections*. Berkeley: University of California Press.

MacDonald, E. 1959. "Outport Medicine in Newfoundland." *Canadian Pharmaceutical Journal* 92: 40–1.

MacDermott, H. 1938. *MacDermott of Fortune Bay Told by Himself*. London: Hodder and Stoughton.

Macknin, M.L., S. Mathew, and S.V. Medendorp. 1990. "Effect of Inhaling Heated Vapour on Symptoms of the Common Cold." *Journal American Medical Association* 264: 989–91.

McLaren, A., and A.T. McLaren. 1986. *The Bedroom and the State. The Changing Practices and Politics of Contraception and Abortion in Canada 1880–1980*. Toronto: McClelland and Stewart.

McNaughton, J. 1989. *The Role of the Newfoundland Midwife in Traditional Health Care 1900 to 1970*. Ph.D. theses, Memorial University of Newfoundland, St. John's, Newfoundland.

McTavish, J.R. 1987. "What's in a Name? Aspirin and the American Medical Association." *Bulletin History Medicine* 61: 343–66.

Mann, C.C., and M.L. Plummer. 1991. *The Aspirin Wars: Money, Medicine and Rampant Competition*. New York: Knopf.

Massing, A.M., and W.L. Epstein. 1963. "Natural History of Warts." *Archives Dermatology* 87: 306–10.

Martindale 1990. *The Extra Pharmacopoeia*. London: Pharmaceutical Press.

Maw, S., Son and Sons. 1925. *A Catalogue of Surgical Instruments, Appliances ... etc.* London: S. Maw, Son and Sons.

*Medicinal Plant Guide. Plants and My Health*. c.1991. (Catalog of Medicinal Plant Distribution), n.p.

Mercer, G.P. 1991. Herbal Medicine and Traditional Remedies Used in the Bay St. George Area of Newfoundland. Unpublished.

Metkoff, J., G.A. Goldsmith, A.J. McQueeney, R.F. Dove, E. McDevitt, M.A. Dove, and F.J. Stare. 1945. "Nutritional Survey in Norris Point, Newfoundland." *Journal Laboratory Clinical Medicine* 30: 475–87.

Mifflen, J.B. 1983. *Journey to Yesterday in the Out-harbours of Newfoundland.* St. John's: Cuff Publications.

Miller, L. 1950. "Public Health in Newfoundland." *Canadian Journal Public Health* 41: 1–6.

– 1958. "Spectacular Change in Public Health Picture." *Newfoundland Journal Commerce* 25: 49–51.

Millspaugh, C.F. 1974 [1892]. *American Medicinal Plants.* New York: Reprint Dover Publications.

Mitchell, H.S. 1930. "Nutrition Survey in Labrador and Northern Newfoundland." *Journal American Dietetic Association* 6: 29–35.

Mitchinson, W. 1991. *The Nature of Their Bodies. Women and Their Doctors in Victorian Canada.* Toronto: University of Toronto Press.

Moerman, D.E. 1986. *Medicinal Plants of Native America.* 2 vols. Ann Arbour: University of Michigan Museum of Anthropology.

Momatiuk, Y., and J. Eastcott. 1988. *This Marvellous Terrible Place, Images of Newfoundland and Labrador.* Camden East: Camden House Publishing.

Money, K.E. 1970. "Motion Sickness." *Physiological Reviews* 50: 1–39.

Morton, J.F. 1990. "Mucilaginous Plants and Their Uses in Medicine." *Journal Ethnopharmacology* 29: 245–66.

Murphy, N.F. 1975. "Medicine in Western Newfoundland." *Newfoundland Medical Association Newsletter* 17(2): 15–7.

Murray, H.C. 1979. *More than Fifty Percent. Women's Life in a Newfoundland Outport 1900–1950,* especially 132–5. St. John's: Breakwater.

Musson, E.E. 1910. "Labrador. Interesting Account of the Country, Its Interests, Hospitals, etc." *Women's Medical Journal* 20: 199–201.

Naphys, G.H. 1875. *The Prevention and Cure of Disease.* Springfield: Holland & Co.

Narváez, P. 1991. *The Good People. New Fairylore Essays.* New York: Garland Publishing.

Nations, M.K., L.A. Camino, and F.B. Walker. 1985. "'Hidden' Popular Illnesses in Primary Care: Residents' Recognition and Clinical Implications." *Culture, Medicine and Psychiatry* 9: 223–40.

Ness, R.C. 1976. *Illness and Adaptation in a Newfoundland Community.* Ph.D. thesis, University of Connecticut, Storrs.

– 1977. "Modernization and Illness in a Newfoundland Community," *Medical Anthropology* 1: 25–53.

*Newfoundland Health Review.* 1986. St. John's: Department of Health.

*Northern Medical Review.* 1943. Editorial. *Northern Medical Review* 1: 17.

Numbers, R.L., and T.L. Savitt, eds. 1989. *Science and Medicine in the Old South.* Baton Rouge: Louisiana State University Press.

"Nutrition in Newfoundland," 1945. *Nutrition Reviews* 3: 251–3.

O'Brien, P. 1989. *Out of Mind, Out of Sight: A History of the Waterford Hospital.* St. John's: Breakwater.

O'Hare, J.P., A. Heywood, C. Summerhayes, G. Lunn, J.M. Evans, G. Walters, R.J.M. Corrall, and P.A. Dieppe. 1985. "Observations of the Effects of Immersion in Bath Spa Water." *British Medical Journal* 291: 1747–51.

Olds, J. M. 1957. "Seal Finger or Speck Finger." *Canadian Medical Association Journal* 76: 455–7.

– 1967. "Routine House Call." *Newfoundland Medical Association Newsletter* 9: 10–2.

Olsson, K. 1989. "Caribou Bones and Labrador Tea." *Canadian Nurse* 85: 18–21.

O'Mara, J. 1982. "Pharmacy in Newfoundland." Unpublished ms.

Omohundro, J. T. 1985. "Efficiency, Sufficiency, and Recent Change in Newfoundland Subsistence Horticulture." *Human Ecology* 13: 291–308.

Onlooker. 1991. *Pharmaceutical Journal* 247: 58.

Opie, I., and M. Tatem. 1989. *A Dictionary of Superstitions.* Oxford: Oxford University Press.

Osler, W. 1985. *Counsels and Ideals from the Writings of William Osler and Selected Aphorisons.* Birmingham: Classics of Medicine Library, Selected Aphorisons section.

Parsons, G. 1936. "Folk Medicine in Newfoundland." *Dalhousie Medical Journal* 1: 18–21.

Parsons, G.T. 1977. "Equal Treatment for All: American Medical Remedies for Male Sexual Problems: 1850–1900." *Journal History Medicine Allied Sciences* 32: 55–71.

Partsch, H. 1890. *Sea-Sickness. A Comprehensive Treatise for Practical Use.* Boston: Cupples.

Patterson, G. 1895. "Notes on the Folk-lore of Newfoundland." *Journal American Folklore* 8: 285–90.

– 1897. "Notes on the Folk-lore of Newfoundland." *Journal American Folklore* 10: 214–15.

Patterson, J.T. 1987. *The Dread Disease Cancer and Modern American Culture.* Cambridge: Harvard University Press.

Pierce, R.V. 1895. *The People's Common Sense Medical Adviser.* Buffalo: Worlds's Dispensory.

Piercey, R.M. 1992. *True Tales of Rhoda Maude,* edited by J. McNaughton. St. John's: Faculty of Medicine, Memorial University of Newfoundland, Occasional papers in the History of Medicine.

Pitt, D.G. 1984. E.J. Pratt. *The Truant Years 1882–1927.* Vol. 1. Toronto, University of Toronto Press.

Pocius, G.L. 1985. "Urban Folk Medicine: Some Thoughts." *Canadian Centre for Folk Culture Studies* 53: 113–18.

– 1991. *A Place to Belong. Community Order and Everyday Space in Calvert, Newfoundland.* Athens: Montreal: McGill-Queen's University Press.

Podgorski, M., and J. Edmonds. 1985. "Non-pharmacological Treatment of Patients with Rheumatoid Arthritis." *Medical Journal Australia* 143: 511–16.

Porter, H. 1979. *Below the Bridge. Memories of the South Side of St. John's.* St. John's: Breakwater.

Porter, R., ed. 1990. *The Medical History of Waters and Spas.* London: Wellcome Institute for the History of Medicine, Medical History Suppl. no. 10.

Porter, R., and D. Porter. 1988. *In Sickness and in Health: The British Experience, 1650–1850.* London: Fourth Estate.

Potter, S.O.L. 1917. *Therapeutics, Materia Medica and Pharmacy.* Philadelphia: Blakiston.

Puller, T., H.A. Capell, A. Millar, and R.G. Brooks. 1982. "Alternative Medicine: Cost and Subjective Benefit in Rheumatoid Arthritis." *British Medical Journal* 285: 1629–31.

Rasky, F. 1988. *Just a Simple Pharmacist. The Story of Murray Koffler, Builder of the Shoppers Drug Mart Empire.* Toronto: McClelland and Stewart.

Reader's Digest. 1986. *Magic and Medicine of Plants.* Pleasantville: Reader's Digest Association.

Renbourn, E.T. 1957. "The History of the Flannel Binder and Cholera Belt." *Medical History* 1: 211–25.

Richler, A. 1979. "A Study of Ocular Refraction in Western Newfoundland." Ph.D. thesis, Faculty of Medicine, Memorial University of Newfoundland, St. John's.

Riddle, J.M. 1970. "Lithotherapy in the Middle Ages. Lapidaries Considered as Medical Texts." *Pharmacy in History* 12: 39–50.

Rieti, B.G. 1989. "The Black Heart in Newfoundland. The Magic of the Book." *Culture and Tradition* 13: 80–93.

– 1990. *Newfoundland Fairy Traditions: A Study in Narrative and Belief.* Ph.D. thesis, Memorial University of Newfoundland, St. John's.

– 1991a. "'The Blast' in Newfoundland Fairy Tradition." In *The Good People New England Essays,* edited by P. Narváez, 284–97. New York: Garland.

– 1991b. *Strange Terrain. The Fairy World in Newfoundland.* St. John's: ISER.

Roberts, K.B. 1986. "Snow Spectacles." *Canadian Bulletin Medical History* 3: 142–3.

Rodahl, K. 1952. "'Spekk-finger' or Sealer's finger." *Arctic* 5: 235–40.

Roeder, B.A. 1988. *Chicano Folk Medicine from Los Angeles, California.* Berkeley: University of California Press.

Rogers, N. 1989. "Germs with Legs: Flies, Disease and the New Public Health." *Bulletin History Medicine* 63: 599–617.

Rompkey, R. 1990. "Philip Henry Gosse's Account of His Years in Newfoundland." *Newfoundland Studies* 6: 210–66.

Ross, J.B. 1969. "Gum-Boot Dermatitis." *World Medicine* 4: 82–3.

– 1969. "Rubber Boot Dermatitis in Newfoundland: A Survey of 30 Patients." *Canadian Medical Association Journal* 100: 13–9.

Rouleau, E. 1978. *List of Vascular Plants of the Province of Newfoundland* (Canada). St. John's: Oxen Pond Botanic Park.

Royal Commission. 1930. *First Interim Report of the Royal Commission on Health and Public Charities, June 1930.* St. John's: King's Printer.

Rubia, G., ed. 1980. *A Poem in my Soup. A Newfoundland Sampler with Selected Poetry of Geraldine Rubia.* St. John's: Jesperson Press.

Saunders, G.L. 1986. *Rattles and Steadies Memoirs of a Gander River Man Retold.* St. John's: Breakwater.

Savitt, T.C., and J.H. Young, eds. 1988. *Disease and Distinctiveness in the American South.* Knoxville: University of Tennessee Press.

Schmitz, R. 1989. "The Pomander." *Pharmacy in History* 31: 86–90.

Schoenthaler, S.J., S.P. Amos, H.J. Eysenck, E. Peritz, and J. Yudkin. 1991. "Controlled Trial of Vitamin-Mineral Supplementation: Effects on Intelligence and Performance." *Personality and Individual Differences* 12(4): 351–62.

Scobie, K., B.S. Burke, and H.C. Stuart. 1949. "Studies of Nutrition in Newfoundland Children." *Canadian Medical Association Journal* 60(3): 233–41.

Scott, P.J. 1978. *Edible Fruits and Herbs of Newfoundland.* St. John's: Breakwater.

– 1987. "Common Names of Plants in Newfoundland." *Regional Language Studies, Newfoundland* no. 11: 1–20.

Sears, Roebuck. 1969 [1902]. *The 1902 edition of the Sears Roebuck Catalogue.* New York: Bounty Books.

Segall, A., and J. Goldstein. 1989. "Exploring the Correlates of Self-Provided Health Care Behaviour." *Social Science and Medicine* 29: 153–61.

Severs, D. 1964. "The Scurvy Problem in Newfoundland." *Canadian Nutrition Notes* 20: 76–8.

– 1975. "Diphtheria – Newfoundland." *Newfoundland Medical Association Newsletter* 17: 15–7.

– 1979. "Immunization in Newfoundland – 1979." *Newfoundland Medical Association Newsletter* 21(1): 19–21.

Sharpe, C.A. 1988. "The 'Race of Honour': An Analysis of Enlistments and Casualties in the Armed Forces of Newfoundland: 1914–1918." *Newfoundland Studies* 4: 27–55.

Shaw, B. 1981. *The Doctor's Dilemma.* New York: Garland.

Shorter, E. 1982. *A History of Women's Bodies.* New York: Basic Books.

Sider, G.M. 1986. *Culture and Class in Anthropology: A Newfoundland Illustration.* N.Y.: Cambridge University Press.

Smallwood, J.R., and R.D.W. Pitt, eds. 1981. *Encyclopedia of Newfoundland and Labrador.* Vol. 1. St. John's: Newfoundland Book Publishers.

Smith, M.C. 1989. *Pharmacy and Medicine on the Air.* New Jersey: Scarecrow Press.

Snow, L.F., and S.M. Johnson. 1977. "Modern Day Menstrual Folklore. Some Clinical Implications." *Journal American Medical Association* 237: 2736–9.

Soucy, P. 1953. "The Proprietary or Patent Medicine Act of Canada." *Food, Drug, Cosmetic Law Journal* 8: 706–16.

Sparkes, R.F. 1983. *The Winds Softly Sigh.* St. John's: Breakwater.

Spitzer, W.O., G.B. Hill, L.W. Chambers, B.E. Helliwell, and H.B. Murphy. 1975. "The Occupation of Fishing as a Risk Factor in Cancer of the Lip." *New England Journal of Medicine* 293: 419–24.

Squire, H. 1974. *A Newfoundland Outport in the Making. The Early History of Eastport Together with an Eye-witness Account of the Greenland Disaster.* n.p.

Stage, S. 1979. *Female Complaints. Lydia Pinkham and the Business of Women's Medicine*. New York: Norton.

Steven, D., and G. Wald. 1941. "Vitamin A Deficiency: A Field Study in Newfoundland." *Journal Nutrition* 21: 461–71.

Strobusch, A.D., and J.W. Jefferson. 1980. "The Checkered History of Lithium in Medicine." *Pharmacy in History* 22: 72–6.

Struthers, G.R., D.L. Scott, and D.G.I. Scott. 1983. "The Use of 'Alternative Treatments' by Patients with Rheumatoid Arthritis." *Rheumatology International* 3: 151–2.

Sugerman, J., and R. Butters. 1985. "Understanding the Patient: Medical Words the Doctor May Not Know." *North Carolina Medical Journal* 46: 415–17.

Sullivan, C. 1984. "Dr. Thomas' Eclectric Oil." *Research Bulletin 218*. Ottawa: Parks Canada.

Tattje, D.H.E., and R. Bas. 1981. "Composition of Essential Oil of Ledum Palustre." *Planta Medica* 41: 303–7.

Thielman, S.B. 1989. "Community Management of Mental Disorders in Antebellum America." *Journal History Medicine Allied Sciences* 44: 351–78.

Thomas, A. 1968. *The Newfoundland Journal of Aaron Thomas, Able Seaman in H.M.S. Boston: A Journal Written during a Voyage from England to Newfoundland and from Newfoundland to England in the Years 1794 and 1795, Addressed to a Friend*, edited by J.M. Murray. London: Longmans.

Thomas, G., and J.D.A. Widdowson, eds. 1991. *Studies in Newfoundland Folklore: Community and Process*. St. John's: Breakwater.

Thomas, S.J. 1982. "Nostrum Advertising and the Image of Women as Invalid in late Victorian America." *Journal American Culture* 5: 104–12.

Tizzard, A.M. 1984. *On Sloping Ground. Reminiscences of Outport Life in Notre Dame Bay*, edited with introduction by J.D.A. Widdowson. St. John's: Breakwater.

Tocque, P. 1878. *Newfoundland as It Was, and as It Is in 1877*. Toronto: Magurn.

Tomes, N. 1990. "The Private Side of Public Health: Sanitary Science, Domestic Hygiene, and the Germ Theory, 1870–1900." *Bulletin History Medicine* 64: 509–39.

Toussaint-Samat, M. 1992. *A History of Food*. Cambridge: Blackwell.

Troake, P. 1989. *No One Is a Stranger. Reminiscences on Tuberculosis, Traditional Medicine, and Other Matters*, edited by J.K. Crellin. St. John's: Faculty of Medicine, Memorial University of Newfoundland, Occasional papers in the History of Medicine.

Tucker, O. 1988. "No Place More Christmas-y Than LaScie Back in 1942!" In *A Christmas Box*, edited by F. Galgay and M. McCarthy, 79–83. St. John's: Cuff Publishers, 1988.

Tyler, V.E. 1982. *The Honest Herbal*. Philadelphia: Stickley.

– 1985. *Hoosier Home Remedies*. West Lafayette: Purdue University Press.

– 1987. *The Honest Herbal*. Philadelphia: Stickley.

Vaughan, W. 1626. *Directions for Health*. London: Beale.

– 1630. *The Newlanders Cure*. London: Constable.

Vaughan, M., and H.S. Mitchell. 1933. "A Continuation of the Nutrition Project in Northern Newfoundland." *Journal American Dietetic Association* 8: 526–31.

Vinikas, V. 1992. *Soft Soap, Hard Sell. American Hygiene in an Age of Advertisement.* Ames: Iowa State University Press.

Viseltear, A.J. 1968. "Joanna Stephens and the Eighteenth Century Lithontriptics: A Misplaced Chapter in the History of Therapeutics." *Bulletin History Medicine* 42: 199–220.

Wainwright, M. 1988. "Maggot Therapy – A Backwater in the Fight Against Bacterial Infection." *Pharmacy in History* 30: 19–26.

– 1989. "Moulds in Ancient and More Recent Medicine." *Mycologist* 3: 21–3.

Wake, D. 1991. "Use of Brown Paper." *Pharmaceutical Journal* 247: 391.

Waldo, F.L. 1920. *With Grenfell on the Labrador.* New York: Revell.

Walker, W. R., and D. M. Keats. 1976. "An Investigation of the Therapeutic Value of the 'Copper Bracelet' – Dermal Assimilation of Copper in Arthritic/Rheumatoid Conditions." *Agents and Actions* 6: 454–9.

Walker, W.R., S.J. Beverage, and M.W. Whitehouse. 1980. "Anti-Inflammatory Activity of a Dermally Applied Copper Salicylate Preparation (Alcusal)." *Agents and Actions* 10: 38–47.

Warren, I., A.E. Small, W. Thorndike, and J.H. Smith. 1903. *The New Warren's Household Physician, enlarged and revised.* Boston: Bradley.

Weil, A. 1990. *Natural Health Natural Medicine. A Comprehensive Manual and Self-Care.* Boston: Houghton-Mifflin.

Whorton, J.C. 1981. "Thallion!!! Anatomy of a Pseudoethical Proprietary." *Pharmacy in History* 23: 114–25.

– 1982. *Crusaders for Fitness. The History of American Health Reformers.* Princeton: Princeton University Press.

– 1989. "Eating to Win. Popular Concerns of Diet. Strength and Energy in the Early Twentieth Century." In *Fitness in American Culture. Images of Health, Sport and the Body, 1830–1940,* edited by K. Grover, 86–122. Amherst: University of Massachusetts Press.

– 1993. "The Phenolphthalein Follies: Purgation and the Pleasure Principle in the Early Twentieth Century." *Pharmacy in History* 35: 3–24.

Wicks, J. N.d. *Embossed Bottles of St. John's. A History and Price Guide.* St. John's: privately printed.

Willmott, W.B. 1860. *Glycerin and Cod Liver Oil.* London: Ballière.

Yonge, J. 1679. *Currus Triumphalis, e Terebintho.* London: Martyn.

Young, J.H. 1961. *The Toadstool Millionaires.* Princeton: Princeton University Press.

– 1967. *The Medical Messiahs. A Social History of Quackery in Twentieth-Century America.* Princeton: Princeton University Press.

– 1974. *American Self-dosage Medicines: An Historical Perspective.* Lawrence: Coronado Press.

– 1984. "The Regulation of Health Quackery." *Pharmacy in History* 26: 3–12.

Zachariah, P.K., and P. Morley. 1977. "Some Reflections on Alcoholism." *Newfoundland Medical Association Newsletter* 19: 15–18.

# Index

Bold numbers indicate Part II main entries.

Warts, 66, 68, 146, 197, **237**
Water: 143, 145, 162; cold, 155; hot, 120; May, 145. *See also* Salt water
Waterford hospital, 26
Water lilies. *See* Beaver-root
Water on the knee, **239**
Water pups (gurry sores), 137, **240**
Watkins Laxative Cold and Grippe Tablets, 169
Weakness, concept of, 32, 39, 229
Wests, 36, 145
Whisky, 60, 169, 222
White, James, 80
Whitlow, 146, **240**

Whooping cough, 235, **241**
Wild cherry, 117, 131, 220, 233, 234, **242**
Wild Strawberry, 132
Willow, 104
Winnipeg, 46
Wintergreen, 78, **244**
Witchhazel, **244**
Witherod, **221**
Women: knowledge of abortion, 57; rights, 47; roles of, 16, 44. *See also* Charmers, Female complaints
Woodwards Gripe Water, 15
Worcestershire sauce, 138
Worms, 22, 167, **245**

Wormwood, 74, 92, 213, **246**
Wyeth's Solution Sage and Sulphur and Lead Acetate, 83

Yarn, strands of, 219
Yarrow, 42, 246
Yellow-mores, 214
Yellow snakeroot, 182, 214
Yucca, 207
Yuck, 36

Zam-Buk, 72, 109, **247**
Zinc: oxide, 72; sulphate, 215
Zylex, 142